"With her new book, Patty Lemer continues her long tradition of providing relevant and up-to-date information as well as making sense of rather complicated issues. Much is known about helping individuals with ASD, and this book is an excellent resource for those on the spectrum, family members, and professionals."

- Stephen M. Edelson, Ph.D.
Director, Autism Research Institute

"We applaud Patricia Lemer who has dedicated her life's work to families of children on the autism spectrum. She holds the hands of the patients and caregivers within the chapters of this new book, walking them through the steps of treatment, guiding them to the best resources.

Patty has been a part of our extended Klinghardt Academy network for over a decade. We are honored that she has included some of our protocols within her loving work, and recommend *Outsmarting Autism* to all. Patty is a vessel of bright light and hope for our future generations."

- Debbie Floyd
Executive Director, Klinghardt Academy & Dietrich Klinghardt, MD, PhD

"*Outsmarting Autism* is a treasure, filled with fascinating, important, up-to-date information. It is a pleasure to read, written to help parents and other non-professionals understand the brain-and-body connection. By any measure, it is destined to be the book that readers seeking answers about autism will turn to first and last."

- Carol Stock Kranowitz
M.A., author, *The Out-of-Sync Child:*
Recognizing and Coping with Sensory Processing Disorder

"The epidemic of new childhood disorders is complex, and figuring out how to help an affected child can be overwhelming. Patricia Lemer provides broad, deep, and accessible guidance to empower parents in taking back their children's health."

- Beth Lambert
Author, *A Compromised Generation:*
The Epidemic of Chronic Illness in America's Children
Executive Director, Epidemic Answers
Executive Producer, The Canary Kids Project

"Continuing an excellent track record of providing unparalleled and timely resources, Ms. Lemer once again has assembled a wealth of up-to-date information about autism in one centralized source. Merging cutting edge approaches with a keen eye for what works, *Outsmarting Autism* is a book that you will find yourself reaching for frequently."

- Dr. Leonard Press
Developmental Optometrist

"*Outsmarting Autism* is essential reading. Its practical, conversational tone makes it very easy to read. Buy two books, one for yourself and the other for someone just starting on this journey. I will be recommending it to all my clients and colleagues."

- Colette Yglesias Silver, MS, OTR/L

"*Outsmarting Autism* is a much-needed practical and comprehensive guide that is a "must read" for every parent and clinician who treats patients with autism. Patty breaks down extremely complicated issues into bite-size explanations that are simple, elegant, and easily understood. *Outsmarting* provides an array of possible options that may not have been considered by mainstream approaches. It is a "must have" for your tool box!"

- Anju Usman, MD

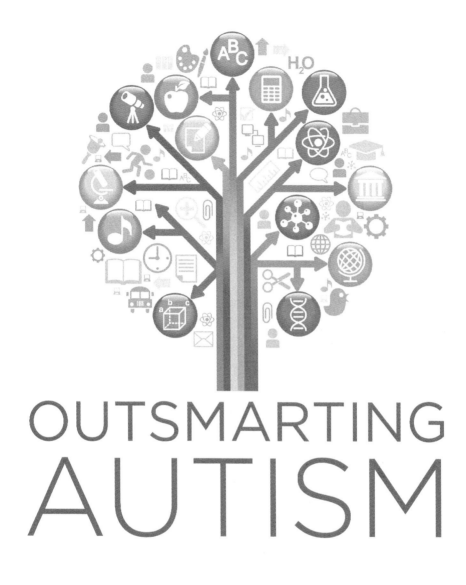

OUTSMARTING
AUTISM

ISBN: 978-1-59571-970-6

Library of Congress Control Number: 2014907761

Designed and published by
Word Association Publishers
205 Fifth Avenue
Tarentum, Pennsylvania 15084

www.wordassociation.com
1.800.827.7903

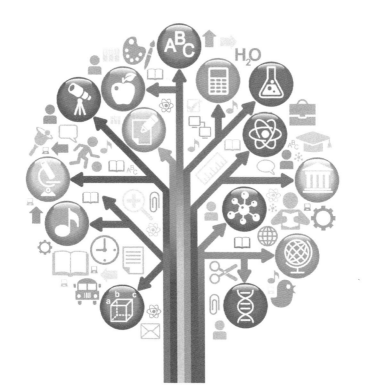

OUTSMARTING AUTISM

The Ultimate Guide to Management, Healing, and Prevention

PATRICIA S. LEMER

Editor of *EnVISIONing A Bright Future*

WORD ASSOCIATION PUBLISHERS
www.wordassociation.com
1.800.827.7903

To parents of children with special needs,
from whom I have learned so much.

Acknowledgements

This book is the culmination of 50 years of learning from my teachers, mentors, clients, colleagues, and friends. To you and the following people, my deep and heartfelt thanks.

The Bloggers who kept me current on the latest research: Teresa Binstock, Larry Kaplan, Elise Miller, Lenny Schafer, Kim Stagliano, and the crew at Thinking Moms Revolution.

Designer for another beautiful cover: Bill Greaves.

Indexer: Cynthia J. Coan, who has made it possible to find everything you are looking for in this tome.

Epidemic Answers, who has given a new home to Developmental Delay Resources (DDR) and me: Beth Lambert, Maria Rickert Hong, and the whole team.

Volunteer Editors and Wordsmiths who taught me how to write, read chapters, and made suggestions for clarity and accuracy: Teresa Badillo, Lynn Balzer-Martin, Kathy Johnson, Eve Kodiak, Carol Kranowitz, Len Press, Mary Rentschler, Scott Thierl, and Deb Wilson.

Optometric Family at OEP, who gave me a voice: Amiel Francke, Irwin Suchoff, and Bob Williams.

Physicians who are in the trenches every day making a difference in the lives of our kids: Ken Bock, Martha Herbert, Dietrich Klinghardt, and Anju Usman.

"Having Healthy Babies" team: Sarah Lane and Janine Burnham Ruth.

Nutritional Gurus: Kelly Dorfman and Donna Gates.

My Personal Wellness Team who have kept me healthy, upright, and happy: Alan, Ann, Caryn, Franne, and Julie.

My Personal Assistant who got the book off the ground and updated material from my first book, Kristen Johanson.

Word Association Team: Tom, April, and editor extraordinaire, Kendra Williamson.

To you all, and to my family and friends for whom I have been too busy and preoccupied for the past two years to be there for you when you were there for me,

My humble gratitude.
Patty

CONTENTS

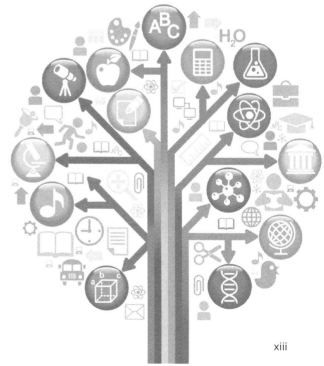

PREFACE

How to Use This Book

Outsmarting Autism is the most comprehensive book available today on managing, healing, and preventing Autism Spectrum Disorders (ASDs). Whether you are a parent, therapist, educator, or an interested consumer, this book is for you!

Don't let its size scare you; I have made it extremely easy to understand. I hope you will read it in sequence, but if you decide not to, at least read chapters 2 and 3 before jumping ahead. Understanding Total Load Theory is so important! Autism did not just show up overnight. Children with autism are sick, and making healthy lifestyle changes—no matter how overwhelming they seem—can be the difference between management and healing. My recommendations derive from over 40 years of experience in the field and can save you time, money, and effort.

Here are a few guidelines for how to approach this book, depending on your background and purpose for reading:

- *For parents or grandparents of a child diagnosed within the past two years:* Please start at the beginning and read chapter by chapter. All children with autism are not the same, and your child deserves an individualized approach to intervention. Which risk factors does your family have? Find a health care practitioner to guide you who knows a variety of approaches and is willing to delve into your family history with pointed questioning and testing.

Be careful of falling into the trap of taking therapies "off the shelf." What your school system offers and what insurance pays for may or may not be all that your child needs. Palliative care and management of symptoms is simply unacceptable for those who are newly diagnosed. Go step-by-step with the goal of healing in mind. Autism may not have to be a lifelong disability! We don't know how much progress we can make for a particular child until we get started and see what happens.

Take care of yourself while you are caring for your family members. Follow this strategy as if you are on an airplane and the flight attendant says to put on your own oxygen mask first—you will need it. As you apply your new knowledge, everyone in the family will become healthier.

• *For families whose member(s) were diagnosed over two years ago and have been involved in interventions for a while:* While your school system and insurance companies may be offering you multiple services, the key to true restoration of your family's health is in your hands. Everything you do at home makes the efforts of your school and outside therapies work better. Read chapter 3 carefully, and share the ideas from Step 2 (Correct Foundational Issues) with your specialists! Find a case manager who can oversee and integrate services. It may be a therapist, teacher, counselor, or family member. Choose someone who has no vested interest in which methods you use.

• *For veterans who have been in the trenches for many years and whose children are approaching adolescence or adulthood:* The world of autism has changed since you entered it in the late eighties or early nineties. I remember those years when we didn't even have the Internet to google "autism"!

In the last five years, since my previous book was published, we have learned about genetic mutations that we can manage through supplementation and detoxification, the importance of certain nutrients to eliminate specific autistic symptoms, and the preferred order of interventions. Please read the chapters in Steps 1 and 2, and revisit sensory problems, especially vision.

Finally, I wrote chapter 15 specifically for *you!* Completing the steps in this chapter will take you at least a year. Revisit some of the therapies you have sampled in the past; approaches are much more sophisticated than they used to be. Technology and social networking have changed the world of disabilities. If you are not using them, now is the time to start.

• *For educators and licensed or certified specialists who provide services to individuals on the spectrum in clinics, schools, or privately:* Put new tools in your tool chest, and approach this book as you would the hardware store. So many brilliant therapists have packaged multidisciplinary programs to address language, social skills, and cognition by focusing on the foundations. These materials are perfect for schools, home therapy, and summer programs.

• *For information mongers who are just curious as to why autism is on the rise and so many kids are sick and delayed:* The information in this book will surprise and amaze you! Our media is not giving you the whole story. Be prepared to have your questions answered. Use political and social networking, and play the role of educator and advocate for those you know who are affected. Read step-by-step to learn what you can do to protect your own health and that of those you love. Many of the approaches recommended for ASDs are also applicable to other chronic conditions, such as Parkinson's, multiple sclerosis, lupus, chronic fatigue, and fibromyalgia.

Outsmarting Autism is meant to challenge a good number of your beliefs. Keep an open mind to exciting new information, some of which goes against mainstream philosophy. If you have questions, please feel free to contact me through my website at www. OutsmartingAutism.com.

Thanks for joining me! Autism is no longer a mystery. We can understand and outsmart it together.

Patricia S. Lemer
June 2014

CHAPTER 1

Autism:
An Epidemic

Diagnosis: Autism. Now what?

Some families can recall the date and time when their toddlers went offtrack and even have home videos to document regression. For others, the advent of autism was a more gradual process. For a handful of adults the diagnosis did not come until midlife. The majority accepted it with relief because it explained their "quirkiness"; a few felt "broken."

Parents of diagnosed young children often go through the sequential steps of denial, anger, bargaining, and finally acceptance. Then they get down to business. "Are we powerless, or can we *outsmart* this thing we don't even understand?"

Growing up, I knew no one who was "autistic." One family down the street had two boys who did not speak and were "different." They attended my school, and we all accepted them in our games. Today they would definitely be labelled. During my college and graduate school in the 1960s, I do not recall ever discussing autism in my psychology, neurology, education, and counseling courses. Is that possible?

Autism is common now. Whenever I lecture or express my passion for working with those with disabilities, someone usually shares, "I have a cousin with autism," or, "My coworker has a child with autism." Almost everyone knows a family that is affected. According to the latest report from the Centers for Disease Control and Prevention (CDC), based on 2010 data, autism occurs in approximately 1 in 68 eight-year-old children in the United States. The number of children identified with ASD ranged from 1 in 175 children in Alabama to 1 in 45 children in New Jersey. We saw a 30% increase in autism from 2006 to 2008, a 78% increase in 10 years, and a whopping 600% increase in the past two decades![1]

The CDC is still unwilling to call autism an "epidemic," defined as "an increase, often sudden, in the number of cases of a disease above what is normally expected in that population in that area."[2] I'm not! Figure 1.1 depicts the statistics:

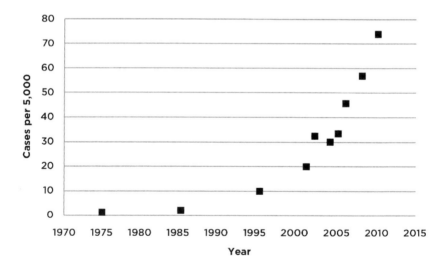

Figure 1.1.

Autism Prevalence in Children in the United States, 1975–2010 (Cases per 5,000)

In an October 2009 study, 1 in 91 American children and 1 in 58 boys between the ages of 3 and 17 carried an autism diagnosis.[3] Boys are 4–5 times more likely than girls to be diagnosed with autism: 1 in 42 boys versus 1 in 189 girls. That's about one and a half million people in the United States. Autism is the country's fastest-growing developmental disability, according to the Autism Society of America, with a 10–17% annual growth rate.[4]

The US government has blindly ignored autism until recently. At the end of 2006, it came out of its slumber and finally recognized the need to focus a little attention on autism by passing Public Law 109–416, better known as the Combating Autism Act. Even though autism was not an "epidemic," maybe it was worth fighting.

Annually, under this law, the Interagency Autism Coordinating Committee draws up a Strategic Plan for Autism Spectrum Disorder (ASD) Research. This plan provides a blueprint for autism research that serves as a basis for partnerships between the Department of Health and Human Services, other government agencies, and private organizations involved in autism research and services. Input from the ASD community, advocacy groups, research funding organizations, and the scientific community all play a critical role in updating funding each year. In 2012, the National Institutes of Health still allocated a puny $169 million for autism research, less than 1% of their $31 billion research budget, according to Autism Speaks.[5]

The autism epidemic is not limited to the United States. The Autism Society of America gives the following global statistics:[6]

- China: 1.1 million or 1.1/1,000
- India: 2 million or 1/250
- United Kingdom: 650,000 or 1/100
- Mexico: 150,000 or 2–6/1,000
- Philippines: 500,000
- Thailand: 180,000
- South Korea: 1/38 children![7]

Who knows about prevalence in countries where statistics are not available?

Even though our government has not declared it so, the autism epidemic is a big deal today. The costs are enormous: $126 billion a year in 2012, or about $60,000 per year per family in the United

States alone.[8] The financial burden falls on school systems, state-financed support programs, and individual families. The wallop affects families, schools, employers, and communities emotionally, sociologically, and psychologically. Autism is not going away. We must stare it in the face, understand it, manage it, heal it, and prevent it. How? By outsmarting it! Let's start with the basics.

The Dawn of Autism

The term "autism" derives from two Greek roots: *auto* (self) and *ismos* (condition). It was first used by psychiatrist Eugen Bleuler in 1913.[9] A few years earlier, however, Theodore Heller, a special educator in Vienna, Austria, wrote about some seemingly normal children whose behavior and learning deteriorated or was arrested in the second year of life. Heller proposed the term "dementia infantilis" to describe these children.[10] The discovery of autism is traditionally attributed to Leo Kanner, who in the 1940s considered it to be a psychiatric disorder, which he called "childhood schizophrenia."[11]

In the 1950s and '60s, we entered a dark time for autism when Freudian psychologist Bruno Bettelheim blamed this condition on poor mothering, giving rise to the "refrigerator mother" theory.[12] In the late 1960s Bernard Rimland, PhD, spoke out loudly in opposition to Bettelheim's ridiculous idea. Rimland, a psychologist and father of a son with autism, would become the voice of a biomedical approach to autism for the next almost 50 years. What began as indefatigable research into the role of vitamin and mineral deficiencies in autism to help his son resulted in his founding of the Autism Research Institute (ARI) and the Defeat Autism Now! movement.[13] Today Rimland's work continues through various streams of private funding.

Disability Law

Discussing autism is impossible without some understanding of two very important federal laws: the Individuals with Disabilities Education Act (IDEA) and the Americans with Disabilities Act (ADA). Entire books have been written about the interpretation of these laws; an overview will have to be sufficient here. To learn about how these laws impact students as they age out of schools and enter the workplace, go to chapter 15.

IDEA and ADA mandate the rights for individuals with a variety of handicapping conditions from birth, in schools, through college, and in the workplace. States have some leeway about how to interpret these federal laws. The scope and breadth of each state's services depends upon both their budgets and numbers of individuals with disabilities. Some offer excellent services with copious numbers of hours of "related services," such as occupational therapy, speech-language therapy, and even one-on-one aides. Others place all students in the mainstream classes, arguing that inclusion is better for everyone and barely supporting teachers and pupils with any related services. Only when parents legally challenge whether services are appropriate and whether the student is placed in the least restrictive environment (LRE) in which he or she can be successful (mandates of IDEA) are changes made.

Some lawyers specialize in disability law. Many have made their reputations by taking school systems and employers to court over violations of their clients' disability rights. For over 20 years I testified as an expert at an untold number of due process hearings, most resulting in my clients obtaining additional services for their children.

Individuals with Disabilities Education Act (IDEA)

In 1975, Congress passed Public Law 94–142 or the Education for All Handicapped Children Act (EHA), which assured a free and appropriate education to school-aged children with over a dozen handicapping conditions, including visual and hearing impairments, physical disabilities, and cognitive deficits, but not autism. Public schools are required to design and implement an Individualized Educational Program (IEP) tailored to each child's specific needs.

EHA was reenacted in 1990 as the Individuals with Disabilities Education Act, which is up for re-authorization every five years.[14] IDEA brought with it two important changes that strongly affected services to students with autism. It extended services to developmentally delayed children under age five, making it possible for young children to receive help even before they begin school.

Most importantly, it added autism as a new category of disability. The timing is of particular interest here, as autism did not show up on the screen in 1975; by 1990, it had reared its ugly head.

Americans with Disabilities Act (ADA)

In 1990 (a banner year for disabilities!) the US government passed the Americans with Disabilities Act, extending services beyond secondary school into college and the workplace. Now individuals with all types of disabilities, including autism diagnoses, could receive special attention beyond high school and age 21.

Post-secondary placements were now required to establish guidelines to accept, hire, and accommodate individuals with disabilities when they graduated from high school and sought further education and jobs. Community colleges, vocational schools, residential colleges, and universities struggled with what to do. They built ramps for wheelchairs—that was a no-brainer. But what types of accommodations were necessary and appropriate for those with autism?

Employers faced the same dilemmas. The law said they must make "reasonable accommodations" to help workers who have any handicap do their job. Such accommodations could include shifting job responsibilities, modifying equipment, or adjusting work schedules. The ADA also guarantees equal employment opportunity for people with disabilities and protects disabled workers against job discrimination. Where do individuals with autism fit under this enormous mandate? A difficult question, no?

Autism Diagnosis

The diagnosis of autism depends on whether the purpose of diagnosis is for medical or for educational purposes. Autism, unlike other chronic problems such as diabetes, has no physiological indicators; thus, an autism diagnosis occurs only when an individual exhibits certain specific behavioral symptoms. While people with an autism diagnosis have specific symptoms, the range of cognitive, social, language, and attentional strengths and deficits is broad.

Experts say, "When you've seen one child with autism, you have seen one child with autism." You cannot generalize about an individual with autism.

The Diagnostic and Statistical Manual (DSM)

The tool of choice for medical purposes is the fifth edition of the *Diagnostic and Statistical Manual of Mental Disorders* (*DSM-5*) published by the American Psychiatric Association.[16] Many parents are shocked to learn that the diagnostic determination for autism is "psychiatric."

According to the *DSM-5*, autism spectrum disorders are characterized by the following impairments in social interaction and communication in the presence of repetitive and stereotyped behavior, interests, and activities. Individuals must meet criteria A–D below, either currently or by history:

A. Persistent deficits in social communication and social interaction across contexts, not accounted for by general developmental delays, including all of the following:
    1. Deficits in social-emotional reciprocity
    2. Deficits in nonverbal communicative behaviors used for social interaction
    3. Deficits in developing and maintaining relationships
B. Restricted, repetitive patterns of behavior, interests, or activities as manifested by at least two of the following:
    1. Stereotypic, idiosyncratic or repetitive speech, motor movements, or use of objects
    2. Excessive adherence to routines, ritualized patterns of verbal or nonverbal behavior, or excessive resistance to change
    3. Highly restricted, fixated interests that are abnormal in intensity or focus
    4. Hyper- or hypo-reactivity to sensory input or unusual interest in sensory aspects of environment
C. Symptoms must be present in early childhood, but may not become fully manifest until social demands exceed limited capacities
D. Symptoms together limit and impair everyday functioning

The following are descriptions of some of the criteria used to determine eligibility:

Impairment in social interaction
- Inappropriate eye contact or facial expression
- Failure to develop peer relationships
- Lack of spontaneous sharing of enjoyment or interests

Impairment in communication
- Delayed or non-existent language development
- Poor conversational abilities if language is present
- Lack of make-believe or social imitative play

Repetitive and stereotyped behavior, interests, and activities
- Abnormally intense preoccupation with one or more interests
- Mannerisms such as hand or finger flapping or twisting or whole body movements
- Preoccupations with object parts

The *DSM-5* arrived to an uproar from the autism community even before its official publication in May 2013. Unlike its predecessor, the *DSM-4*, published in 2000, it includes all degrees of autism—mild, moderate, and severe—under one umbrella term: autism spectrum disorder. After reassessing all diagnostic criteria and definitions of the *DSM-4*, an expert panel appointed by the American Psychiatric Association had made the decision in 2012 to eliminate the previously discrete diagnoses and clump them.

With this landmark revision, individuals with previous diagnoses of autism, Pervasive Developmental Disorder (PDD), and Pervasive Developmental Disorder not otherwise specified (PDD-NOS) became simply "autistic." Childhood Disintegrative Disorder (CDD) and Rett syndrome, diagnoses in *DSM-4*, are no longer considered to be forms of autism. Patients with Rett Syndrome (a genetic abnormality) who have autistic symptoms might still be described as having ASD "with known genetic or medical condition" to indicate symptoms related to Rett's. The rarity of a CDD diagnosis made evaluation difficult, so it was eliminated altogether.

Asperger syndrome also lost its status as an autism spectrum disorder. This change raised the most ruckus among mental health professionals. Researchers fear that removing the diagnosis will affect long term research on that population. Also of great concern is that many high-functioning individuals will lose their much-needed support and services.

The *DSM-5* decision to capture all of autism under one huge category turned the autism world upside down. Many believe that one of the reasons for the changes was to bring down the numbers. Excluding Rett's, Asperger's, and CDD from the autism spectrum would allow the Food and Drug Administration (FDA) to continue to deny an epidemic. Fewer people on the spectrum translates into less money spent on services from the government, insurance companies, and school systems.

The most common use of the *DSM* diagnosis is, not surprisingly, by health insurance companies to allow or deny coverage for a given treatment. Often, an autism diagnosis is a death sentence for insurance coverage because most companies recognize how expensive and extended such services would be.

Remember that a *DSM* diagnosis of ASD is medical, and it does not guarantee educational services. Each school system has its own procedures for determining placement and eligibility for services. Some may just review medical and other reports and qualify a student for services. In large, complex school districts, the process often must start over to diagnose and qualify a student because IDEA now has 14 categories of disability. A school system's multidisciplinary team could decide that a young student diagnosed as ASD by his doctor is "speech-language impaired," "developmentally delayed," or "other health impaired." It's even possible for a highly functioning student that the school will deny services altogether. Quite confusing, isn't it?

Autism as a Spectrum of Disorders

The idea of an autism spectrum is not new. Lorna Wing, a British psychiatrist, first used this term almost 20 years ago.[17] One can even argue for including attention deficit hyperactivity disorder (ADHD), learning disabilities (LD), nonverbal learning disabilities (NLD), and the previously recognized diagnosis of Asperger syndrome on the spectrum. The figure below illustrates this concept:

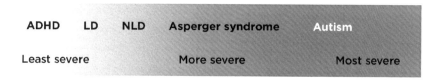

ADHD	LD	NLD	Asperger syndrome	Autism
Least severe			More severe	Most severe

Figure 1.2.

The Autism Spectrum of Disorders

These diagnoses result from an infinite number of subjective characteristics that make their precise placement on a linear chart difficult and debatable. Imagine the frustration of a parent searching for the "right" diagnosis. Having only one possibility, ASD, solves that problem also.

What a Diagnosis Says

A diagnosis of autism can be so overwhelming and confusing! What everyone must understand is that it merely says that an individual's symptoms match a specific cluster of behaviors; it does not prescribe treatment. Individuals with the same diagnosis may have similar symptoms; however, they do not necessarily require the same treatments. Prescribing treatment requires identifying a cause.

Consider the following example:

Symptom: A pounding pain in the right front temporal lobe
Diagnosis: Headache

Possible Causes	Treatment for that cause
Tension and Stress	Aspirin, bed rest
Brain tumor	Surgery
MSG poisoning	Alka-Selzer Gold
Nagging spouse	Divorce

If a person with a headache has not ingested Chinese food, bottled salad dressing or another food containing MSG, or is unmarried, causes can be narrowed down to stress and a brain tumor. While this example might seem frivolous, it clearly demonstrates the difficulty in determining cause and prescribing treatment for to those with autism spectrum disorders.

Is Autism Over-Diagnosed?

Many cynics and some scientists actually believe that the rise in autism cases is not real. Frankly, I find that astounding! Clearly the public is far more aware of autism today than in the past, and we are probably doing a better job of identifying those whose symptoms fit the criteria. I will also go as far as agreeing that we are including some higher-functioning individuals such as Einstein, Thomas Jefferson, and Bill Gates, brilliant "geeks" who may not have been labeled as autistic in the past.

But even a combination of increased awareness, better identification, and more inclusive diagnostic criteria is insufficient to explain the numbers occurring worldwide. It simply is not possible that so many children with a seriously debilitating condition would go unnoticed for so long, that well-educated parents would remain silent for so long, and that professionals would suddenly wake up — and all at the same time!

The autism epidemic is real. When I began my career in the late sixties, no laws even existed to mandate services. I was part of teams that determined eligibility for services at all levels of education from preschool through college. We focused almost solely on those with learning disabilities at first, then those with attention deficits. Not until the late 1980s was the word "autism" even mentioned.

Yes, autism may be slightly over-diagnosed, but the worldwide epidemic of autism is real!

What Causes Autism?

Many factors contribute to autism; most experts agree that it does not have a single cause. However, the multitude of possible causes of autism can all be captured under a single umbrella: STRESS! Stressors come from our genetic makeup; our personal lifestyle choices; toxins in our air, food, and water; insufficient exercise and sleep; inappropriate expectations; family relationships and events; and more. Figure 1.3 depicts some of these stressors in six general categories: Biological, Emotional, Physical, Environmental, Educational, and Behavioral.

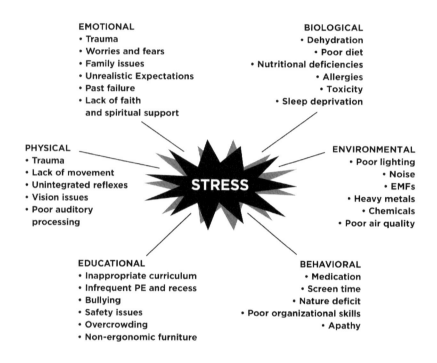

Figure 1.3.
Sources of Stress

Every person has a unique load limit, as does a bridge. Each individual with an autism diagnosis has a different combination of stressors that mount up and gradually overload the bridge to its breaking point. What we call "autism" may very well be the end product of many systems of the body being stressed to their limits. The larger the load of problematic factors on an individual's body, the more severe the attention, behavior, and cognitive difficulties.

Envision a wellness threshold, below which individuals are "healthy" and above which they are "sick." As load factors accumulate and take a person closer and closer to the line, only a single assault may be necessary to go over the top. An autism spectrum diagnosis occurs as the number of stressors rises above the threshold.

Immunological, digestive, respiratory, skin, language, motor, and attention symptoms occur as an individual's body approaches its personal limit and eventually exceeds it. These issues coexist with developmental, cognitive, sensory, and social/emotional problems, and their relationship is very complex. Every biological, psychological, environmental, sociological, and other stressor adds to a body's burden or "Total Load."

Your will learn more about the Total Load Theory of Autism and about oxidative stress in the next chapter. For now you just need to know that the answer to "what causes autism?" is super complicated. But if you want one umbrella that covers it all, the word is *stress*. Let's look at where some of those stressors come from.

Genetics

Since the early 1990s, the bulk of the scant autism research has been on the genetics of autism. About 10 to 20 times more research dollars are spent on studies of the genetic causes of autism than on other areas, including environmental ones (see below), according to Irva Hertz-Picciotto, PhD, an epidemiology professor at University of California Davis.[18]

Still, millions of dollars have gone toward finding *the* gene for autism. Until recently, researchers have made little headway toward understanding the causes of autism through the avenue of genetics alone. So far scientists have been able to identify several hundreds of loci that are likely to contribute to the complex genetic heterogeneity in autism; together, they account for only 5–8% of the cases.[9]

We now know that about 98% of children with autism carry at least one gene mutation for **M**ethylenetetrahydrofolate **R**eductase (MTHFR), a genetic polymorphism.[20] This gene cannot convert folic acid into its active form L-5 Methyltetrahydrofolate, leaving the body incapable of detoxifying heavy metals.[21] If your eyes are not rolling back yet and you want to know about MTHFR, go to www.MTHFR. net and www.MTHFRsupport.com.

Another genetic polymorphism commonly seen in autism is a gene mutation for Sulfite Oxidase or SUOX. While the MTHFR polymorphism inhibits a step of detoxification called methylation, the SUOX gene mutation impedes another step called sulfation. When this marker is present, an individual cannot properly process sulfur-containing foods and turn the sulfites into less-toxic sulfates.

Other possibly genetically-based differences between the brains of typical and autistic individuals show up with sophisticated brain imaging techniques. Differences in structure,[22] brain and head size,[23] and activity level,[24] but not the etiology of their neurological differences, are apparent. Viewing autism as simply a genetic condition is now diminishing.

Bottom line: An epidemic due to genetics alone is biologically impossible, as it takes a generation of approximately 20 years for changes to show up. For families affected by autism, genetics loads the gun. However, something has to pull the trigger.

The Environment

That something is the environment. By "environment" I mean more than the trees and the sky. Our environment is everything tangible and intangible outside our body that affects our physical, psychological, and biological status. Air, trees, water, and all they bring with them, are a part of it, but so is the food we eat, the clothes we wear, the products we use, the people we interact with, and the invisible energies that emanate from them. Any and all of these can affect us both positively and negatively. More and more, scientists are pointing a finger at the environment.

Good news: we have some control over our environment. On a small scale we can buy positive products, hang out with positive people, and let our kids watch only positive shows. On a large scale, we can work for and donate to campaigns for healthy air, food, and water, and strive for a healthier planet. See more about this subject in chapter 3.

Looking at the role environmental insults play in illness is not new. Rachel Carson shocked the world in her 1962 classic, *Silent Spring*.[25] This frightening exposé about how pesticides, chemicals, and other poisons have disrupted the bodies of all creatures on earth was a wake-up call to everyone. Theo Colburn disrupted our sleep again in 1997 with *Our Stolen Future*,[26] which confirmed that a generation later, things were getting worse, not better. The newest "thriller" is *Only*

One Chance: How Environmental Pollution Impairs Brain Development – and How to Protect the Brains of the Next Generation, by Phillippe Grandjean.[27]

Mercury was and continues to be highly suspect in autism. One study found that proximity to sources of mercury pollution was positively related to autism prevalence. For every 1,000 pounds of industrial release, there was a corresponding 2.6% increase in autism rates; a 3.7% increase was associated with power plant emissions. For every 10 miles from industrial or power plant sources, there was an associated decrease in autism.[28]

Robert F. Kennedy, Jr., a staunch environmentalist, calls children with autism "the canaries in the coalmine" as medical and manufacturing interests have mounted an assault on human health and covered their tracks along the way.[29] In their impeccably researched exposé of how "medicine has made reckless use of one of Earth's most toxic substances," investigative reporter Dan Olmstead and autism-dad Mark Blaxill declare autism a man-made epidemic. Their book, *The Age of Autism,* reads like a mystery novel that you cannot put down.[30] Learn more about mercury's devastating role in autism in chapter 2.

Environmental chemicals are now not the only stressors polluting newborns and young children. At no point in history have there been such dramatic changes in the physical environment. The 21st century has also brought genetically-altered and preserved foods, polluted air, electromagnetic fields, treated and tainted water, depleted soil, and a myriad of practices that undermine development. While positive early experiences in general serve to reinforce emotional resilience, negative ones diminish it, compromising a child's ability to adjust to stress in the future.[31]

Scientists will continue to look at autism "hot spots," such as those in California and New Jersey, and discover that they are downstream from chemical plants. The environment is clearly the trigger that activates the loaded gun.

Epigenetics: Genetics *and* Environment

Epigenetics is the biology of how external modifications to an individual's DNA can turn genes "on" or "off" with environmental triggers. Epigenetics is so important that it has made the cover of *Time*[32] and *Scientific American*.[33] In 2012, the *International Journal of Epidemiology* devoted an entire issue to it, calling epigenetics "the next big thing."[34]

Epigenetics is at the heart of the matter in autism. Epigenetics explains why all young children exposed to today's environmental chemical, electromagnetic, and sociological soup don't end up with autism. Why do some and not all children regress into autism? Individuals with ASDs appear to have a genetic propensity or predisposition that manifests itself only when triggered by the "right" combination of environmental factors.[35] Any of the environmental exposures mentioned above can change gene expression, resulting in MTHFR or SUOX mutations.[36]

Related to the SUOX mutation is another environmental impact: the coincidental timing during the 1980s of a recommendation by the medical community for replacing aspirin with acetaminophen for pain. Acetaminophen is the main ingredient in Tylenol™ and some other popular painkillers. According to recent research, acetaminophen toxicity can overload the defective sulfation pathway catalyzed by phenol sulfer-transferase (PST), which is deficient in autism (see chapter 4), leading to overproduction of the toxic metabolite N-acetylp-benzoquinone imine (NAPQI). Increased levels of NAPQI reduce an individual's ability to detoxify toxic chemicals, thus increasing oxidative stress and cascading into protein, lipid, and nucleic acid damage from free radicals.[37] Read more about these detoxification problems in chapter 7.

Ultimately, the more "right" the genetic material combined with the more "right" environmental insults, the more severe the disability. Those on the lesser end of the spectrum have fewer genetic variables combined with fewer environmental insults. Those with severe autism are unfortunate enough to have a larger number of each factor.

How is Autism Treated Today?

After getting an autism diagnosis, most parents hope and pray that the next step is easy: just treat autism like a headache, and it will go away. Unfortunately, autism treatment is extremely complex. The relationship between symptoms and cures is not always linear, but rather a synchronistic matrix with multiple variables. Every family of someone with autism, just like a patient with chronic headaches, tenaciously searches for the right combination of "magic bullets" that will provide relief, and money to cover the costs.

What interventions can jumpstart language, extinguish self-stimulatory behaviors, or normalize social interactions? And who is going to pay? Three choices: an insurance company, the school system, or the family; most often money comes from all three pockets. As autism numbers have risen—surprise—all three are becoming bankrupt. Nobody wants this hot potato!

Old Thinking: Manage Autism by Eliminating Symptoms

Historically, medical, psychological, and educational approaches *manage* autism by trying to eliminate symptoms. Tools are pharmaceutical intervention, special education, counseling, and applied behavior analysis (ABA). These treatments focus on eliminating undesirable behaviors while increasing desirable outcomes. The ultimate goal is to replace hyperactivity, attentional difficulties, anxiety, depression, mood swings, agitation, aggression, self-injurious behavior, insomnia, perseveration, and impulsivity with relatedness, eye contact, self-control, a longer attention span, and confidence.

Medications can alleviate behavioral and attentional symptoms, but often with undesirable side effects. While behavior management and special education provide external methods of monitoring and handling behavior, they may fail to allow the child's own sensory systems to learn from experience how to modulate and integrate information and to develop internal controls. Counseling programs help parents cope with issues such as fecal smearing, picky eating, and sleep problems but do not address possible causes.

The benefits of these symptom-alleviating treatments are short term at best. At worst, benefits may not outweigh side effects. Also of great concern is the huge long-term financial burden placed on both the health care and the educational systems, which were not designed to manage so many children.

Medications. According to C. T. Gordon, MD, a psychiatrist who for many years has treated individuals with autism pharmacologically and the father of an adult son with autism, "The ultimate goal of medication in an individual who has autism is to prepare the brain's physiology to take optimal advantage of other aspects of treatment. In other words, pharmacologic intervention should typically be viewed as only one part of a multi-modal treatment plan for an individual with autism. The goal of medication, as well as all other treatments in autism, is to maximize the individual's functioning."[38]

Gordon suggests that medications be prescribed one at a time so that effectiveness and side effects can be accurately determined. Unfortunately, clinicians often use several drugs together to balance out one another's side effects.

Since they were introduced over 60 years ago, medications for autism have become more specialized and powerful. Table 1.1 lists drugs that are being prescribed for children on the autism spectrum at the present time. This chart will, most likely, be outdated as soon as it is printed and new medications hit the market.

CLASS	DRUGS	BENEFIT	SIDE EFFECTS
Anti-psychotics or Neuroleptics	Clozapine Stelazine	Reduce agitation, anxiety, aggression, hyperactivity, stereotypic and self-stimulatory behaviors, temper outbursts	Addiction, agitation, blurred vision, dyskinesia, psychosis, heart problems, sedation, tremors
Typical Neuroleptics	Geodon Naltrexone Risperdal	Reduce aggression, agitation, self-injurious behavior	Agitation, increased appetite, low white blood cell count, tardive dyskinesia, elevated blood sugar, nausea, weight gain
Anti-depressants	Abilify Anafranil Desipramine Effexor Luvox Paxil, Prozac Tofranil Zoloft	Raise serotonin levels, reduce anxiety, reduce obsessive-compulsiveness and ritualistic behaviors	Arhythmias, blurred vision, constipation, dry mouth, dizziness, fatigue, headache, hyperactivity and impulsivity, lowered threshold for seizures, nausea, sleep disturbances

CLASS	DRUGS	BENEFIT	SIDE EFFECTS
Anti-hypertensives	Clonidine Halcion	Calm and improve sleep, decrease hyperactivity and impulsivity	Constipation, dizziness, irritability, low blood pressure, sedation, nausea, weakness
Anti-histamines Anti-fungals Anti-convulsants/ Mood stabilizers	Atarax Benadryl Phenergan Diflucan Nystatin Nizoral Depakote Felbatol Lithium Phenobarbitol Tegretol Zarontin	Treat allergic reactions like sneezing, hay fever, and hives Treats fungus and mold infections such as thrush, candida, and ringworm Calm behavior, lessen mood swings and outbursts	Constipation, diarrhea, dizziness, insomnia excitability, headache, drowsiness, loss of appetite, nausea, nervousness or anxiety, upset stomach, vomiting, weakness. Changes in taste, diarrhea, dizziness, headache, indigestion, nausea, stomach pain, vomiting Confusion, clumsiness, diarrhea, poor kidney function, stomach pain, tremors, vomiting, weakness, weight changes, vision impairments such as rapid eye movements
Stimulants	Adderall Cylert Ritalin	Increase levels of dopamine and norepinephrine, improve focus and regulation, monitor arousal system, decrease impulsivity	Abdominal pain, appetite suppression, depression, fever, perseveration and repetitive behaviors, insomnia, irritability, nausea, nervousness, palpitations, vomiting

Table 1.1.

Common Medications Used for Children with Autism by Class[39]

The only two drugs on this list that the FDA has approved to treat symptoms related to *autism* are *Risperdal* and *Abilify*.[40] All others are used off-label. Minor to severe health-related side effects are inevitable with almost all drugs, so use of all medications must be monitored by a physician.

Some behavioral issues of individuals with autism are secondary to drug side effects. It is imperative that all health care providers evaluate a patient's medications when taking a health history and become familiar with the side effects of individual drugs by reading the latest *Physicians' Desk Reference*. They must then decide whether sleep disturbances, constipation, seizures, and potentially fatal heart problems are acceptable trade-offs for increased attention and decreased aggression.

Since 1967, the ARI has been collecting parent ratings of the behavioral effects of over 40 drugs on individuals with autism. Table 1.2 shows statistics from 2009 that represent responses from over 27,000 parents. With the majority of drugs, parents reported improved behavior less than 50% of the time. Seeking safer solutions has become their quest.

PARENT RATINGS OF BEHAVIORAL EFFECTS OF BIOMEDICAL INTERVENTIONS
Autism Research Institute ● 4182 Adams Avenue ● San Diego, CA 92116

The parents of autistic children represent a vast and important reservoir of information on the benefits—and adverse effects—of the large variety of drugs and other interventions that have been tried with their children. Since 1967 the Autism Research Institute has been collecting parent ratings of the usefulness of the many interventions tried on their autistic children.

The following data have been collected from the more than 27,000 parents who have completed our questionnaires designed to collect such information. For the purposes of the present table, the parents responses on a six-point scale have been combined into three categories: "made worse" (ratings 1 and 2), "no effect" (ratings 3 and 4), and "made better" (ratings 5 and 6). The "Better:Worse" column gives the number of children who "Got Better" for each one who "Got Worse."

DRUGS	Got Worse[A]	No Effect	Got Better	Better: Worse	No. of Cases[B]
Actos	19%	60%	21%	1.1:1	140
Aderall	43%	26%	31%	0.7:1	894
Amphetamine	47%	28%	25%	0.5:1	1355
Anafranil	32%	39%	29%	1.1:1	440
Antibiotics	33%	50%	18%	0.5:1	2507
Antifungals[C]					
Diflucan	5%	34%	62%	13:1	1214
Nystatin	5%	43%	52%	11:1	1969
Atarax	26%	53%	21%	0.8:1	543
Benadryl	24%	50%	26%	1.1:1	3230
Beta Blocker	18%	51%	31%	1.7:1	306
Buspar	29%	42%	28%	1.0:1	431
Chloral Hydrate	42%	39%	19%	0.5:1	498
Clonidine	22%	32%	46%	2.1:1	1658
Clozapine	38%	43%	19%	0.5:1	170
Cogentin	20%	53%	27%	1.4:1	198
Cylert	45%	35%	19%	0.4:1	634
Depakene[D]					
Behavior	25%	44%	31%	1.2:1	1146
Seizures	12%	33%	55%	4.6:1	761
Desipramine	34%	35%	32%	0.9:1	95

DRUGS	Got Worse[A]	No Effect	Got Better	Better: Worse	No. of Cases[B]
Dilantin[D]					
Behavior	28%	49%	23%	0.8:1	1127
Seizures	16%	37%	47%	3.0:1	454
Fenfluramine	21%	52%	27%	1.3:1	483
Haldol	38%	28%	34%	0.9:1	1222
IVIG	7%	39%	54%	7.6:1	142
Klonapin[D]					
Behavior	31%	40%	29%	0.9:1	270
Seizures	29%	55%	16%	0.6:1	86
Lithium	22%	48%	31%	1.4:1	515
Luvox	31%	37%	32%	1.0:1	251
Mellaril	29%	38%	33%	1.2:1	2108
Mysoline[D]					
Behavior	41%	46%	13%	0.3:1	156
Seizures	21%	55%	24%	1.1:1	85
Naltrexone	18%	49%	33%	1.8:1	350
Low Dose Naltrexone	11%	52%	38%	4.0:1	190
Paxil	34%	32%	35%	1.0:1	471
Phenobarb.[D]					
Behavior	48%	37%	16%	0.3:1	1125
Seizures	18%	44%	38%	2.2:1	543

DRUGS	Got Worse[A]	No Effect	Got Better	Better: Worse	No. of Cases[B]
Prolixin	30%	41%	28%	0.9:1	109
Prozac	33%	32%	35%	1.1:1	1391
Risperidal	21%	26%	54%	2.6:1	1216
Ritalin	45%	26%	29%	0.6:1	4256
Secretin					
Intravenous	7%	50%	43%	6.4:1	597
Transderm.	9%	56%	35%	3.9:1	257
Stelazine	29%	45%	26%	0.9:1	437
Steroids	34%	30%	36%	1.1:1	204
Tegretol[D]					
Behavior	25%	45%	30%	1.2:1	1556
Seizures	14%	33%	53%	3.8:1	872
Thorazine	36%	40%	24%	0.7:1	945
Tofranil	30%	38%	32%	1.1:1	785
Valium	35%	42%	24%	0.7:1	895
Valtrex	8%	42%	50%	6.7:1	238
Zarontin[D]					
Behavior	34%	48%	18%	0.5:1	164
Seizures	20%	55%	25%	1.2:1	125
Zoloft	35%	33%	31%	0.9:1	579

A. "Worse" refers only to worse behavior. Drugs, but not nutrients, typically also cause physical problems if used long-term.
B. No. of cases is cumulative over several decades, so does not reflect current usage levels (e.g., Haldol is now seldom used).
C. Antifungal drugs and chelation are used selectively, where evidence indicates they are needed.
D. Seizure drugs: top line behavior effects, bottom line effects on seizures.
E. Calcium effects are not due to dairy-free diet; statistics are similar for milk drinkers and non-milk drinkers.

Table 1.2.

Parent Ratings of Behavioral Effects of Drugs
Autism Research Institute March, 2009 (Reprinted with permission)

New Thinking: Heal Autism by Treating Underlying Causes

New thinkers want to *heal* their children. New thinkers believe that what we are calling "autism" is the outward manifestation of an accumulation of stressors on the body — including exposure to toxins, malfunctioning digestive systems, and immune system failures — which I will address throughout this book.

New-thinking parents believe strongly that their kids' digestive issues, allergies, vaccine reactions, and behavioral and learning issues deserve closer attention. They *know* there is a relationship between their kids' health problems and their behavior. They recognize that traditional medical treatments and educational management techniques can certainly have palliative affects, but they are looking for better outcomes than simply helping children compensate.

One amazing group of these parents has banded together to form The Thinking Moms' Revolution. Their website is chock-full of great information, and they publish a daily newsletter to which readers can subscribe on www.thinkingmomsrevolution.com.

In the past 10 years, some new-thinking doctors have written helpful guides to understanding the biological issues in autism. These groundbreaking books are not by a group of "quacks," but rather by well-respected physicians with impeccable credentials:

- *Changing the Course of Autism: A Scientific Approach for Parents and Physicians*, by Bryan Jepson, MD[41]
- *Healing the New Childhood Epidemics: Autism, ADHD, Asthma, and Allergies*, by Kenneth Bock, MD[42]
- *Healing and Preventing Autism*, by Jerry Kartzinel, MD, and outspoken autism mom, Jenny McCarthy[43]
- *The Autism Book: What Every Parent Needs to Know about Early Detection, Treatment, Recovery, and Prevention*, by Robert Sears, MD[44]

The latest voice and one of the most respected and leading proponents of new thinking is Martha Herbert, MD, a pediatric neurologist and professor at Harvard Medical School. For Herbert, autism is not a "thing." It is an outcome of an assault on the brain when the body is in poor health. She believes that autism is a not a "brain disorder" but rather a "disorder that affects the brain." In her book *The Autism Revolution*, she takes a whole-body approach that targets foundational systems like immunity, gut function, and detoxification.[45]

California physician Michael J. Goldberg, MD, agrees that autism is a medical disorder. In his book *The Myth of Autism*, he argues that autism is a misunderstood epidemic that can be healed.[46]

Many other doctors, like these outspoken pioneers, are treating thousands of patients, many of whom experienced regressive development; all believe that recovery may be possible. Grassroots movements such as Cure Autism Now, Defeat Autism Now!, and Prevent Autism Now have put on conferences, designed websites, offered webinars, published books, made movies, recorded DVDs, founded schools, started camps, and produced programs with an endless potpourri of exciting, innovative techniques and methods to outsmart this thing called autism. The vast quantity and cost of these programs could make a parent's head spin!

Because they understand individual variability, new thinkers believe that subscribing to a generic treatment plan is just plain stupid. So they evaluate each individual's unique history, identify possible causes, and set priorities. As interventions address causes one by one, stressors fall away, freeing up new energy for the body to address others.

Where Can I Turn? Who Can Be Trusted?

Autism has become big business in a thriving marketplace of interventions delivered by talented and experienced practitioners, most of whom have something to offer a child with an autism diagnosis. New approaches are emerging every day, claiming to be the missing link. Hurry up — early intervention is crucial, according to experts. Seek therapy, advice, support. Do it *now*!

This is sage advice — people with autism do need help, but from whom? The first of many difficult choices looms.

- *Pediatrician?* Most families suspect that "something" is wrong with their children well before getting a formal diagnosis. Many beg their pediatricians to make a referral for an autism screening or for early intervention.

    In the past, parents' pleas often fell on deaf ears. Since 2007, however, the American Academy of Pediatrics (AAP) has strongly urged their member physicians to routinely screen babies for autism at 18 and 24 months, and not to wait for a diagnosis before referring them for services.[47] Unfortunately, those screenings have two drawbacks: they come just at the time that the vaccine schedule accelerates, and the recommended referral is for palliative therapies that treat symptoms, not underlying causes.

    The good news is that doctors are urged to work together with their patients as partners and to take parents concerns seriously. The AAP suggests that physicians consider requests for alternative treatments and individualized vaccine schedules, rather than "fire" families from their practices if they do not conform. While these mandates should help toward the goal of early diagnosis, some fear they may also lead to *over*diagnosis.

• *Developmental pediatrician?* These children's doctors are specialists for kids with a myriad of genetic, language, motor, and behavioral disorders. Some developmental pediatricians may be old thinkers who suggest a trial of medication, behavioral management, and special education that provides intense language, motor, and social-emotional therapies for a child with autism. In the past five years, however, more and more are suggesting treatments that focus on physical symptoms, like immunological, dermatological, digestive, sensory, neurological, respiratory, cognitive, psychological, and developmental markers that preceded the diagnosis.

• *Friends and family?* Well-meaning relatives and parents encourage each other to try therapies that they have heard about or personally found helpful. This buffet-dining approach, which includes many side dishes and has no main course, can waste both time and money. Simply taking therapies off the rack like a dress in a department store is like going into the wilderness without a map and compass.

• *Conferences?* Informative conferences take place at airport hotels and auditoriums in warm places almost every weekend. In addition to learning from national experts in powerful educational sessions, parents learn from and network with each other. At the hundreds that I have attended, I am always amazed at the incessant buzz about the latest treatment option that resonates throughout the halls as parents share their latest experiences, successes, and failures.

The exhibit halls are akin to buffets at casinos; the smorgasbords and stakes are similar, as well. Both venues offer promising options, which sometimes are not as rewarding as they look. Space in these marketplaces sells out quickly to vendors with payment plans that make their wares accessible to everyone. Few companies are pedaling snake oil; careful screening of exhibitors assures that products have efficacy. However, taking therapies off the shelf at these events can waste valuable time and money, and can even be dangerous. The looming question is, will it work for *my* child?

- *The Internet?* The Internet offers a global society, and everyone has a website. The discovery of new, exciting therapies with the potential to change children's lives spreads faster than California wildfires. How do you know who is legitimate and who is not?

- *Case manager?* Some mental health professionals and developmental pediatricians can serve as professional case managers; ask around. For almost 30 years I was a case manager to families of children with special needs. I was proud that I had no vested interest in any particular area because I did not offer treatment.

This book? Why do we need yet another book on healing autism, written by neither a physician nor a parent? Because discoveries are occurring very rapidly, and much of the information in this book is not in the resources listed above. Because we need a step-by-step model that includes not only biological, but also sensory, motor, language, social-emotional, academic, and vocational areas across the lifespan. Because we need an up-to-date, practical, easy-to-read guide that is appropriate for parents, professionals, and lay persons, complete with resources on where to get help in each area.

Reading this book is a great beginning to outsmarting autism, whether you are a parent with a newly diagnosed child or one who has "tried everything" with a teenager or young adult. Use it with confidence along with your hand-picked healthcare team. Autism is *not* an immutable psychiatric brain disorder for which no cure exists. Those who perpetuate this myth should be silenced!

Outsmarting Autism

Every child with an autism spectrum diagnosis deserves and requires a set of basic principles to manage healing, many of which are good for anyone interested in recovering good health. The general principles form a strong, unbendable foundation for disease-free living. They are appropriate no matter whether the diagnosis is at the mild, moderate, or severe end of the autism spectrum, or is even a degenerative disease of modern society.

In addition, they need and deserve a customized therapy plan tailored to that individual's unique needs. Each plan must be monitored by a qualified health care professional or a case manager, and will change daily, weekly, monthly, and yearly as the child responds, regresses, progresses, and heals.

This book's model provides a hierarchy of therapies based on the premise that those with autism are physically sick. Autism did not just happen overnight. It took some time for Load Factors from a variety of sources to accumulate, overload, and overwhelm their bodies. Biological functions, such as digestion, respiration, circulation, and immunity, must take precedence over talking, looking, and listening at least for a short time as the body heals. Eventually, focusing on language, social skills, and academics makes sense.

Healing autism is a process that starts with examining a family's lifestyle and making changes in daily practices before seeking therapies. Which therapies should take priority? How long should they take? Everyone wants to see instant improvement, but healing take time. Too many at once can overburden an already stressed-out system. What occurs inside the gut, the immune system, and brain are slow processes that may not be apparent.

In order to outsmart autism, I will guide you through five steps, each of which has several parts:

1. Take away the bad stuff, and add back the good stuff.
2. Correct foundational issues in structure and reflex integration.
3. Address sensory problems.
4. Focus on interacting, communicating, and learning.
5. Plan for the future.

These steps are prioritized for a reason—they tackle the various causes of autism at the source. If you just treat symptoms, it is impossible to heal. While complete healing may not be possible for everyone, what is possible without a doubt is improved function.

That said, I don't expect that most people buying this book will read through sequentially. Familiarize yourself with the structure, and use what works for you. Every individual with autism is different.

This book is a road map from today to the future. Looking back and feeling guilty only wastes energy. The road is long and sometimes bumpy. Put on your seatbelt and join me for the ride. By using Total Load Theory as a guide, we can *outsmart autism* together!

---

[1] Centers of Communicable Disease and Prevention. Prevalence of Autism Spectrum Disorder among Children Aged 8 Years—Autism and Developmental Disabilities Monitoring Network, 11 Sites, United States, 2010. Morbidity and Mortality Weekly Report Surveillance Summaries, Mar 2014, 63:2.

[2] Centers for Disease Control and Prevention. Lesson 1: Introduction to Epidemiology, Section 11: Epidemic Disease Occurrence. http://www.cdc.gov/osels/scientific_edu/ss1978/lesson1/section11.html. Accessed Dec 10, 2013.

[3] Maternal & Child Health Bureau of Health Resources and Services Administration (HRSA), US Department of Health and Human Services. The Prevalence of Parent-Reported Diagnosis of Autism Spectrum Disorder among Children in the United States, 2009.

[4] McAuliffe J. CDC: Autism rates growing 10–17% annually. The Times-Tribune.com, Oct 23, 2011.

[5] http://www.autismspeaks.org/what-autism/facts-about-autism. Accessed Dec 11, 2013.

[6] Grossman L, Barrozo P. The Next Global Human Rights Issue: Why the Plight of Individuals with Autism Spectrum Disorders Requires a Global Call to Action. Autism Advocate, 4th ed., 2007; Monarch Center for Autism. Around the World. http://www.monarchcenterforautism.org/about-autism/around-the-world. Accessed Apr 14, 2014.

[7] Kim YS, et al. Prevalence of Autism Spectrum Disorder in a Total Population Sample, American Journal of Psychiatry online, May 9, 2011.

[8] Autism Speaks. New Research Finds Annual Cost of Autism Has More Than Tripled to $126 Billion in the U.S. and Reached £34 Billion in the U.K. www.autismspeaks.org. Accessed Dec 10, 2013.

[9] Bleuler E. Autistic Thinking. Am J Insanity, 1913, 69, 873–886.

[10] http://info.med.yale.edu/chldstdy/autism/cdd.html. Accessed Jan 2, 2008.

[11] Kanner L. Autistic Disturbances of Affective Contact. Nervous Child 2, 1943, 217–250.

[12] Bettelheim B. The Empty Fortress—Infantile Autism and the Birth of the Self. New York: The Free Press, 1967.

[13] Rimland B. Infantile Autism. Upper Saddle River, NJ: Prentice-Hall, 1964, 43.

[14] Individuals with Disabilities Education Act (IDEA). 20 U.S.C. § 1401 (3) (26) §300, 1997.

[15] Americans with Disabilities Act. (ADA) 42 U.S.C. §§12101–12213, 1990.

[16] American Psychiatric Association. Diagnostic and Statistical Manual of Mental Disorders, 5th ed. Washington, DC: American Psychiatric Association, 2013.

[17] Wing L. The Autistic Spectrum: A guide for parents and professionals. Philadelphia: Trans-Atlantic Publications, 1996.

[18] Hertz-Picciotto I, Delwiche L. The rise in autism and the role of age at diagnosis. Epidemiology, Jan 2009, 20:1, 84–90.

[19] Schaaf CP, Zoghbi HY. Solving the Autism Puzzle a Few Pieces at a Time. Neuron, Jun 2011, 70:5, 806–808.

[20] Boris M, Goldblatt A, Galanko J, James SJ. Association of MTHFR Gene Variants with Autism. Jrnl American Physicians and Surgeons, Winter 2004, 9:4.

[21] Liu X, Solehdin F, Cohen IL, Gonzalez MG. Population- and family-based studies associate the MTHFR gene with idiopathic autism in simplex families. J Autism Dev Disord, Jul 2011, 41:7, 938–44.

[22] Casanova MF, Buxhoeveden DP, Switala AE, Roy E. Minicolumnar pathology in autism. Neurol, 2002, 58, 428–32.

[23] Hazlett H, et al. Early brain overgrowth in autism associated with an increase in cortical surface area before age 2 years. Arch Gen Psychiatry, May 2011, 68:5, 467–76; Courchesne E, Carper R, Akshoomoff, N. Evidence of brain overgrowth in the first year of life in autism. JAMA, Jul 2003, 290:3, 337–44.

[24] Anagnostou E, Taylor MJ. Review of neuroimaging in autism spectrum disorders: What have we learned and where we go from here. Molecular Autism, Apr 2011, 2:1, 4.

[25] Carson R. Silent Spring. Boston: Houghton Mifflin Co., 1962.

[26] Colburn T, Dumanoski D, Myers JP. Our Stolen Future. New York: Penguin Books, 1997.

[27] Grandjean P. Only One Chance: How Environmental Pollution Impairs Brain Development—and How to Protect the Brains of the Next Generation. New York: Oxford Univ Press, 2013.

[28] Palmer RF, Blanchard S, Wood R. Proximity to point sources of environmental mercury release as a predictor of autism prevalence. Health Place, Mar 2009, 15:1, 18–24.

[29] Kennedy RF. Robert F. Kennedy Jr. Interviews Dr. Boyd Haley on Mercury Toxicity Alzheimer's and Autism. http://www.ageofautism.com/2011/03/robert-f-kennedy-jr-interviews-dr-boyd-haley-on-mercury-toxicity-alzheimers-and-autism.html.

[30] Olmstead D, Blaxill M. The Age of Autism: Mercury, Medicine, and a Man-Made Epidemic. New York: St. Martin's Press, 2010.

[31] McGowan PO, et al. Epigenetic regulation of the glucocorticoid receptor in human brain associates with childhood abuse. Nature Neuroscience, 2009, 12:3, 342–48.

[32] Cloud J. Why your DNA is not your destiny. Time Magazine, Jan 6, 2010.

[33] Rusting R. Epigenetics Explained. Scientific American, Nov 22, 2011.

[34] Ebrahim S. Epigenetics: The next big thing. Int. J. Epidemiol, Feb 2012 41:1, 1–3.

[35] Insel T. The New Genetics of Autism—Why Environment Matters, Apr 4, 2012. http://www.nimh.nih.gov/about/director/2012/the-new-genetics-of-autism-why-environment-matters.shtml. Accessed Jan 11, 2013.

[36] Baccarelli A, Bollati V. Epigenetics and environmental chemicals. Curr Opin Pediatr, 2009, 21:2, 243–51.

[37] Shaw W. Evidence that Increased Acetaminophen use in Genetically Vulnerable Children Appears to be a Major Cause of the Epidemics of Autism, Attention Deficit with Hyperactivity, and Asthma. Journal of Restorative Medicine, 2013, 2, 1–16.

[38] Gordon CT. Pharmacological Treatment Options for Autism: Part 1. J National Alliance for Autism Research, Spring 2003, 8.

[39] http://www.autism.com/index.php/pro_adversereactions. Accessed Dec 10, 2013.

[40] http://www.fda.gov/NewsEvents/Newsroom/PressAnnouncements/2006/ucm108759.htm. Accessed Dec 10, 2013.

[41] Jepson B. Changing the Course of Autism: A Scientific Approach for Parents and Physicians. Boulder, CO: Sentinent Publishing, 2007.

[42] Bock K, Stauth K. Healing the New Childhood Epidemics: Autism, ADHD, Asthma, and Allergies. New York: Ballantine Books, 2008.

[43] McCarthy J, Kartzinel J. Healing and Preventing Autism. New York: Dutton, 2009.

[44] Sears RW. The Autism Book: What Every Parent Needs to Know about Early Detection, Treatment, Recovery, and Prevention. New York: Little Brown, 2010.

[45] Herbert M. The Autism Revolution. New York: Ballantine Books, 2012.

46 Goldberg MJ, Goldberg E. The Myth of Autism. New York: Skyhorse Publishing, 2011.

[47] Johnson C, Myers S. Identification and evaluation of children with autism spectrum disorders. Elk Grove Village, IL: American Academy of Pediatrics, Oct 29, 2007.

CHAPTER 2

Total Load Theory:
Why So Many Children Have Autism

Have you ever had a bad day at work, gotten caught in traffic on the way home, yelled at your kids for something insignificant, and, as you fell into bed, felt a cold coming on? You experienced "Total Load": the cumulative effect of multiple individual assaults that overload the body.

Total Load Theory is a concept from engineering that explains why, as a heavy truck travels over a bridge, the structure collapses. Who or what is to blame? The truck driver? The trucking company? The engineer who designed the bridge? The weather? The ship captain whose tanker bumped into the moorings endless times? Obviously, not any of them is a single cause, even though each stressor contributed to the outcome. An accumulation of dozens of stressors caused the bridge to collapse. About 20 years ago my colleagues and I realized that this engineering theory could apply to autism.

The Total Load Theory of Autism brings together many possible etiologies: biological, environmental, immunological, neurological, psychological, and toxicological. As these and other stressors mount, they cause sensory, motor, language, social-emotional, and other systems to collapse.

Researchers are investigating the causes of "emerging symptoms" of autism:

- gastrointestinal abnormalities, such as reflux, diarrhea, constipation, and abdominal pain;[1]
- altered metabolic processes, such as the impaired ability to metabolize toxic chemicals;[2] and
- immune system abnormalities,[3] such as allergies to common foods[4] and the emotionally-charged possible relationship between immunological status and vaccines and their adjuvants, including aluminum[5] and thimerosal, the mercury-containing preservative still in some vaccines.[6]

Scientists are only beginning to understand the complex synergy among all of these stressors and how they affect causation.[7] One, Helen V. Ratajczak, PhD, provides a detailed, coherent, and straightforward explanation of how a buildup of load factors causes autism. Her findings are discussed in two articles published together in the esteemed *Journal of Immunotoxicology*. Dr. Ratajczak, whose doctorate is in molecular biology, spent part of her career working for a pharmaceutical company. She applied her scientific knowledge to recovering her grandson from autism after he was diagnosed at age three; he is a young adult today. Ratajczak's exhaustive review supports the premise of this book, a theory I hatched in the early 1990s.

In Part 1 Ratajczak writes, "Autism could result from more than one cause, with different manifestations in different individuals that share common symptoms. Documented causes of autism include genetic mutations and/or deletions, viral infections, and encephalitis following vaccination. Therefore, autism is the result of genetic defects and/or inflammation of the brain. The inflammation could be caused by a defective placenta, immature blood-brain barrier, the immune response of the mother to infection while pregnant, a premature birth, encephalitis in the child after birth, or a toxic environment."[8]

In Part 2, after reviewing the literature from 1943 to 2011, Ratajczak adds the gastrointestinal, immunologic, neurologic, and toxicological biomarkers, such as increased vulnerability to oxidative stress, immune dysfunction, and more. Ratajcak's exhaustive research supports the idea that many factors can influence a person's vulnerability, resulting in a collapse of systems from all types of stress.[9]

Esteemed Harvard neurologist Martha Herbert, MD, agrees. In her groundbreaking book, *The Autism Revolution*, she says, "the child's brain and body have been battered so much by the world that they have lost the resources to protect themselves."[10]

Load Factors

Remember the chart of stressors in chapter 1? Any stressor — biological, physical, environmental, behavioral, educational, or emotional — can be a load factor for anyone. Internal stress from a poor diet, toxins, or pathogens occurs at a cellular level and affects vulnerable organs and systems. External factors, such as academic demands and family problems, further stress our bodies and their ability to function properly.

The following section lists load factors that occur in individuals with autism. The possible combinations of accumulated load factors making up an individual's Total Load is infinite!

Oxidative Stress

One of the most significant biological stressors is oxidative stress, which is stress that occurs at a cellular level. Through a chemical process called "oxidation," toxic substances known as "oxidants" overwhelm a cell's natural defenses. During oxidation, oxidative stress gradually disrupts a cell's basic function, eventually contributing to DNA damage or even cell death.

Oxidants enter the body either from the environment or as by-products of the body's normal metabolism. Because most cells in the body are vulnerable to oxidation, limiting oxidants through diet and using natural products are extremely important interventions included in the upcoming chapters.

The body fights off oxidants with compounds called "antioxidants," which include vitamins and minerals from food and special enzymes that the body makes. When antioxidants outnumber oxidants, health is good. When oxidants prevail, cells suffer oxidative stress. In individuals with autism, high levels of toxins overpower low levels of antioxidants, allowing their bodies continuously to accumulate more toxins, thus causing chronic oxidative stress.[11]

Scientists are just beginning to understand the far-reaching effects of oxidative stress in autism. Pat Levitt, PhD, Director of Developmental Neurogenetics at The Saban Research Institute of Children's Hospital Los Angeles, believes that one of the most important outcomes of comprehending the impact of oxidative stress is that it will allow us "eventually to be able to individualize therapies in order to achieve the best possible outcomes for children with ASD."[12]

Immunological Stress

Of all the possible load factors associated with autism, dysfunction of the immune system is the one that has received the most attention. Jane El-Dahr, MD, the Head of Pediatric Immunology and Allergy at Tulane Medical Center, likens the immune system to the United States Department of Defense (DOD). Just as the DOD acts to keep the country safe from invaders, the body's immune system acts to defend it against harmful substances. The "ideal" immune system recognizes all foreign organisms efficiently, rapidly destroys invaders, prevents further infection, and never causes damage to itself.[13]

Children on the autism spectrum clearly have less-than-ideal immune systems. Their histories almost always include several of the following indicators of immune system dysfunction:

- mother with chronic fatigue, fibromyalgia, or low thyroid
- mother who received vaccine(s) prior to or during pregnancy or while nursing
- family history of auto-immune disorders and allergies, especially to cow's milk
- sensitivity to dyes, chemicals, perfumes, or medications
- yeast infections, such as severe diaper rash or thrush
- digestive problems, including colic, reflux, vomiting, constipation, and diarrhea

- skin problems, including eczema and pallor
- dark circles under the eyes (allergic "shiners")
- red ears or "apple" cheeks
- recurrent ear, sinus, or strep infections
- history of vaccine reaction(s) or vaccines given simultaneously with antibiotics and/or acetaminophen (Tylenol™)
- chronic unexplained fevers
- respiratory problems, including asthma and bronchitis
- repeated use of antibiotics
- febrile seizures associated with vaccination reaction and ingesting Tylenol™
- regression in function between 15 and 30 months
- seizures in puberty
- hyperactivity
- sleep disturbances

An immune response is appropriate against invaders like bacteria, yeast, viruses, parasites, and toxins, but the immune systems of children with autism respond to almost anything, including, but not limited to, molds, pollen, chemicals, metals, common foods, food additives, and incompletely digested particles of food.[14] In fact, their immune overreaction is being recognized as a hallmark of autism.

Toxins

Over two billion pounds of toxic chemicals are released into the air, land, or water each year. The Toxic Substances Control Act (TSCA) of 1976 grandfathered some 62,000 chemicals on the market, despite the lack of safety data to support this policy. Another 20,000 chemicals have come into the market since, also with little or no information about their possible consequences for human health. More than 80,000 chemicals are registered for use in the United States today.[15]

Compared to previous generations, today's children are significantly more exposed to toxic metals, chemicals, drugs, pesticides, plastics, and food additives that are foreign and toxic to living systems.[16] Exposure to these toxins, called "xenobiotics," starts prenatally and continues after birth.

In May 2000 the Greater Boston Physicians for Social Responsibility released the 140-page booklet, *In Harm's Way: Toxic Threats to Child Development*, now available as a free download from www.psr.org. This comprehensive report details how overexposure to toxic substances has caused millions of American children to exhibit learning, behavioral, and developmental disabilities, including AD(H)D and autism.[17] Even though it is a little dated, this booklet still contains valuable information about toxic exposures and their outcomes.

Toxins that primarily affect the nervous system are called "neurotoxins" because they destroy the nervous system's ability to develop and function normally. They can also alter and suppress immune system function, and even be carcinogenic. A review of the top 20 chemicals reported on in the 2000 Toxics Release Inventory reveals that nearly half are known or suspected neurotoxins.[18]

Dietrich Klinghardt, MD, PhD, an expert on diagnosing causes and determining treatments for those with autism spectrum disorders categorizes suspect neurotoxins into four groups: heavy metals, environmental toxins (from manufacturing, plastics and consumer products), mycotoxins (from mold), and the nasty endo- and exotoxins created by pathogenic microbes in the body.

Heavy metals. Prenatal exposures to toxic metals are highly suspect as causes of autism spectrum disorders. The metals most implicated are the following:

- **Mercury from dental amalgams, excessive fish consumption, vaccines, power plants, light bulbs, cleansers, cosmetics, Rhogam, and other sources.**[19] Mercury is the second most toxic metal on the planet, next to plutonium. An Rh-positive baby born to an Rh-negative mother who received Rhogam containing thimerosal and who has a mouth full of mercury-containing amalgams is exposed to many micrograms of mercury prenatally.[20] Even before leaving the womb, its Total Load of mercury alone is nearing its body's threshold. Add to this infant's load a few more micrograms of mercury within hours of birth, from the hepatitis B vaccine, and that baby has a high chance of having an autism diagnosis by age two.

- **Lead from the soil, food products, and chipping paint.** According to the CDC and the US Public Health Service, the devastating effects of lead on the mental and physical development of young children is one of society's most shameful environmental tragedies.[21]
- **Aluminum from cans, cookware, antacids, antiperspirants, and vaccines.** Aluminum has no recognized biological function. Studies relate elevated aluminum to memory and learning impairments.[22]
- **Antimony from flame-retardants in sleepwear, bedding, carpets, and textiles.** Over 70% of crib mattresses contain toxic chemicals and metals.[23] All mattresses are required by law to be fireproof, which necessitates the use of antimony.[24] Ever wonder why legislation mandated that mattresses be made fireproof in the first place? Rumor has it that it was to protect everyone from the dangers of smoking in bed! That was when most parents smoked and before we had smoke detectors. Maybe it's time to update this law and prohibit known toxic chemicals from being next to our bodies for one-third of our lives as we sleep!
- **Arsenic from flame-retardants, pressure-treated wood used in playgrounds, fungicides, herbicides, corrosion inhibitors, and lead and copper alloys.** Arsenic is also high in some seafood and rice (and its byproducts, such as baby cereal and rice milk) grown in areas where arsenic is in the water, both in the US and abroad.[25] It may also come from animals, such as chickens, that ingest arsenic in their feed.[26]
- **Cadmium from cigarette smoke[27] and alloys used in plumbing.[28]**

Before leaving the topic of heavy metals, readers should hear the now-legend story of how mercury was implicated in autism. In late 1999, three families, all with children who regressed into autism, started delving into the possible sources of their children's illnesses. Sallie Bernard, Lyn Redwood, and Albert Enayati had never met, but corresponded, comparing notes about their children. After attending a conference on biomedical approaches to autism, they came away convinced that their children were suffering from mercury poisoning. After much research, they wrote a joint paper with a physician and scientist, entitled "Autism: A Unique Type of Mercury Poisoning."[29]

The authors formalized their relationship with the founding of The Coalition of SafeMinds (Sensible Action For Ending Mercury-Induced Neurological Disorders). SafeMinds is a private, nonprofit organization whose mission is to restore health and protect future generations by eradicating the devastation of autism and associated health disorders induced by mercury and other toxicants.

Environmental toxins. We all have several hundred chemicals in our bodies that were unknown before the 20th century.[30] Synthetic chemicals, such as Polychlorinated biphenyls (PCBs) and Polybrominated Diphenyl Ethers (PBDEs), add to the body's toxic load.

PCBs, which are chemicals used in coolants, plasticizers, electrical coatings, and for other purposes, have been banned for the past 25 years, yet they remain in the soil, water, and air forever. The higher the levels of PCBs in the mother's blood and breast milk, the larger the deficits in children's intelligence, memory, and attention.[31]

PBDEs, the "sons" of PCBs, are flame retardants that have been used in hundreds of everyday products since the 1970s. Children's sleepwear, furniture, computers, TV sets, automobile parts, polyurethane foam, plastics for computers and electronics, and stain-proofing for textiles such as Scotchgard® all contain PBDEs. These products look like PCBs chemically, behave like PCBs environmentally, and have the same toxic effects as PCBs biologically. They are in dumps everywhere, persistently contaminating the food chain and making their way into human bodies, where they act as endocrine disrupters.[32] (See more on endocrine disruption below.)

PBDEs, like PCBs, showed up in breast milk, first in Sweden and then in the United States. A frequently referenced study by the Environmental Working Group (EWG) examined 20 American babies born to first-time mothers; it showed average levels of flame retardants to be 75 times greater than the average found in European studies. Milk from two study participants contained the highest levels of fire retardants ever reported in the United States, and milk from several of the mothers had among the highest levels of these chemicals yet detected worldwide.[33] Minute doses of PBDEs can cause deficits in sensory and motor skills, learning, memory, and hearing, as well as impair attention, learning, and behavior in laboratory animals.

Other xenobiotics that can invade breast milk are chlordane, DDT, lindane, dioxins, and furans. American babies appear to be exposed to far higher amounts of fire retardants than babies in Europe, where some of these chemicals have already been banned.[34] In the United States, so far Alaska, California, Hawaii, Illinois, Maine, Maryland, Michigan, New York, Oregon, Vermont, and Washington State restrict the use of PBDEs.

Some chemicals are endocrine disruptors, meaning that they set off a cascade of unnatural reactions interfering with the synthesis, transport, binding, action, or elimination of hormones.[35] Endocrine disruptors are ubiquitous, creeping up not only in food and water, but in an extremely diverse collection of consumer products, including cosmetics, shampoos, detergents, sunblocks, perfumes, and pharmaceuticals. Did you know that the magic that makes some medications, including prenatal vitamins, "time-released" is an endocrine disruptor? These chemicals enter the body through inhalation, absorption, ingestion, and placental transfer.[36]

Much current research is focusing on how PBDEs and other chemicals such as perchlorates in drinking water, Bisphenol A (BPA — a by-product of making plastic), and phthalates, solvents, and plasticizers, disrupt the entire endocrine system in individuals with autism.[37] The Endocrine Disruption Exchange Inc. (TEDX) provides a searchable database with more information about the activity of approximately 870 endocrine disruptors to help professionals identify possible culprits in various types of dysfunction.[38] Read more about the endocrine system in chapter 6.

In 2010 and again in 2011, the late Senator Frank R. Lautenberg (D-NJ), chairman of the Senate Subcommittee on Environmental Health, declared that "America's system for regulating industrial chemicals is broken." In his efforts to protect our children from dangerous chemicals in everyday products, he introduced the Safe Chemicals Act to bring the aforementioned Toxic Substances Control Act up-to-date for the first time since 1976.[39] It did not pass, probably due to heavy lobbying against it by the powerful chemical lobbies.

One of TSCA's only pluses is that it has allowed states to develop their own chemical policies and restrictions. Many states have banned particularly toxic chemicals like mercury, cadmium, and BPA from particular categories of products. Some forward-thinking states, including California, Maine, Washington, and Minnesota, have developed even more comprehensive policies that address broader classes of chemicals designed to improved public health and environmental quality.

The latest effort to protect our children from toxic chemicals is the bipartisan Chemical Safety Improvement Act (CSIA), which has been languishing in hearings since Lautenberg's death in June 2013. Some strong anti-chemical advocates refuse to support it because CSIA would preempt state restrictions and not hold chemical companies liable for harm caused by their products.[40] Female senators Kirsten Gillibrand (D-NY), Barbara Boxer (D-CA), and Barbara Mikulski (D-MD), among others, continue trying to protect our kids.

Mycotoxins from mold. Many homes in the US have elevated levels of mold, including aspergillus, cladosporium, and stachybotrys, caused by poor building plan and materials.[41] Molds are spore-forming organisms. Their spores travel quickly and hatch in warm places in buildings as well as in warm, moist places in the body, such as the nasal passages. They are extremely resistant to complete removal, and they release potent neurotoxins that can damage many aspects of gastrointestinal, respiratory, hematological, immunological, and neurological function.

Endo- and exotoxins from pathogens. **Toxins found within the cell are called "endotoxins," while those secreted by the cell are called "exotoxins." Bacteria and other pathogenic microbes produce secondary toxins as they undergo their biological processes.**

How do these pathological bugs get into our bodies? We eat, drink, and breathe them! If doctors have prescribed multiple rounds of antibiotics to kill them, as has occurred with **many** individuals on the spectrum, the balance of good and bad bacteria in the gut can become disrupted, in a process called "dysbiosis." An imbalanced gut is a favorable environment for colonization by opportunistic pathogens, such as clostridium, a ubiquitous type of bacteria that produces a potent neurotoxin.[42]

The following are red flags for possible toxic stressors com
the histories of those diagnosed with autism:

- mother with exposures to mercury from amalg;
  excessive fish consumption, vaccines before or during
  pregnancy, Rhogam shots, and occupational hazards
- sensitivity to dyes, chemicals, perfume, or medications
- hyperactivity
- mood swings
- self-injurious or violent behavior
- aggression at puberty

When assessing toxic exposure, questions about timing, duration,
levels, routes, agents, and interactions are all crucial in history-
taking, and make pinpointing a relationship between exposures and
outcomes extremely complex. In general, the most sensitive time for
toxic assaults is during critical periods of rapid brain development,
such as the pre-, peri-, and post-natal periods, because the blood-
brain barrier is not fully developed in the infant to protect it against
toxins. Mothers who have had years of toxic exposure pass two-
thirds of their toxic load through the placenta into their babies during
pregnancy. The firstborn child is often more severely affected than
subsequent ones.[43]

Pound for pound, young children eat, drink, and breathe more
than adults, making their exposure to toxins disproportionately high.
What constitutes toxicity depends upon a person's weight. Experts
continually revise "safe" thresholds of exposure downward as our
knowledge about neurotoxic chemicals increases. The legal standard
for lead poisoning was well over 10 micrograms per deciliter (mcg/
dl) in most states 10 years ago. Research shows that levels as low
as 5 or 6 mcg/dl can decrease a child's ability to read, write, and
calculate.[44] In May 2012, the CDC officially established 5 mcg/dl as its
new reference level. Many toxicologists now believe that *no* amount
of lead is safe.[45]

Excitotoxins. Substances added to foods and beverages, such
as aspartame (Equal™ and NutraSweet™), hydrolyzed vegetable
protein, and monosodium glutamate (MSG), are "excitotoxins."

These ubiquitous additives are in almost all processed foods; their sole purpose is to alter taste. Both solid and liquid forms are toxic, but the liquids are worse because the body absorbs them more rapidly.

In solid form excitotoxins are sometimes disguised as "natural flavoring," "spices," "yeast extract," "textured soy protein," and a host of other non-food products. As liquids they are added to soups, gravies, diet sodas, ice cream, candy, cigarettes, cheese products, chewing gum, gelatin, and infant formulas. They also show up in some "secret" places, such as vaccines, in the form of processed free glutamic acid, described as a "stabilizer," an ingredient used to keep the virus alive. According to Dr. Joseph Mercola, at one time the chicken pox and measles/mumps/rubella (MMR) vaccines made by Merck & Co. contained the excitotoxin "free glutamic acid."[46]

In adults, the negative effects of excitotoxins are subtle and develop over a long period of time. MSG, aspartame, and other excitotoxins gradually stimulate neurons to death (a process called apoptosis), causing varying degrees of damage to all parts of the nervous system, including the brain, resulting in neurodegenerative diseases. However, in unborn babies the effects of excitotoxins can be immediate and dramatic because of the unprotected blood-brain barrier. Continuous stimulation of children's unprotected and immature neurons can cause seizures, inflammation, oxidative stress, endocrine disruption, hyperactivity, sleep deprivation, head banging, and eventually cell death.[47] Excitotoxins and their chemical reactions are an important part of the Total Load of children with autism spectrum disorders.

The best way to avoid toxins of all types is to eat organic food, use natural cleaners, choose natural alternatives to antibiotics, buy natural personal care products, and filter air and water. Read more about this subject in chapter 16.

Structural and Reflex Abnormalities

The early histories of individuals later diagnosed with autism include a number of physical and developmental abnormalities, which may be additional load factors, including the following:
- premature or traumatic birth
- low birth weight

- skipped developmental steps
- large head size

These characteristics could indicate possible trouble in the structural integrity of the body, which affects the ability of inborn reflexes to emerge, become active, and integrate properly.

Babies are more at risk for later developmental problems if they endured pregnancy complications or subtle birth trauma (such as oxygen deprivation, breech presentation, or were born by Cesarean section) and if their mothers had a large toxic load (including a number of silver dental amalgams) or conditions such as thyroid problems, severe allergies, chronic fatigue syndrome, or fibromyalgia. Babies born to mothers confined to bed rest for long periods during their pregnancies area also at risk, as they might miss important stages of reflex integration, with harmful effects on their motor development.

The end of the second year of life is a particularly vulnerable period, when development in all areas is taking place at a rapid rate. That autism is often diagnosed at this time should be no surprise. Chapter 3 enumerates these and other physical stressors, such as sleep deprivation, dehydration, positioning, and lack of movement opportunities.

The Sensory Connection

The mainstream world is now familiar with the severe sensory issues individuals with autism experience because of the Emmy-winning film, *Temple Grandin*, starring Claire Danes, arguably the most famous adult autistic. As a young girl, Temple calmed herself using a branding machine on her relatives' farm. She experienced hearing sensitivities, relating that certain noises "sounded like a dentist's drill going through my ears."[48]

Others with autism describe visual issues or the need for deep pressure, movement, and touch, as well as an abhorrence of certain smells, tastes, and sounds.[49] Clearly, those with autism are living in a sensory world that is too loud, too tight, or too bright.

The source of these sensory sensitivities is as varied and complex as the individuals themselves. Maybe they stem from problems in the cerebellum, the brain's center of sensory perception and motor control, which is very sensitive to thyroid disruption.[50] Other possible sources and symptoms of sensory problems seen in the histories of children diagnosed with autism are:

- recurrent ear, sinus, or strep infections
- sensory deprivation
- skipping crawling developmentally
- lack of eye contact
- sleep disturbances
- mood swings

Whatever the source of sensory problems, tactile, auditory, visual, and other sensory issues are additional load factors. When piled on top of oxidative, toxicological, immunological, environmental, and physical stress, regression into autism is inevitable.

Every Child Is Unique

Remember, those with autism spectrum disorders vary markedly biologically despite similar behavioral symptoms. It is worth repeating that health care professionals must treat each patient as a unique individual with a unique health and developmental history.

One family traced their son's autism back to mold exposure during gestation. Another found the same chemicals in their child's blood as the exterminator sprayed to rid their house of termites. Yet another discovered a new cell phone tower not far from their home. While no chemical or electro-magnetic field alone is the "cause" of autism, in an immune-compromised body, any one exposure could be the "straw that breaks the back" of a child's body's ability to cope.

Determining appropriate treatments and their sequence requires knowing the multiple causes of symptoms in each patient. The only way to determine possible causes of an individual's autism is to take a complete history of all possible Total Load factors, including genetic, prenatal, natal, environmental, developmental, and medical concerns. This process could take many hours, a sharp memory, and significant understanding of biochemistry. Laboratory tests can frequently assist in pinpointing individual needs in each case.

Testing for Load Factors

Doctors usually run traditional laboratory tests, such as a complete blood count (CBC) and sometime even IgE allergy scratch tests. Obviously, results from these tests can be helpful. Looking for answers with only these tests, however, is like looking in the kitchen for your underwear: you are in the wrong room.

If autism is indeed a "unique form of mercury poisoning," as SafeMinds contends, then testing children with autism for mercury as well as for aluminum, lead, pesticides, preservatives, solvents, and other pollutants is imperative. Proving that a particular child has toxic levels of a specific poison can be extremely difficult, however, even in clear cases of overexposure, such as mercury-loading from vaccinations.

Measuring accurate levels of toxicity via laboratory testing has thus been elusive until recently. Fortunately, many specialized laboratories have developed hundreds of very sophisticated tests that look at both genetic and environmental factors to pinpoint exactly what has gone awry with the immune, digestive, respiratory, and endocrine systems, as well as the detoxification pathways. Simplified methods, such as tape-on bags for urine samples from those who are not potty-trained, and home blood test kits complete with a lance to prick a finger, make sample collection fairly easy. Only with certain tests, in which doctors use a chelator that binds to the toxic metals, were scientists able to show that those with autism also had high levels of toxic metals hiding in their bodies.[51]

Each health care professional has his or her favorite lab for each test. Some labs specialize in one of the tests and do not offer others. Other labs offer all the tests. Most physicians order tests that measure the following:
- strength of both immediate and delayed systemic responses to various common foods
- presence of gluten and casein peptides
- overabundance of abnormal organic acids associated with yeast, fungal, and clostridia metabolism
- undesirable invaders such as intestinal parasites, bad bacteria, yeast, and viruses

- levels of amino and fatty acids
- efficiency of thyroid function
- unusually high antibody titers resulting from markedly abnormal responses to childhood immunizations, including MMR, DPT, and oral polio
- the presence of genetic mutation(s), including MTHFR and SUOX
- deficiencies of essential minerals
- excessive levels of toxic metals

Deciding which tests to do and which labs to use is a balancing act weighing the expense of tests with their usefulness in diagnosis. Convenience, time, and expense all play a role. A doctor's prescription is necessary to run most tests. Because one approach never fits all cases, listing a "standard" test protocol is impossible.

Blood, Stool, and Urine Tests

Uncovering what toxins are lying deep in the cells is tricky since most blood, stool, and urine tests pinpoint only recent exposures. Furthermore, blood levels do not always yield answers because metals are stored in fat tissue, not blood. Still, many tests using blood and excretory products can yield highly useful results about digestion, pathogens, immune status, and allergic reactions.

Hair Analysis

Once considered unreliable, analyzing minerals and toxins excreted through the hair is now better understood. This testing method is most useful for the detection of recent exposure to toxic metals. In a landmark hair analysis study completed on children with autism and their typical siblings, researchers were astounded to find that the unaffected children showed higher levels of toxic metals in their hair than the affected ones. Why? Because the bodies of the non-autistic kids had a strong ability to detoxify and excrete the poisons, while those with autism still harbored the metals in their bodies.

Several labs have recently developed some extremely innovative tests that can identify molecular damage in blood and urine that only toxins can cause.

Mercury Speciation Analysis

The new kid on the block is Christopher Shade, PhD, with his Colorado-based laboratory Quicksilver Scientific, founded in 2005. An environmental scientist, Shade became interested in the unique qualities of mercury when assessing the impacts of mercury release from natural gas drilling in Southeast Asia. He developed the patented Liquid Chromatographic Mercury Speciation technology that separates and measures the different forms of mercury: methylmercury, ethylmercury, and inorganic mercury.

- *Methylmercury,* commonly found in fish and other animal tissues, is the most highly researched form of mercury. Methylmercury is mobile and easily absorbed in the human organism. In fact, human intestines absorb about 95% of the methylmercury that enters the digestive tract. Methylmercury easily crosses the placental and blood-brain barriers, exposing the fetus and often resulting in debilitating neurological effects. Methylmercury is difficult for organisms to eliminate, so it accumulates in biological tissues.

- *Ethylmercury* is present in sediments and petroleum hydrocarbons. Importantly, the most common exposure route for this form of mercury is through vaccinations containing the preservative thimerosal. Like methylmercury, ethylmercury can move easily into biological tissues. Ethylmercury tends to break down into inorganic mercury more rapidly than methylmercury.

- *Inorganic mercury* occurs in sediments, soils, and some food sources, but is not very mobile, nor does it bioaccumulate to the same degree as organic mercury. It gathers in tissues when one of the more mobile forms of mercury above enters the tissue and breaks down into inorganic mercury. In biological tissues, most organic forms of mercury will eventually break down into inorganic mercury. However, when inorganic mercury is absorbed into biological tissues, it becomes an immediate toxic threat. Once inside, inorganic mercury is very difficult to remove.

Having this information is vital for those with autism because total mercury analysis alone cannot provide an adequate representation of an individual's mercury level. The Quicksilver method analyzes methylmercury, inorganic mercury, and total mercury in one simultaneous procedure. Only through speciation analysis can health care providers gain understanding of the ratio of methylmercury to inorganic mercury; this is critical data that facilitates understanding of toxic effects on the human body and how to remediate them. For more information on speciation analysis, go to www.quicksilverscientific.com.

Porphyrin Testing

Have you ever noticed that the complexions of some children with autism and other developmental delays appear unusually pale and pasty? That is because of a defect in hemoglobin production, either from inadequate iron or because mercury is interfering with their porphyrin.

Porphyrins are a group of pigments, occurring in a ring structure, that the body uses for various purposes. Hemoglobin is an example of a porphyrin ring with iron in the middle. Because of the presence of iron, blood, which contains hemoglobin, is red. Mercury and other toxins disrupt porphyrin production, resulting in malformed or incompletely formed porphyrins that the body excretes because they cannot be used to build hemoglobin.

By measuring the presence of porphyrins in urine, laboratories can detect some specific incomplete, unusable porphyrins that the body has discarded. These specific porphyrins are present only in urine because of mercury and other toxins in the body. In the United States, LabCorp and Quest Laboratories offer tests measuring porphyrins in plasma and urine. Both domestic labs still have limited experience with the test, and they do not report all of the by-products. Laboratoire Philippe Auguste in Paris, France, has broader experience with the testing and provides clear results. Patients can send a urine sample via air mail; the test takes about 10 days to process. Go to www.labbio.net for more information.

Outsmart Autism by Removing Total Load Factors

In his brilliant book, *The Four Pillars of Healing*, Leo Galland, MD, likens bringing a body back to health to restoring a fine painting.[52] In both cases, you must know the history. In the book's introduction, Galland takes the reader to an art restoration center in Florence, where experts are learning about the environmental history of a 15th-century masterpiece. How many damp basements and fires did it survive? What pigments did the artist use to paint it? What solvents did historians apply during its last restoration?

A child diagnosed with autism demands and deserves at least as careful a look as a painting. In order to reveal a child's true abilities and allow them to emerge, one must know his or her history. Galland views disease as the appearance of symptoms related to an accumulation of load factors in the body. Peel back and treat each layer, one by one, until the person is well.

A large subgroup of kids demonstrates physical illnesses before they "have" autism. Many doctors now recognize that their ear infections, allergies, sleep disturbances, constipation, diarrhea, skin problems, or other symptoms are risk factors for autism. These kids have usually gotten sick from the outside-in: first skin, then digestive, respiratory, and nervous systems, and finally cognitive factors show imbalances.

Wellness usually progresses from the inside-out. During treatment, parents often report that their children become more cognitively aware and begin speaking better long before their respiratory and gut symptoms resolve. The final phase of healing usually includes some skin eruptions, such as pimples and even boils, along with growth in complex cognitive skills such as abstract thinking and relating socially.

Recall The Autism Spectrum of Disorders presented in chapter 1, figure 1.2. This continuum can easily look like alphabet soup to a confused parent. Usually, the broader the exposure to Total Load factors, the more severe the diagnosis. As problems accumulated and were possibly exacerbated by medical treatments and practices (such as antibiotics, back sleeping and positioning that restricted movement, and self-limited diets) outward manifestations appeared.

47

This process could have taken months, even years. Getting well will take at least as long as getting sick. Outsmarting autism takes a different path for each child because of biological uniqueness.

The following chapters address eliminating important load factors:

- **Chapter 3: Reducing everyday stress factors** with lifestyle changes such as establishing daytime and nighttime routines; limiting screen time; buying organic and nontoxic products for the home, school, and workplace; teaching a developmentally appropriate curriculum; and resolving chronic family problems
- **Chapter 4: Modifying the diet** by eating in-season, locally-grown, organic foods, as well as repopulating the gut with good bacteria and adding special diets that remove problematic foods containing gluten, casein, soy, grains, sugars, nuts, and identified allergens
- **Chapter 5: Boosting the immune system** by addressing the role of antibiotics and vaccinations, and using nutritional supplementation to tame inflammation and fight infections
- **Chapter 6: Regulating the endocrine system** through hormone testing and balancing
- **Chapter 7: Detoxification** of the bodies and minds of affected children and their families, as well as their home, school, and general environments, using various methods including homeopathy
- **Chapter 8: Reducing and eliminating structural problems** through innovative methods including chiropractic, osteopathic, and cranial-sacral therapy
- **Chapter 9: Reflex integration** to enhance all aspects of development
- **Chapter 10: Ameliorating sensory issues**, such as problems with touch, smell, taste, balance, and pressure
- **Chapter 11: Correcting vision dysfunction**, such as difficulties using the two eyes together efficiently and integrating vision with motor skills and the brain.

The ultimate goal is to remove the largest load factors first so the energy can be redirected toward healing. Patience is essential. At first, sensory, language, social-emotional, and academic development must take a backseat to biological issues. Once the body is putting less energy into digestion, circulation, respiration, and detoxification, a team of experts can develop the specifics of a hierarchy of adjunct therapies.

While it may sound crazy to wait, even for a short time, this plan will waste less time and money in the long term. Allowing the body to use its own wisdom to heal may result in bypassing some therapies altogether. We *can* outsmart autism together! Let's get started.

---

[1] Krigsman A, Boris M, Goldblatt A, Stott C. Review of Clinical Presentation and Histologic Findings at Ilepcolonoscopy in Children with Autism Spectrum Disorder and Chronic Gastrointestinal Symptoms. *Autism Insights, 2010, 2, 1–11;* Buie T, et al. Recommendations for evaluation and treatment of common gastrointestinal problems in children with ASDs. *Pediatrics, Jan* 2010, 125:Suppl1, S19–29.

[2] Alberti A, Pirrone P, Elia M, et al. Sulphation deficit in low functioning autistic children: A pilot study. Biological Psychiatry, 1999, 46, 420–4; James SJ, Cutler P, Melnyk S, Jernigan S, Janak L, Gaylor DW, Neubrander JA. Metabolic biomarkers of increased oxidative stress and impaired methylation capacity in children with autism. Am J Clin Nutr, Dec 2004, 80:6, 1611–7.

[3] Russo, AJ, Krigsman A, Jepson B, and Wakefield A. Generalized Autoimmunity Related to Severity of Disease in Autistic Children With GI Disease. *Immunology and Immunogenetics Insights, 2009, 1, 37–47.*

[4] Singh V, Fudenberg H, Emerson D, Coleman M. Immunodiagnosis and immunotherapy in autistic children. Annals NY Acad Sci, 1988, 540, 602–604; Gupta S. Immunological treatments for autism. J Autism Dev Dis, 2000, 30, 475–9.

[5] Tomljenovic L, Shaw CA. Do aluminum vaccine adjuvants contribute to the rising prevalence of autism? Journal of Inorganic Biochemistry, Nov 2011, 105:11, 1489–99.

[6] Geier MR, Geier DA. Neurodevelopmental disorders after thimerosal-containing vaccines: A brief communication. Silver Spring, MD: The Genetic Centers of America, 2002.

[7] Lemer P. Total Load Theory: How the cumulative effect of many factors causes developmental delays. New Developments newsletter, Summer 2007, 12:4, 2.

[8] Ratajczak HV. Theoretical aspects of autism: Causes: A review. Jrnl of Immunotoxicology, 2011, 8:1, 68–79.

[9] Ratajczak HV. Theoretical aspects of autism: Biomarkers: A review. Jrnl of Immunotoxicology, 2011, 8:1, 80–94.

[10] Herbert M, Weintraub K. Autism Revolution: Whole-Body Strategies for Making Life All It Can Be. New York: Ballantine Books, 2013, 12.

[11] McGinnis W. Oxidative stress in autism. Altern Ther Health Med, Nov–Dec 2004,10:6, 22–36.

[12] Researchers Unravel Role of Oxidative Stress in Autism Spectrum Disorder. The Wall Street Journal, July 13, 2013. http://online.wsj.com/article/PR-CO-20130703-908403.html. Accessed Dec 11, 2013.

[13] El-Dahr JM. Immunologic Issues in Autism. Lecture delivered at the Defeat Autism Now! Conference, April, 2004, Washington, DC.

[14] Children with autism have distinctly different immune system reactions compared to typical children. Press release, May 5, 2005. www.EurekAlert.org. Accessed Dec 11, 2013.

[15] www.epa.gov. Accessed Dec 11, 2013.

[16] Grandjean P. Only One Chance: How environmental pollution impairs brain development — and how to protect the brains of the next generation. New York: Oxford University Press, 2013.

[17] Greater Boston Physicians for Social Responsibility. In Harm's Way: Toxic threats to child development. Boston, 2000.

[18] http://www.epa.gov/tri/. Accessed Dec 11, 2013.

[19] Palmer RF, Blanchard S, Wood R. Proximity to point sources of environmental mercury release as a predictor of autism prevalence. *Health Place*, Mar 2009, 15:1, 18–24.

[20] Geier DA, Geier MR. A prospective study of thimerosal-containing Rho(D)-immune globulin administration as a risk factor for autistic disorders. J Matern Fetal Neonatal Med, May 2007, 20:5, 385–90.

[21] McCandless J. Children with Starving brains, 2nd ed. Putney, VT: Bramble Books, 2005.

[22] Agency for Toxic Substances and Disease Registry (ATSDR). ToxFAQs for Aluminum, 1993.

[23] Clean and Healthy New York and American Sustainable Business Council. The Mattress Matters: Protecting Babies from Toxic Chemicals While They Sleep. 2011.

[24] ATSDR. ToxFAQs for Antimony, 2005.

[25] Surprisingly high concentrations of toxic arsenic species found in U.S. rice. http://www.speciation.net/News/Surprisingly-high-concentrations-of-toxic-arsenic-species-found-in-US-rice-;~/2005/08/03/1561.html. Accessed Nov 3, 2011.

[26] ATSDR. ToxFAQs for Arsenic, 2007.

[27] British-American Tobacco Company Limited. The Cadmium Content of Tobacco and Smoke, 2005. http://legacy.library.ucsf.edu/tid/lib34a99. Accessed Nov 2, 2011.

[28] ATSDR. ToxFAQs for Cadmium, 2008.

[29] Bernard S, Enayati A, Binstock T, Roger H, Redwood L, McGinnis W. Autism: A novel form of mercury poisoning. Medical Hypotheses, 2001, 56:4, 462–71.

[30] www.ourstolenfuture.org. Accessed Dec 11, 2013.

[31] Jacobson JL, Jacobson SW. Intellectual impairment in children exposed to polychlorinated biphenyls in utero. N Engl J Med, Sep 1996; 335:11.

[32] Vos JG, Becher G, Van den Berg M, de Boer J, et al. Brominated flame retardants and endocrine disruption. Pure and Applied Chemistry, 2003, 75:11–12, 2039–46.

[33] Darnerud PA, Eriksen GS, Johannesson T, Larsen PB, et.al. Polybrominated diphenyl ethers (PBDEs): Occurrence, Dietary Exposure, and Toxicology. Environmental Health Perspectives, Mar 2001, 109:Suppl1, 49–68.

[34] Williams F. Toxic Breast Milk? New York Times Magazine, Jan 9, 2005.

[35] Colburn T. Dumanoski D, Meyers JP. Our stolen future. New York: Plume/Penguin, 1997.

[36] Engel SM, Miodovnik A, Canfield RL, Zhu C, Silva M, Calafat AI, Wolff MS. Prenatal Phthalate Exposure is Associated with Childhood Behavior and Executive Functioning. Environmental Health Perspectives, 2010, 118, 565–71.

[37] Miodovnik A, Engel SM, Zhu C, Ye X, et al. Phthalates, BPA linked to atypical childhood social behaviors. NeuroToxicology, Mar 2011, 32:2, 261–7; Kim Y, Ha EH, Kim EJ, Park H, et al. Prenatal Exposure to Phthalates and Infant Development at 6 Months: Prospective Mothers and Children's Environmental Health (MOCEH) Study. Environ Health Perspect, Oct 2011, 119:10, 1495–500; Williams R. Phthalates Affect Child Development. Environment Report, Sep 2011.

[38] TEDX List of Potential Endocrine Disruptors. www.endocrinedisruption.com/endocrine.TEDXList.overview.php. Accessed Mar 28, 2014.

[39] http://www.ewg.org/kid-safe-chemicals-act-blog/kid-safe-chemicals-act/. Accessed Oct 31, 2011.

[40] http://www.saferchemicals.org/safe-chemicals-act/. Accessed Dec 13, 2013.

[41] Greenberg E. Practical Solutions for Autism Recovery. Explore! Publications, July 2007, 16:4.

[42] Bolte ER. Autism and clostridium tetani. Med Hypotheses, Aug 1998, 51:2, 133–44.

[43] Klinghardt D. Klinghardt Academy Conference: Healing the Brain, New York, May 2013.

[44] Lanphear BP, Dietrich K, Auinger P, Cox C. Cognitive deficits associated with blood lead concentrations <10 μg/dL in US children and adolescents. Public Health Reports, Nov 2000, 115, 521–9.

[45] http://www.consumerreports.org/cro/2012/03/cdc-advisers-call-for-less-allowable-lead/index.htm. Accessed Dec 11, 2013.

[46] Samuels. J. The danger of MSG and how it is hidden in vaccines. www.mercola.com. Accessed Dec 11, 2013.

[47] Blaylock RL. Excitotoxins: The taste that kills. Santa Fe, NM: Health Press, 1997.

[48] www.brainyquote.com. Accessed Jan 24, 2013.

[49] Tomchek SD, Dunn WS. Sensory processing in children with and without autism: A comparative study using the Short Sensory Profile. *American Journal of Occupational Therapy*, 2007, *61*, 190–200.

[50] Berbel P, Obregón MJ, Bernal J. Thyroid Hormone Action in Cerebellum and Cerebral Cortex Development. J Endocrinology, 2010, 95:9, 4227–34.

[51] Holmes AS, Blaxill MF, Haley BE. Reduced Levels of Mercury in First Baby Haircuts of Autistic Children. Int J Toxicol, 2003, 22, 277–85.

[52] Galland L. The Four Pillars of Healing. New York: Random House, 1997, xiii–xvi.

STEP 1

Take Away the Bad Stuff,
and Add Back the Good Stuff

CHAPTER 3

Reducing Load Factors
through Lifestyle Changes

As soon as an autism spectrum disorder is suspected, the very first step is to reduce as many stressors as possible. This chapter enumerates the common stressors that accumulate as load factors in families with autism, eventually affecting everyone's health, learning, and behavior. Creating lifestyle changes improves the health and well-being of each family member—sick, well, diagnosed, or not. Diet and nutrition are important major stress factors included only minimally in this chapter; they deserve a chapter of their own, which follows.

Remember, these are general ideas, as all those with autism are not the same! Some of the suggestions in this chapter may not yet be applicable for families of children who are still nonverbal, families with significant global challenges, or even some generally higher-functioning kids with isolated severe challenges. Keep ideas on the shelf for a later date. Regardless of the severity of autism, lessening everyday load factors *before* embarking on expensive and time-consuming therapies can immeasurably improve future outcomes and quality of life, as well as save considerable time, effort, and expense.

Environmental and Chemical Stressors

The air we breathe, the water we drink, the foods we eat, the products we use, and the invisible energies that penetrate our nervous systems can all be toxic. Most people are aware that outdoor air pollution can damage their health, but few know that indoor air pollution can also have significant health effects. Studies of human exposure to air pollutants by the Environmental Protective Agency (EPA) found levels of about a dozen common pollutants to be two- to five-times higher inside homes than outside, regardless of whether the homes were located in rural or highly industrial areas. While using products containing chemicals, people can expose themselves and others to very high pollutant levels, and elevated concentrations can persist in the air long after the activity is completed.[1]

Tobacco exposure remains a significant problem despite extraordinary measures to educate the public about the dangers of smoking. Environmental tobacco smoke is a major source of indoor air contamination, and thus unintentional, passive inhalation of tobacco smoke by nonsmokers is unavoidable. Environmental tobacco smoke is a dynamic, complex mixture of more than 4,000 chemicals. This single air pollutant can be contributing significantly to the epidemic of childhood asthma and allergies.[2]

Building materials are major sources of airborne neurotoxins from off-gassing. "Sick building syndrome" — discomfort, "allergies," or illness that result from living or working in a building with airborne contaminants or inadequate ventilation — is not just limited to office buildings. Some people reside in "sick" homes.[3] Siding, cabinets, carpeting, glue, insulation, and other materials can off-gas for days, months, and even years. I once visited a school where, upon entering, I was knocked over by the new carpet smell. When I met the principal, I commented on how lovely her new carpeting was. She exclaimed,

"Oh that carpeting isn't new; it's been down for almost a year!" If I could smell it, the fumes were significant. You don't have to smell fumes to inhale poisons.

Pest control traditionally uses toxic chemicals to kill bugs in all stages of life, from larva to adult. Most people are afraid of bugs and assume they carry diseases. In truth, the dangers of pesticides far outweigh the dangers of most insects. Even a slight exposure to pesticides can have negative effects on children's well-being.[4]

Pesticides are everywhere. Even if you don't use them at home, everyone is exposed to them through non-organic foods, landscaping, and the routine spraying of office buildings and even doctors' offices!

Cleaning products are notoriously toxic. Did you know that Ajax powder, Comet cleanser, Dove soap, Ivory liquid, Joy Dishwashing liquid, and Murphy's Oil soap all contain mercury?[5] Dryer sheets and fabric softeners contain a toxic brew of chemicals that can cause allergic reactions, central nervous system disorders, headaches, loss of muscle coordination, and even cancer.[6]

Art supplies from abroad often contain toxins. Crayons, paints, magic markers, and anything with color could contain mercury, asbestos, lead, and other poisons.

Personal care products and their plastic containers contain heavy metals such as lead and mercury and phthalates, which are plasticizers used to add texture and luster to hair spray, deodorant, nail polish, lipstick, perfume, and other products. Lotions and creams are especially problematic. Phthalates can be absorbed through the skin, inhaled through off-gassing, and ingested by children mouthing products.

Hundreds of studies show that phthalates can damage the liver, kidneys, lungs, and reproductive system.[7] In pregnant women, phthalates pass through the placenta to be absorbed by the fetus. Later they show up in breast milk of nursing mothers, whose babies ingest them. In exposed males, phthalates can cause testicular atrophy, leading to a reduced sperm count.[8] Plastic containers for food and drink can also be harmful to health, especially if microwaved.[9]

Heavy metals such as mercury, antimony, and cadmium are in the earth where our food grows, in the ground water and wells where our drinking water comes from, and in the air we breathe. Refer back

O

to chapter 2 to recall the sources of these ubiquitous toxin
drinking, and breathing poisonous metals are now an inevi
of life. As we have seen, toxicity from mercury, aluminum,
cadmium, and lead can profoundly affect the health and development
of children.

I know one child with autism who was found to have arsenic
poisoning. He had bloody splits between his toes, large callouses on
his hands, and "rainbow" skin on his back. None of the health care
professionals who had examined him through the years recognized
these physical signs of arsenic poisoning. If he had not been eating
such a clean diet, and if his other toxic load factors were not so low,
he probably would have died. Rather, he "only had autism." With
detoxification of arsenic, his language and behavior both improved.

Electro-smog is millions of times more abundant than it was just
10 years ago, emerging as one of today's major stressors on the body
and its nervous system. This umbrella term refers to electromagnetic
fields (EMFs) and radio frequency radiation generated from power
lines, cell phone towers, and wireless devices. It includes high-
frequency radiation from microwaves, cellular phones, and wireless
devices; intermediate frequencies from "dirty electricity" emanating
from transformers, fluorescent lighting, computers, and plasma
televisions; and low-frequency fields from computers, copiers, clock
radios, and electric heaters. Other sources of smog are cordless
telephones, laptop keyboards, treadmills, and poor electric wiring in
the home.

Wireless technology has become a way of life, and the evidence
that information- carrying radio waves from cell phones in
particular is a risk to health is getting stronger and stronger.[10]
EMFs damage cell membranes, thus decreasing intracellular
communication by disrupting microtubular connections that allow
biophotons to communicate among cells. If that is insufficient to
scare you, the damaged cell membranes allow heavy metals to
enter the cells, resulting in intracellular production of free radicals,
which can significantly decrease cellular production of energy and
cause great fatigue.[11]

Bacteria, viruses, and other bugs do not like EMFs either; high-frequency waves cause them to respond as if they are being attacked. They react by stepping up their output of toxins and thus become even more virulent when exposed. A European colleague of Dietrich Klinghardt did an experiment on microbial cultures in which he compared the growth and endotoxin production of microbes shielded in special cages to cultures subjected to typical EMF exposure without protection. The proliferation and endotoxin production went up 600% when subjected to ambient EMFs.[12]

Geopathic stress is the negative effect of the earth's energies on human well-being. Vibrations emitted by these stressors do not directly cause disease; however, they are significant load factors that stress the body. Stressors such as underground formations, subterranean water currents, specific mineral deposits, and fault lines can emit electromagnetic radiation. Living and sleeping in the energetic field of natural geological stressors could be as damaging to health as man-made sources. The bedroom is our refuge for healing and cellular regeneration. Some individuals with autism could be sleeping in "unsafe" spaces during the very time their bodies are supposed to be on the mend.

In areas of fracking or natural gas drilling, health advocates are very concerned about effects on the health of individuals living nearby. Drilling could not only affect the quality of the water, air, and food, but also release natural radiation that has been deep under the earth's surface for millions of years.[13]

Lighting options have changed dramatically in the past decade. The incandescent light bulb will soon be extinct, replaced by compact fluorescent bulbs, which are energy efficient and neither environmentally friendly nor good for our health. Each of these new bulbs is an environmental and health time bomb emitting radio frequencies and holding three to five milligrams of mercury.[14] The mercury is not a problem until the bulb breaks — either in your home or in the landfill where it eventually ends up.

The audible buzz emitted by fluorescent lights and visible flickering as a bulb burns out can be problematic for many students with special needs. One student I know had her first seizure in fourth

grade. When the father, an optometrist, came to the school to pi
up, he noticed that the fluorescent light had a strobe effect. Ren... .
her from that classroom cured her "seizure disorder."

For reading and writing, lights should not have too much blue.
Full spectrum lights, according to lighting expert Robin Mumford, are
"like the whole orchestra playing off-key." Good lighting offers the
few notes that make a chord. Mumford has designed ergonomically
validated ceiling, floor, and desk lighting systems that can increase
the speed with which students perform reading and writing tasks.[15]
Find out more at www.mumfordinstitute.org.

Eliminating and Reducing Environmental and Chemical Stressors

Eliminating environmental and chemical stressors starts by
identifying sources of exposure to any and all toxins. Toxins can
come from anything a child eats, drinks, breathes, and puts on his or
her skin or in the mouth, whether it happens in the home, school, or
other locations that the child frequents.

Monitor tobacco exposure. If any family members are still smokers,
insist that they smoke well away from the house. Boycott restaurants
and bars that permit smoking. Minimize contact with adults wearing
clothes saturated with secondhand smoke, which transfers to others
through touch and movement.

Choose building and remodeling materials carefully. Ensure that
school buildings have no asbestos or lead paint. Buy recycled or
chemical-free products that do not off-gas for renovations. Choose
cork, bamboo, and other natural flooring instead of carpet with
chemicals. Use no-VOC paints and wood that is not treated with
formaldehyde, especially when preparing a baby's room. Be sure that
renovation doesn't occur while people are in residence.

Practice safe pest control. The best way to control pests is to keep
them outside. Since shoes track in outside dirt as well as pesticides,
imitate the Japanese and leave shoes at the door. Try using herbs and
other natural products, such as bay leaves for cockroaches, black
pepper to deter ants, or lavender, cedar oil, and camphor to repel
rodents. Choose integrated pest-management systems instead of
chemicals, even when treating head lice. Protect pets with natural
bug repellants, such as diatomaceous earth—a fine, white powder

made from ground-up, fossilized remains of diatoms, a sea algae. For information on how to institute a nontoxic approach in your school and home go to http://schoolipm.ifas.ufl.edu or www.headlice.org.

Use nontoxic cleaning products. Wash clothes with perfume-free laundering products. Minimize dry cleaning, which also uses toxins. If clothes must be dry cleaned, air them out to let the chemicals dissipate before bringing them indoors. Buy "green," toxin-free dishwasher soaps, bathroom cleaners, and detergents. Try Deirdre Imus' Greening the Cleaning® products, Mrs. Meyer's Clean Day, and Seventh Generation items, now widely available. Seventh Generation also manufactures many paper products, bath and facial tissue, diapers, baby wipes, and other essentials that are good both for you and your family and for the environment.

Best of all, simply use common household products like vinegar, baking soda, and lemon juice to make your own. Learn how from the mistress of the green household and expert on chemical poisoning, Annie B. Bond. Her book, *Home Enlightenment: Practical Earth-Friendly Advice for Creating a Nurturing, Healthy, Toxin-Free Home and Lifestyle*, is your all-purpose handbook.[16]

Read labels on art supplies and toys. Purchase only products with the Art and Creative Materials Institute (ACMI) Nontoxic Seals. Use only lead- and asbestos-free crayons, water-based glues and paste, and magic markers denoted "nontoxic." Around children, avoid using chalk (which contains talc), oil-based paints (which contain toxic metals), and spray adhesives (which contain other poisons). To learn more, read Healthy Child Healthy World's "What's on the Label: Art and Hobby Supplies," available online.[17]

Seek out toys made of natural materials like wood. Look for terms like "nontoxic" and "eco-friendly" on plastic toys.

Go outside. Since outdoor air is significantly healthier than indoor air, the best possible antidote to breathing toxic air is to spend more time outdoors. Second best is opening the windows, even in winter, to bring the outside in. Being outside exposes us to the sunshine's vitamin D, the benefits of which are extensive.[18] The relationship ʳitamin D deficiency and autism is well documented.[19] Read ʳe about it in chapter 5.

Use 100% natural clothing and bedding. Buy organic whenever possible. Avoid flame retardants in mattresses and sleepwear. A good way to avoid this problem is to buy a futon, which can be made of 100% organic cotton because it is not officially a "mattress," and 100% cotton outfits that are not officially "pajamas." Replace electric and synthetic blankets with natural bedding. Three safe mattress brands are Vivetique, White Lotus, and Naturepedic. Some other sources of bedding are www.lifekind.com, www.greensleep.com, and www. nontoxic.com.

Watch those phthalates and plastics. Some trusted companies that are committed to safe personal care products are Aubrey Organics, Desert Essence, Dr. Bronner's, Pangea Organics, and Terressentials. Read numbers carefully on plastic products. Avoid #3, #6, and #7, which can leach harmful chemicals into food and drinks. These numbers occur in some bags, wraps, toys, Styrofoam cups, to-go containers, metal can liners, and clear plastic bottles.

Reduce exposure to EMFs. Buy a Gauss meter and take measurements of EMFs at home and school. Stay out of "hot rooms" such as computer labs in schools. Purchase filters that block dirty electricity in electrical outlets. Remove all electrical and wireless appliances from everyone's bedrooms, including plasma TVs, treadmills, computers, cordless phones, routers, cell phones, and their chargers. Use a battery or wind-up alarm clock. Turn off Wi-Fi at night or, better yet, switch to DSL. Make sure you know what is on the other side of the wall from the head of all beds. If a TV is on that wall, move it or the bed. Never use laptops on the lap. Keep cell phone use to an absolute minimum. Try not to use cellphones in the car, and at home use only corded phones. Attach an external keyboard to laptops to reduce the amount of radiation sent to the hands.

Learn whether your home is affected by geopathic stress by having it inspected by a trained Building Biology Inspector (see www. buildingbiology.net). To learn more, read *Zapped: Why Your Cell Phone Shouldn't Be Your Alarm Clock and 1,268 Ways to Outsmart the Hazards of Electronic Pollution,*[20] *Electromagnetic Fields: A Consumer's Guide to* the Issues and How to Protect Ourselves,[21] *BioGeometry: Back to a Future for Mankind*,[22] and *Disconnect: The truth about cell phone radiation, what the industry has done to hide it, and how to protect your family.*[23]

Change your lighting. Stock up on incandescent bulbs or switch to LEDs. Compact fluorescent light bulbs give off high levels of EMFs!

Invest in a good air filter. After taking all of the above steps to reduce and eliminate toxins at home and school, then investigate a good air filter for your home. However, remember that spending money on air filters and purifiers is a waste unless the toxins are eliminated in the first place.

Replace toxic with nontoxic. Every time you run out of something and need to replace it, think nontoxic. Upgrade gradually, and within a year or so your home will be "green."

Physical Stressors

Air, water, food, and sleep are the basics for survival. The last section contains strong recommendations for ensuring that the air our children breathe is healthy and that they are not unnecessarily exposed to other outdoor toxins. This section emphasizes the vital importance of good hydration, deep breathing, and sound sleep, all habits lacking in many individuals with autism spectrum disorders.

Dehydration is an often-overlooked contributor to stress in kids with autism; it could be the hidden culprit in fuzzy thinking, behavioral issues, and poor memory. Human bodies are at least 50% water, and the brain up to 85% water.[24] Every bodily function from cellular communication to digestion depends upon good hydration.

Efficient breathing is essential for both mind and body. Natural, spontaneous, relaxed, deep breathing supplies oxygen to our blood, cells, and brain, giving us energy and strength, reducing tension, and releasing energy that allows us to pay attention to the environment.

When we habitually hold our breath or breathe in a shallow way due to stress, we are more likely to experience exhaustion. We literally "lack inspiration." According to optometrist Mel Kaplan, a high percentage of patients on the autism spectrum exhibit dysfunctional breathing patterns. Their inability to integrate movement and breathing stresses their muscles and nervous systems, and reduces attention. The resulting tension impairs vision, leading to mismatches in how the brain interprets where things are relative to where they appear to be.[25] Read more about vision issues and more of Dr. Kaplan's contributions in Chapter 11.

Some symptoms of inefficient breathing in those with autism spectrum disorders include the following:

- **poor blowing skills**, such as with candles on a cake, bubbles, or a musical instrument;
- **yawning and/or sighing** in an attempt to get more oxygen;
- **rocking**, which compensates for lack of synergistic neural control of the eyes, head, and body;
- **holding of the breath** when giving effort to motor and visual activities as well as reading and writing; and
- **hyperventilation** related to fear and anxiety.

Poor sleeping practices are a hallmark of this millennium. Kids stay up late and fall asleep at their desks in school while their parents try to function on five to six hours per night. Virtually *everyone* is sleep-deprived!

Sleep is essential. A biologically restorative state of consciousness, sleep replenishes the body on all levels: cellular, endocrine, immune, metabolic, physical, and emotional. During restorative sleep, the brain and body produce serotonin, a chemical necessary for mood stabilization, coping, attention, and memory. The less serotonin available, the less able one is to deal with the stressors of life.

When sleep deprived, the body and brain begin a slow deterioration that impacts all areas of health and function. Sleep deprivation impairs metabolism, immune function, and motor skills. It increases stress hormones and cripples sugar metabolism. One study of non-medicated adults showed symptoms of ADHD when deprived of sleep.[26]

Although the body can survive for a month or more without food, death can occur in a week without sleep. Three nights without restorative sleep can produce a state known as "sleep deprived psychosis," in which rational thinking is impossible. Seizures can occur after 24 hours without sleep.

Exercise is now something one does at a gym or on a playing field, not by walking to school or joining a pick-up game of ball. Schools are decreasing opportunities for movement, and some are eliminating recess and physical education altogether. Parents are enrolling kids in group sports and lessons to replace free play, even for our youngest and least coordinated children. Our busy, over-scheduled days allow little time for kids to engage in unstructured play. Children must make playdates instead of picking up games spontaneously and building forts out of cushions at home or stones in the woods. Free play, without adults hovering over kids, is where social skills begin to develop.

By requiring children's bodies to conform to motor poses and their minds to rules of the game, few are learning how to control their bodies spontaneously and by trial and error. Instead, they are acquiring "splinter" athletic skills and playing games by rote.

In attempts to keep our kids safe, we have severely restricted their movements from the day they are born. We squish them into molded plastic Bumbo seats, strap them into car seats, back packs, playpens, and walkers. In addition to further impeding the emergence and integration of reflexes (see chapter 9), these modern-day pieces of equipment are limiting children's natural sensory needs to touch and move. Touch and movement deprivation impedes kids' innate abilities to know where they are in space and to use their bodies purposefully. Read more about sensory issues in chapter 10.

Cortisol levels rise in the presence of large amounts of stress, continuous stress, or both, negatively affecting thyroid hormone availability. Read more about this stress hormone in chapter 6. Thus, ongoing stress can be physical as well as emotional.

Diet and nutrition are covered in depth in the next chapter. Obviously, poor diet and malnutrition are stressors on the body. Today's kids are drinking gallons of sodas and eating colored cereals and baked goods that have virtually no nutritional value. As kids eat increasing amounts of processed foods, their consumption of fresh fruits and vegetables wanes.

Even fruits and vegetables cannot be assumed to be safe! Many are sprayed with pesticides, some more than others. The Environmental Working Group (EWG) has declared the following "The Dirty Dozen" because they have the largest pesticide residues: apples, celery, strawberries, peaches, spinach, nectarines, grapes, bell peppers, potatoes, blueberries, lettuce and kale.[27]

Eliminating and Reducing Physical Stressors

Drink good quality water frequently. Drinking water throughout the day can cut off many problems before they show up. What kind of water should kids drink? Only clean, fresh, mineral-rich, natural spring, filtered, non-fluoridated, unadulterated water. Not coffee, not tea, not juice, not flavored water, and certainly not soda. The body identifies these water-based products as food, not water.

Much of the water that comes out of the tap, is sold in bottles, or drawn from wells does not meet the above criteria.[28] These waters can be mineral-deficient, toxin-laden, or home to bugs that can cause tummy problems. In fact, the presence of chlorine, fluoride, and parasites in tap water are all contributors to the toxic load. Fluoride is a neurotoxin that increases the possibility that the water will leach heavy metals from cookware and foods.[29] Elevated aluminum and lead from old plumbing and city water supplies are often overlooked as possible causes of hyperactivity, violent behavior, and subtle learning disabilities.[30]

Dietrich Klinghardt, MD, PhD, recommends using a reverse osmosis water filter that uses pressure and a fine membrane to remove all impurities, such as bacteria, pesticides, and other particulates. He then adds electrolytes, liquid minerals, and a special mineral formulation called "M water" that increases absorption and utilization of nutrients, oxygen availability to the cells, and the body's ability to detoxify.[31]

Breathe deeply. Recognizing the importance of efficient breathing, therapists from many disciplines add breathing exercises to their remediation programs to improve movement, language, vision, cognition, learning, and behavior. Remind kids throughout the day to take long, deep breaths, especially when they are upset. Introduce them to yoga and martial arts that emphasize breathing.

Check your cortisol levels. Ask your health practitic best way to do this. Lessen other stressors to decrease th stress hormone, about which you can learn more in chap

Catch your zzzs by establishing a sleep hygiene program, just as you have grooming hygiene. Create strict bedtime routines with a set schedule. Begin at least 30 minutes before lights out; follow the same routine every single night, especially with kids on the autism spectrum.

- Establish bedtime—7:30 p.m. for preschoolers and 8:30 p.m. for school-age.
- Banish TV, computer, or video games for at least an hour before bedtime.
- Draw a 10–15 minute warm bath, followed by a deep towel massage. Add Epsom salts for detox and calming. Speak quietly and soothingly. Put on pajamas and get straight into a warm bed.
- Read or tell a story and turn out the lights.

According to experts, school-aged children need 10–12 hours of sleep a night, teenagers 8½ –9 hours, and adults 7–8½ hours. Put infants and toddlers on their tummies when awake and sleeping in the presence of an adult. Make sure that your sleeping area is safe from EMFs and all electro-smog. If your home is exposed to cell phone towers, televisions in neighboring apartments, or geopathic stress, consider buying special netting, sheeting or other mitigators from Safe Living Technologies (www.slt.co) to deflect the EMFs.

Bedrooms are for sleeping! Make sure the bedroom is not a home to electronic devices, including computers. Klinghardt believes that EMF exposure is especially dangerous during sleep. Pregnant women sleeping in EMF-rich environments are jeopardizing the developing fetus. Klinghardt performed a small study showing that children whose mothers slept in strong electromagnetic fields during pregnancy began to exhibit neurological abnormalities within the first two years of life.

Move and play. In his best-selling book, *The Last Child in the Woods: Saving Our Children from Nature-Deficit Disorder*, Richard Louv describes the disconnection between today's children and nature.[32] Let kids go outside to play, even in bad weather. Do your exercise outside (not on a treadmill), walk, play ball; teach them to bike and swim—both essential life skills and great exercise!

Outdoor play has many advantages over playing computer games and watching TV. Playing outdoors antidotes sedentary activity. Developmental specialists recognize that young students' bodies need movement as much as a nutritious breakfast. Let kids play freely, make up games with found objects, walk on walls, ride their bikes around the neighborhood (with a helmet, of course!), and engage in freestyle motor activities instead of just group sports.

Cook! In his book, *Cooked: A Natural History of Transformation*, food activist Michael Pollan states that cooking is the single most important thing that a family can do to improve health and general well-being.[33] He notes that watching top chefs cook on television for 27 minutes has replaced the 30 minutes of actual cooking time his mother spent on dinner. He likens the outsourcing of cooking to paying a seamstress to alter clothes or a mechanic to change your car's oil. In American households today, the amount of time spent cooking is half of what it was in the 1960s. In fact, Americans spend less time cooking than any other nation!

Cooking food distinguishes humans from other animals. In *Catching Fire: How Cooking Made Us Human*, Harvard anthropologist Richard Wrangham develops the "cooking hypothesis."[34] Cooking is the evolutionary prerequisite that allowed us to transcend animals by using fire in the place of bodily energy to break down complex carbohydrates and make proteins more digestible. Eating cooked food releases more bodily energy for other functions, such as thinking. Obviously, raw food enthusiasts would disagree!

Use gas or electric stoves. Minimize use of the microwave, or better yet, throw it out. Never, ever microwave food in plastic containers. Find your grandmother's recipes and cookbooks, and ask your mother for her favorites. Go online and find new recipes using vegetables, grains, and fruits your children will eat. Take some cooking classes and learn how to use unfamiliar nutrient-rich foods such as quinoa, amaranth, seaweeds, and parsnips. Serve a variety of seasonal home-cooked foods. Limit sugar, wheat, and dairy products, as well as kid- and fast-food.

Eat together at least once a day—and in the car doesn't count! Choose one meal per day and give it the respect it deserves. Sit together without stress for at least 10 minutes. Make meals an enjoyable experience. Turn off the TV and computer; do not answer the telephone. Let kids take their time to accept or not eat what is put in front of them. Don't force-feed, prod, plead, or bribe.

Share cooking with children, who are more apt to eat something they made themselves. Grow a vegetable garden; go to local farmers' markets. Buy organic when you can. Use the outdoors as a classroom for science and social studies.

Social Stressors

The sociological environment in which kids are growing up today shows both subtle and significant changes from past generations. This section focuses on how some of these changes are stressing out our kids.

Families have changed; they are no longer like the traditional Ozzie and Harriet model with Mom at home and Dad at the office. When a child has two parents, both most likely work; both parents may or may not be the same sex, race, culture, or religion. Home life is less structured, with fewer routines and rare family meals. More time engaged with electronic devices cuts down on interpersonal interactions.

Consequently, grandparents, nannies, day-care centers, and babysitters have assumed parenting roles. Research shows that children in day care are as emotionally well-adjusted as those who are raised at home with both parents.[35] The problems stem from the stress that arises from parents of children with special needs who worry about their children while at work, and who attend to work responsibilities while at home.

Distance separates close relations, offering less support than having relatives in the same town. Many children of this generation hardly know their parents' siblings and parents because few aunts, uncles, and grandparents live nearby. Spending a few precious days with them during holidays and school vacations in a whirlwind of ice cream, pizza, movies, and other Disneyland treats is not the same as developing a day-to-day relationship.

Food is available almost everywhere, not just at home, in the grocery store and at school. Vending machines are ubiquitous, and dining at bookstores and sports events constitutes a "meal." The number of meals eaten out doubled from 16% in 1978 to over 30% in 2005.[36] In 2013, Americans ate approximately 40% of their meals at restaurants![37] The rare family eats more than three meals a *week* together at home, according to my informal surveying. Compare that to the three meals a *day* I ate with my family when growing up.

Children are missing out on home-cooked foods and all the nutrients they contain, as well as on the experiences that accompany them, such as waiting for dessert, passing the peas, and seeing who gets the last bite of mashed potatoes. One kindergarten teacher suggested that sitting through a 15-minute dinner with the family should be a prerequisite to circle time at school.

Eating microwaved Chinese beef and broccoli from a take-out container in front of the television or in the car on the way to soccer is not the same as a sharing meat loaf and broccoli at the table. Mom's version is made with organic virgin olive oil, fresh onions, and love. The whole family's relationship with food mirrors how everyone interacts with those they love. Pass love on through both the food you eat and the lifestyle you live.

Regular family meals provide much more than companionship. Eating together lowers the risk of obesity and heightens school achievement. One commonality of National Merit Scholars is eating family dinners. You might be asking, what do National Merit Scholars and kids on the autism spectrum have in common? Good question. They both can take advantage of family dinners to build vocabulary, learn how to listen, copy good manners, and pass on family history.[38] The ritual of family meals is transforming!

Screens have replaced human baby sitters. Instead of playing ball against the steps, today's kids are entertained by playing games on a computer or phone, or watching a movie or a sitcom. Our children and grandchildren have shorter attention spans because they are constantly being entertained by moving objects on screens. Few are permitted to venture out into the woods (if they can find any woods) for safety reasons. Even if they were, they would be connected to home by a cell phone, "just in case." Gone are the days when kids would disappear into a safe neighborhood and come home when the street lights came on.

Another issue with TV is that it replaces imaginary play and real-life, hands-on play with on-screen images of characters and action. Susan Johnson, MD, an anthroposophical physician and Waldorf-educated teacher and mother, observes that children who have a great deal of screen time have difficulty making mental images in their mind's eye. Creating pictures is not just entertaining, but the foundation of dreams and higher thoughts, such as intuition, inspiration, and imagination. Everyone dreams, thinks, and imagines future possibilities in pictures.[39] See more about helping our kids participate in imaginary play in chapter 12.

Jane Healy, PhD, psychologist and author of several books on children's brain development, believes that while "educational" television like Sesame Street does teach concepts, it cannot replace real life experiences. Most alarming is that studies show that watching television anesthetizes higher brain functions and disrupts the balance and interaction between the left and right hemispheres.[40]

Eliminating and Reducing Social Stressors

Establish day- and night-time routines; think seasonally. Introduce time concepts to kids early. Use words like "next week, tomorrow, in 5 minutes." Keep the same sequence of events for meals, homework, and bedtime rituals. Kids like the safety and security of routines. They do not push limits if they know you are serious. Be stalwart in sticking to them, except in very special circumstances, such as on a birthday or holiday.

Build seasonal routines and traditions like my daughter has with my granddaughter. They go strawberry picking in May and apple picking in September. Every year, they visit a pumpkin patch, go on a hayride, build a gingerbread house. They attend local annual festivals and volunteer at social service organizations so she can understand how to help those who are less fortunate.

Read and tell stories. Share books and stories, especially as a bedtime ritual. Jane Healy's classic, *Endangered Minds: Why Our Children Don't Think and What We Can Do About It*, includes a chapter

"Sesame Street and the Death of Reading." Reading with children has the same advantages of the family dinner: vocabulary building, visual imaging, waiting, and listening. While listening to stories, children's minds create their own pictures, which lead to ideas that lead to action.

Making up imaginary stories is great fun for kids. In her book, *See It, Say It, Do It*, Denver-area optometrist Lynn Hellerstein, OD, FCOVD, recommends taking kids on hot air balloon rides over their day each night before bed.[41] Looking down upon people, places, and things, they conjure up colors, sounds, textures, temperature, and feelings.

Find alternatives to TV that encourage creativity. Limit screen time and computer games, especially close to bedtime. Kids need free time to use their imaginations and find something to do when nothing grabs their imagination. Encourage them to dig for worms in the garden, paint, make crafts, sing songs, and play instruments. Healy's recommendation is that, for TV viewing to be constructive, parental discretion and involvement are essential.

Separate home and work duties. The most successful families I know keep strict boundaries between the two main areas of their lives. If they do not, they are not fully present in either place.

Educational Stressors

For many kids with autism, their schools are sources of stress, especially if they are being pushed prematurely into academics. What was once taught in first grade is now part of the kindergarten curriculum. Many kindergarteners still have poor control over their own bodies, let alone pencils and scissors. Despite the fact that they have not had the experience of sitting through a 15-minute meal, they are expected to sit through 45 minutes of circle time in kindergarten and a 60-minute lesson in first grade. Many stare out the window for visual relief, or wiggle and squirm to keep alert.

When are children really ready to read, write, and do mathematics? When all sensory systems are strong, and they show interest in and begin to participate in those activities spontaneously. Children who are ready for reading have strong motor foundations, can move their eyes across the page without upper body or head movements, and can not only recognize words, but also read with understanding. They use their eyes together as a team, change focus easily from the book to the teacher, and perceive just-noticeable differences among visually similar objects and words.

Some children with autism read very early. Extremely early reading, called hyperlexia, is a sign of uneven development, especially in the area of vision. Early reading should be discouraged; it is not a sign of a budding genius.

Here are some aspects of the educational system that are stressing out our kids:

Early reading initiatives, as a result of the ill-conceived No Child Left Behind Act, have hastened the teaching of reading and writing to a generation of children who cannot sleep through the night, tie their shoes, or speak in complete sentences. The lack of understanding of normal childhood development among some of today's educators and politicians has resulted in unrealistic expectations for young children. Pushing kids ahead academically without first establishing a strong foundation of motor, sensory-motor, and language skills forces them to learn by rote, at best.

Decreased time for the creative arts is common in schools today. Music and art are becoming extinct as we focus on academics. After-school lessons in playing an instrument and painting still lifes are not the same as providing art materials, keyboards, or drums and allowing freedom of expression.

Computers, tablets, and SMART Boards are replacing people. Our excitement about the technology that allows those with autism to communicate is accelerating as fast as the technology itself. Toddlers now know how to use a mouse or touchscreen on phones, tablets, and computers. Learning handwriting and keyboarding are becoming unnecessary as technology takes their place. Calculators have replaced many students' needs to do simple math in their heads.

iPads and computers with all their new apps certainly have their place, but not for our youngest children with autism. Kids under five still need to look at and interact with humans and stimulate their brains by moving and touching the real thing, not by staring at a screen.

Class size is increasing. Today's teachers must contend with up to 30 children of varying abilities and achievement levels in their classrooms, often without assistance. The common solution of hiring an aide or "shadow" for a student with autism can help unburden the teacher. However, sometimes aides act as policemen, keeping students with ASD "on task," further squelching their needs to move and touch.

As schools are cutting back on their budgets, classes can also span two or more grades. If a system has 40 first graders and 20 second graders, they might make a one-two combination. Placing higher-level first graders with lower-functioning second graders is a questionable practice.

Increase in safety concerns for children on the **autism** spectrum is a huge issue. Some are "runners," others climb, jump, and otherwise put themselves in harm's way, and some just wander off. Schools have to hire one-on-one aides to watch individual children, and some parents have resorted to tagging their kids with electronic devices.

Eliminating and Reducing Educational Stressors

Advocate. While parents cannot control most of the stressors at school, they *can* make a difference. Get involved and know what's going on. Join committees and attend school board meetings. Be active against bullying and for getting junk food out of the schools.

Have a summer cut-off for school entrance. Make sure that children are fully five-years-old before entering kindergarten. Give the gift of time to those with summer and fall birthdays, so they develop foundational skills before being introduced to academics. A tremendous amount of learning precedes reading and writing. Make sure children have good motor control of both the upper and lower parts of their bodies before asking them to sit still and pay attention.

Discourage unnecessary labeling as "disabled." Work at children's varying developmental levels. Extra time in pre-academic pursuits avoids lengthy, expensive testing and IEPs for those who could catch up if permitted. Respect for kids' development will reduce the number of children in special education.

Provide a developmentally-appropriate curriculum. Meet children at their developmental stages and levels. For instance, if a child with autism is chronologically eight, but has the language and social skills of a five-year-old, reading, writing, and arithmetic instruction should be at a kindergarten, not third-grade, level. This is not dumbing kids down. It is being respectful of their need for time to develop foundational skills in the motor, sensory-motor, and language areas before asking them to tackle higher-level academics. It also does not mean that content must be babyish. Adults, like children, can build blocks, play with trains, and perform science experiments—just at a higher level. Educators must learn to adjust the content to meet the cognitive needs of each child while keeping the reading and writing demands appropriate, too.

Incorporate movement and sensory activities into the school day. Learning is not all in your head! Whatever the goal, adding movement gives the body muscle memory, which reinforces all the other senses. Engage the help of occupational therapists to determine the "just right" amount of touch, movement, pressure, and sound for each child. Perform science experiments and use hands-on materials for math.

Try out a variety of seating options, swings, and irregular surfaces. Kids love three-legged stools, balls, and beanbags for chairs. Avoid hard, unforgiving plastic and wooden chairs. Consider partially inflated seat cushions if only hard chairs are available. Encourage teachers to use Brain Gym® or other warm-up activities first thing in the morning before academics begin. Ensure that kids are getting adequate food for their nervous systems by including as much time for recess and physical education as for computer lab.

Use games to encourage number learning. Count money; estimate time and distance. Use the language of time freely during the day: "We will clean up in ten minutes," or "Recess is only a half hour away." Use clocks and calendars to help kids see the passage of time. One family I know underwrote a store in their child's school so that each class could "purchase" supplies of pencils, paper, blocks, and art materials daily. Kids actually had to pay for the supplies and make change.

Provide teachers with in-service training and extra hands. Support teachers to attend at least two workshops per year to learn new skills and recharge their batteries. Burnout among special education teachers is rampant. Teach them new skills that help them deal productively with difficult behaviors. Give them parent volunteers and aides whenever the pupil-teacher ratio exceeds 10:1.

Offer healthy sensory and food diets. Promote a varied sensory diet. Watch for sensory overload. Wear simple clothing; avoid too many visual distractions from hanging and reflective objects. Be careful of the use of noisy machines during lessons. Play quiet, calming music; dim the lights, avoiding fluorescents that hum. Eliminate smells such as disinfectant, perfumes, and markers. Add calming scents like lavender. Serve healthy snacks and reinforcers free of gluten, dairy sugar, or sugar substitutes. Include raw fruits and vegetables — no candy, trans fats, or artificially colored foods.

Support inclusion. Research shows that both students with disabilities and those without benefit from being in classes together.[42] For students with autism inclusion satisfies placement in the least restrictive environment in which they can attain success. All students enjoy meaningful friendships, increased appreciation, acceptance and understanding of others, and enhanced social skills. Students with autism also gain:

- peer role models
- increased achievement of Individualized Educational Plan (IEP) goals
- greater access to the general curriculum
- enhanced skill acquisition and generalization
- increased inclusion in future environments
- higher expectations
- increased parent participation
- more integration of their families into the community

Many safeguards must be in place for inclusion to be successful. These include various types of teacher training and support. I could not find *any* research showing negative effects of inclusion when school systems implemented it appropriately.

Observe behaviors and teach diagnostically. Emulate Sherlock Holmes. Try to figure out the cause of a child's behavior. Is it sensory overload? Off-gassing from the carpet? Too much gluten for lunch? A need for movement? A stressed visual system? A family in crisis? What can you do to lessen the stressor(s)?

Write realistic, measurable IEP goals. The Individualized Education Plan (IEP) is the prescription for academic services for all students with special needs. Its goals and objectives are the guidelines for teachers and related service providers. As a team, these adults, along with the student's parents, need to set achievable goals each year for a child.

IEP goals are aimed at success! Establishing appropriate goals drive an appropriate placement. Together the IEP goals and objectives along with the proper placement increase a child's ability to have successful outcomes. Nothing is more frustrating for a parent than to see the same unachieved goals year after year in a child's IEP.

One suggestion to help ensure success is to remove behavioral goals for compensatory techniques, such as increasing eye contact and lessening repetitive, self-stimulatory behaviors. Poor eye contact and "stimming" are a child's attempts at coping with stress. These undesirable behaviors usually disappear spontaneously when the stressors are lessened or removed.

Emotional Stressors

While we used to think that kids with autism could not show or feel different emotions, we now know that isn't true. They have fears, worries, phobias, and anxiety about all kinds of things. Knowing what is bothering them is challenging, especially if they have difficulty expressing themselves verbally. Some possible emotional stressors for kids can include the following.

Ridicule and bullying are genuine fears for those with ASD. They are particularly easy targets for bullies because of their combination of naiveté, poor communication skills, and loyalty to the rules. They rarely tattle on the bully because of their additional fears of ridicule, embarrassment, or retaliation. Unlike their typical peers, they may not recognize bullying and instead think that a bully is a friend. They can thus be lured into compromising positions or places and convinced to do dangerous things.

Worries, anxiety, and phobias abound about visiting a dentist's or eye doctor's office, an upcoming fire drill, or bugs on the playground. Any of these can be emotional stressors for children with autism. Unfortunately, parents and teachers cannot anticipate every possible scary or over-stimulating experience.

Young children with autism can be terrified of the swirl of water in a toilet, an ambulance siren, or the roar of a vacuum cleaner, hair dryer, or lawn mower. Parents and teachers can work on these unpredictable assaults on the sensory systems when they are *not* happening.

Stress on the family system related to having a child with autism is immeasurable. Families who have two or more children with varying degrees of autism encounter significantly increased stress. The divorce rate among families with autism is estimated at 80%.[43] Relationships with siblings can be trying. Most siblings are quite tolerant and protective of their brother or sister with ASD. However, sometimes siblings feel resentful of the child with autism taking up so much of the parents' time, and they may lash out.

Adults who do not understand autism can also be emotionally trying at times. Incidents in public places, such as the grocery store, airplanes or buses, or a shopping mall, behaviors such as stimming, tantruming, and self-talk may seem to the uneducated as signs of bad parenting. Some parents carry cards to hand to adults who appeared annoyed or angry, explaining that their child is autistic and not badly behaved. Others choose to communicate this through a sticker or button that a child can wear.

Feelings of inadequacy and being "broken" can last a lifetime, resulting in poor self-esteem. Sometimes kids who have been going to therapies for years and have improved to the point of being included with typical peers balk as they approach puberty; they demand that "enough is enough!" They want to be accepted as they are, and refuse any more appointments to "fix" their inadequacies.

Eliminating and Reducing Emotional Stressors

Teach your child how not to be a victim. School psychologist Izzy Kalman has developed an anti-bullying program that teaches kids how to deal with bullies. It is unlike any other bullying program you have ever encountered. Once kids learn to recognize bullying, Kalman teaches them how to disarm the bully without retaliation and while retaining their self-respect. Go to www.bullies2buddies. com.

Use sensory techniques to calm down emotions. Joint compression and brushing are two simple interventions that can desensitize a child's overwhelmed nervous system. Parents can easily learn how to release serotonin into a child's body with these and other tools, thus giving an overwhelming feeling of peace. Refer to chapter 10 for more on this important subject.

Prepare kids for new situations, people, and places. Just talking through what's coming up, even when it is routine, can be comforting and make a child with autism feel more secure. Scoping out new people and places and seeing what possible sensory or other traps may be lurking there can avoid meltdowns some of the time. Use role playing and social stories for fears of the unknown. Practice tolerating sirens and loud noises, or providing headphones to mask them can also be useful.

Take advantage of local and online autism support systems. Many parent support systems are available for families living with autism. Some groups now have programs for siblings, too. Check out www. siblingsupport.org to see what is available near you.

Love children with autism unconditionally. Many parents have told me that having a child with autism is the best thing that ever happened to them; it helped them grow and learn more about themselves. They learn how to experience joy not only in the special moments, but also day to day. Many have the ability to see beyond the tragedy and embrace this whole different world that connects them to so many other parents with the same struggles, hopes, and dreams. It is always imperative to love children with autism unconditionally, but puberty is a time when this goal is even more important.

Be fully present when interacting with your child. Turn off the cell phone or computer and interact fully. That sends a message to your child that what he or she is doing and saying is important to you; you are modeling for your child to do the same.

Support Environmentally Healthy Practices

One important way to reduce stressors of all kinds is by supporting and joining national nonprofits that are working to keep us and our kids safe. Here are some organizations you may want to look into:

Green America is the oldest, largest, and most diverse network of socially and environmentally responsible businesses in America. They support an environmentally sustainable society and link green businesses of all kinds to the consumers. Membership includes a subscription to Green American magazine, which has recent articles on such varied and timely subjects as "Eco-friendly Children's Clothing," "Look for Earth Friendly School Supplies," "CFLs vs LEDs: The Best Bulbs," and "Beyond Lead: Toxins in Toys." See www. greenamerica.org.

Healthy Child Healthy World empowers parents with information to find the products and companies that help create a safer, greener, healthier life. They publish a book, pocket guides (also available as apps) on buying everything from food to cleaning materials, videos, and an extremely deep and informative website, www.healthychild. org.

Healthy Schools Network is the leading national voice for children's environmental health. They support three core facets of environmental health at school:

- child-safe standards for school design, construction, and siting;
- child-safe policies for housekeeping and purchasing (targeting indoor air pollutants, mercury, pesticides and other toxins, and the use of safer substitutes); and
- environmental public health services for children in harm's way.

Healthy Schools/Healthy Kids Clearinghouse©, offers dozens of fact sheets, guides, and peer-reviewed reports. Its first two parent guides (on indoor air and green cleaning) have been nationally distributed since 1999. See www.healthyschools.org.

The Safe Cosmetics Campaign at www.safecosmetics.org is a coalition of women's, public health, labor, environmental health, and consumer-rights organizations that work with manufacturers to encourage reformulations and safer ingredients. In 2012, they released an app for the iPhone to look up any product and learn its ingredients instantly! Of course, this information is also available on their website.

The True Food Network at www.truefoodnow.org is the grassroots arm of the Center for Food Safety. Get updates and action reports on food labeling, and download their pocket-sized Shopper's Guide — either as an app or a document — on how to avoid genetically modified products.

Take-Home Points

Making some serious lifestyle changes can reduce load factors substantially, resulting in cleaner homes and schools, healthier and happier kids, closer and more accepting relationships, easier learning, and a generally better quality of life. No matter how well we manage our stress, new stressors lurk just around the corner as environments and relationships change.

Stay ahead of the game by reading books, listening to webinars, going to conferences, and subscribing to newsletters. While we cannot control *everything*, we can at least try!

Books
- *Chemical-Free Kids: How to Safeguard Your Child's Diet and Environment*[44]
- *Chemical-Free Kids: The Organic Sequel*[45]
- *Healthy Child Healthy World*[46]
- *Squeaky Green: The Method Guide for Detoxing your Home*[47]

Newsletters and Online Magazines

- *Green Chi Café* — celebrate green lifestyle and culture with best-selling green living author, Annie B. Bond (www.anniebbond.com)
- *Green Living Tips* — earth-friendly advice for going green and reducing costs, consumption, and environmental impact (www.greenlivingtips.com)
- *Care 2* — eco-friendly health and wellness tips (www.care2.com/greenliving)
- *Low Impact Living* — a great guide for finding green home products (www.lowimpactliving.com)
- *Mothering* — *the* resource for *everything* natural from pregnancy through elementary age; join forums, ask questions, search past issues of print magazine, and find new recipes (www.mothering.com)

Make health a priority before investing in costly therapies. You will be surprised what a difference some simple lifestyle changes can make in your road to outsmarting autism!

---

[1] American Lung Association. Indoor Air Pollution Fact Sheet — Biological Agents. 1991. Publication No. 1186C.

[2] Gold D. Environmental Tobacco Smoke, Indoor Allergens, and Childhood Asthma. Environmental Health Perspectives, Aug 2000, 108(S4).

[3] May JC. My house is killing me. Baltimore: Johns Hopkins University Press, 2001.

[4] Grandjean P. Only One Chance: How environmental pollution impairs brain development — and how to protect the brains of the next generation. New York: Oxford University Press, 2013.

[5] http://www.ericsissom.com/health_alternative/mercury_in_products.htm. Accessed Nov 7, 2011.

[6] Steinemann AC, Gallagher LG, Davis AL, MacGregor IC. Chemical Emissions from Residential Dryer Vents During Use of Fragranced Laundry Products. Air Quality, Atmosphere and Health, 2011.

[7] Schettler, T. Human exposure to phthalates via consumer products. Int J Androl, Feb 2006, 29:1, 134–39.

[8] Swan S. Environmental phthalate exposure in relation to reproductive outcomes and other health endpoints in humans. Environmental Health Perspectives, 2008.

[9] Ferrel J. Are Plastic Food and Beverage Containers Safe? http://ezinearticles.com/?Are-Plastic-Food-and-Beverage-Containers-Safe?&id=57347. Accessed Nov 20, 2011.

[10] Swerdlow AJ, et al. Mobile phones, brain tumors, and the Interphone study: Where are we now? Environ Health Perspect, 2011, 119:11, 1534–38.

[11] www.electromagnetichealth.org. Accessed Nov 20, 2011.

[12] Klinghardt D. The Unavoidable Hidden Factor that Greatly Contributes to Autism, presentation. http://articles.mercola.com/sites/articles/archive/2008/12/25/. Accessed Nov 10, 2011.

[13] Williams R. Fracking and geopathic stress. www.househealing4you.com. Accessed Dec 14, 2013.

[14] www.energystar.gov. Accessed Nov 20, 2011.

[15] Mumford, RB. Improving visual efficiency with selected lighting. JOVD, Fall 2002, 3:3, 1–7.

[16] Bond AB. Home Enlightenment: Practical Earth-Friendly Advice for Creating a Nurturing, Healthy, Toxin-Free Home and Lifestyle. New York: Rodale Books, 2008.

[17] http://healthychild.org/blog/comments/whats_on_the_label_art_and_hobby_supplies/. Accessed Nov 16, 2011.

[18] www.vitamindcouncil.org.

[19] Cannell JJ. Autism and vitamin D. Med Hypotheses, 2008, 70:4, 750–59.

[20] Gittleman AL. Zapped: Why Your Cell Phone Shouldn't Be Your Alarm Clock and 1,268 Ways to Outsmart the Hazards of Electronic Pollution. New York: Harpers, 2011.

[21] Levitt BB. Electromagnetic Fields: A Consumer's Guide to the Issues and How to Protect Ourselves. www.backinprint.com, 2011.

[22] Karim I. BioGeometry: Back to a Future for Mankind. Egypt, 2010.

[23] Davis D. Disconnect. New York: Dutton Books, 2010.

[24] www.answers.yahoo.com. Accessed Nov 14, 2011.

[25] Kaplan M. Seeing through New Eyes. Philadelphia: Jessica Kingsley Publishers, 2006.

[26] Mahajan N, Hong N, Wigal TL, Gehricke JG. Hyperactive-impulsive symptoms associated with self-reported sleep quality in non-medicated adults with ADHD. *Journal of Attention Disorders, Sep* 2010, 14:2, 132–37.

[27] Environmental Working Group. EWG's 2011 Shopper's Guide to Pesticides in Produce. Washington, DC, 2011.

[28] Ingram C. The Drinking Water Book: How to Eliminate Harmful Toxins from Your Water. Berkeley, CA: Celestial Arts, 2006.

[29] Tennakone K, Wickramanayake S. Aluminum leaching from cooking utensils. Nature, Jan 1987, 325:6101, 202.

[30] Guillete EA. Examining childhood development in contaminated urban settings. Environ Health Persp, Jun 2000, 108:Suppl3, 389–93.

[31] Klinghardt D. "Biological Medicine 2012 Conference." New York. Klinghardt Academy, February, 2012. (http://www.klinghardtacademy.com/images/stories/event/biological_medicine_2012_speaker_schedule.pdf

[32] Louv R. The Last Child in the Woods: Saving our children from nature deficit disorder. Chapel Hill, NC: Algonquin Books, 2008.

[33] Pollan M. Cooked: A Natural history of transformation. New York: Penguin Books, 2013.

[34] Wrangham R. Catching Fire: How Cooking Made Us Human. New York: Basic Books, 2009.

[35] Ceglowski D, Bacigalupa C. Keeping Current in Child Care Research, Annotated Bibliography: An Update. Early Childhood Res and Pract, 2002, 4:1.

[36] Farner B. Eating Out Healthy, June 2005. www.urbanext.uiuc.edu. Accessed Dec 9, 2007.

[37] Wolfe J. Eating Out is a Diet Killer, May 14, 2013. www.discovery.com. Accessed Dec 14, 2013.

[38] David L. Changing the Way We Eat. TEDx Manhattan, Feb 12, 2011.

[39] Johnson SR. TV and Our Children's Minds, 2007. www.youandyourchildshealth.org.

[40] Buzzell K. *The Children of Cyclops: The Influence of Television Viewing on the Developing Human Brain.* Boulder, CO: Assoc of Waldorf Schools of North America, 1998.

[41] Hellerstein L. See It, Say It, Do It. Centennial, CO: HiClear Publishing, 2009.

[42] http://www.kidstogether.org/inclusion/benefitsofinclusion.htm. Accessed Nov 16, 2011.

[43] http://www.nationalautismassociation.org/htmlpages/divorce.htm. Accessed Oct 30, 2011.

[44] Magaziner A, Bonvie L, Zolezzi A. Chemical-free kids: How to safeguard your child's diet and environment. New York: Kensington Publishing Group, 2003.

[45] Zolezzi A, Bonvie L, Bonvie B. Chemical-Free Kids, the Organic Sequel. La Hambra, CA: ASM Books, 2008.

[46] Gavigan C. Healthy Child Healthy World: Creating a Cleaner Greener Safer Home. New York: Dutton, 2008.

[47] Ryan E, Lowry A, Suqi R. Squeaky Green. San Francisco: Chronicle Books, 2008.

CHAPTER 4

Diet and Digestion Dos and Don'ts

The relationships among diet, digestion, and behavior are hotly debated, and opinions on these subjects are mixed. One gastroenterologist with a waiting room full of candy once told me that diet had nothing to do with digestion! Does he *really* believe that? I don't! To me, *nothing* is more fundamental to health than eating well.

The goal for all children is optimal nutrition. How can you tell if your child is well-nourished? Nutritionist Kelly Dorfman makes these comparisons:[1]

A well nourished child:	*A poorly nourished child:*
Has good coloring	Has a pasty complexion / yellow or grey pallor
Is well most of the time	Has three or more illnesses a year
Is interested in a variety of foods	Has restricted eating habits
Has fairly consistent responses to therapy	Is erratic and unpredictable
Has clear eyes	Has dull eyes
Has good breath	Has sour or bad breath

Bottom line: A child who *looks* unhealthy probably *is* unhealthy.

This chapter begins with an overview of the dietary modification process, and then a short course in digestion is followed by the many dietary complications and culprits common in autism. Next is a detailed description of many of the special diets that are helping those with autism digest more efficiently. Finally, we look at picky eating, one of the banes of keeping a family member with autism well-nourished.

Where does one begin?

Getting Started on Dietary Modification

Clean Up the Existing Diet

The first step in improving the diet for a child on the spectrum is to evaluate your definition of food. What is "food"? Do goldfish crackers, Twinkies, and organic tofu dogs qualify as food? According to food guru Michael Pollan, author of six books on food, "If your grandmother didn't eat it, if it was made in a plant instead of grown on a plant, you and your kids probably shouldn't eat it either."[2]

For the past 50 years, artificial colors, flavors, preservatives, excitotoxins, and sugar have hidden in foods to enhance their taste, smell, and shelf life. Flavoring foods is an industry that employs thousands of people and tries to addict us to tastes that sell their products. Processed and genetically modified (GMO) foods have crept into our refrigerator and onto our tables; processed and GMO foods are not real food.

Fruit juice, often considered "healthy," is one of the most common and overlooked sources of sugar. Many children with autism consume up to a quart of juice each day. Dilute all fruit juices and limit to one cup a day, keeping in mind that one cup of fruit juice is a very concentrated amount of fruit. Apple and grape juice both contain salicylates, so these products give susceptible children a double dose of potential poisons. Apple juice also contains arabitol, a derivative of arabinose, a toxic by-product of yeast; applesauce does not.

Furthermore, for kids with autism, unprocessed foods are much less likely to cause problems than processed ones with many ingredients, including additives. Strive for a diet based on a balanced variety of unrefined, unprocessed food. Buy and eat fresh, mostly organic foods in season. Minimize eatables that come in jars, boxes, bags, or cans. Canned foods leach BPA, a byproduct of the container's plastic lining.[3] Read labels. *Real* food requires no labels, except perhaps to tell us the country of origin.

Vary high-quality proteins, carbohydrates, and fats. Eat plants — fruits and vegetables, which are complex carbohydrates. Eliminate trans fats and include good fat sources like cold-water fish, nuts, seeds, and vegetables that supply essential omega-3 fats. Rotate different grains, meats, fruits, and vegetables.

Pollan synthesizes what a good diet entails into seven simple words: "Eat food . . . not too much . . . mainly plants." Unfortunately, it's not as simple as it sounds, especially when attempting to outsmart autism with a picky, picky eater.

Expensive, you say? Not if you eat *real* food: protein from beans and animal sources, vegetables, and grains. *Hard to do?* Maybe a little at first, but *so* much support is available online and at local food co-ops and grocery stores.

Remove Targeted Offending Foods

One of the pioneers in targeting foods as problematic is Doris Rapp, MD, author of *Is This Your Child?*[4] For at least 50 years Rapp has been an active advocate for dietary modification as first-line therapy for improving learning and behavioral outcomes. She has developed easy-to-follow, clear guidelines for implementing week-long elimination diets for the most common offenders: dairy products and other casein-containing foods, gluten- and wheat-containing foods, eggs, and sugar. Not convinced? Watch some of her videos showing angelic children turn into devils after ingesting a food to which they react.

In her brilliant book, *Cure Your Child with Food*, "nutrition detective" Kelly Dorfman states that food problems with most kids follow what she calls the "Binary Law of Nutrition": either something is bothering the body or something is missing.[5] The next sections in this chapter look at what might be bothering your child's body and brain, and steps to take for elimination. Chapters 5–7 educate about possible missing nutrients.

The late Dr. Jacqueline McCandless, author of *Children with Starving Brains* and grandmother of a young girl with autism, believes that restricting the diets of those with autism is the number-one choice for healing: "When I first started working with kids, I had two groups of parents. One, the parents were very conscientious . . . they took away the wheat, they took away the milk, they took away the soy, and finally they took away the sugar. These kids were starting to get well. I had another group of parents who were resistant. They couldn't believe that a little bit of sugar, bread, or a cookie here and there could hurt. And those kids would keep getting infections and have regressions."[6] McCandless finally refused to work with any parent who was unwilling to follow an elimination diet strictly.

Digestion 101

A short course on the normal digestive process is necessary before understanding what goes wrong in the digestion of those on the autism spectrum. Digestion starts in the mouth. Each bite of food that enters the mouth mixes with saliva and is swallowed. A process of muscle contraction called peristalsis moves the partially digested food into the stomach, small intestines, and colon, where enzymes and other juices work it further.

Enzymes, which are proteins responsible for many essential biochemical reactions, are vitally important for proper digestion. Enzymes act as catalysts, breaking down carbohydrates, proteins, and fats into simple forms that the body can absorb, burn for energy, or use to build or repair itself. As the body absorbs nutrients, toxins and other waste products finish the journey and exit through the rectum as fecal matter.

This very complex process could take hours to days, depending upon many factors. Ideally food should not tarry too long in the intestines, as the digestive organs then reabsorb wastes. Ideally, the contents of a healthy, well-fed gastrointestinal tract, assisted by an adequate supply of food and water, break down food into usable particles, pick up wastes, and produce at least one significant bowel movement per day without any effort.

The entire digestive tract is a living ecological community of good, bad, and ugly microorganisms, called our "microbiome," that share our body space for the purpose of assisting food absorption and waste elimination.[7] The average person carries around over three pounds of more than 100 trillion bacteria to do the job![8] The microbiome was discovered in the late 1990s and is now believed to potentially have an overwhelming impact on human health.

Some of the gut's bacteria are "friendly," whereas others are considered "bad." The good guys are beneficial to the digestive process and much more. The bad guys disrupt the digestive process and health in general. Good and bad bacteria compete for space in the digestive tract, but the goal, of course, is for the good to outnumber the bad.

The gut and the brain are both branches of the body's autonomic nervous system that communicate not only with each other but also with the immune system. At least 70% of the immune system is located in the digestive tract, according to Michael Gershon, MD. He has dubbed the subdivision of the autonomic nervous system that directly controls the gastrointestinal system, known scientifically as the enteric nervous system, "the second brain."[9] A modern pioneer in the emerging field of neurogastroenterology, Gershon has enhanced our understanding of the complex interactions among the damaged gut, the immune system, and the brain. Nowhere is this connection clearer than in the bodies and minds of those with autism.

Digestion and Autism

Dysbiosis

Children with autism have higher levels of bad bacteria and lower levels of good bacteria,[10] a condition known as dysbiosis.[11] An out-of-balance gut is like a garden full of too many bad bugs that eat the plants, and too few bees, snails, and worms to pollinate the flowers and make good soil. A balance of intestinal flora is crucial to many biological processes, including our nutritional status, detoxification abilities and our ability to think and feel.

Dysbiosis contributes further to health and behavioral issues because the overgrowth of bad microorganisms alters an individual's resistance to infection and general immune response. In other words, unwanted bugs wreaking havoc in the gut is *big* trouble because the body must deal with additional toxins produced as waste by-products from their metabolism.

One nasty bug, clostridia, which causes diarrhea and colitis, also produces a potent neurotoxin that could be responsible for some kids' very erratic behavior, according to Sydney M. Finegold, MD at UCLA Medical Center. He and his colleagues found clostridia in the guts and feces of some children with regressive autism.[12]

Want to see gut bugs in action? Watch *The Autism Enigma*, a documentary on gut issues as a major contributor to autism. In this film an international group of scientists examines the gut's amazingly diverse and powerful microbial ecosystem and its efforts toward healing.[13]

Phenol Sulfur-Transferase (PST) and Phenols

When enzyme production is off, other digestive and behavioral functions can also go awry. One missing enzyme, phenol sulfur-transferase (PST), is necessary for the body to break down and remove certain chemicals and toxins, called phenols, from the body. PST is key to the digestive problems of some kids with autism. Dr. Rosemary Waring, a British scientist who discovered the role of PST, found that as many as 90% of those with autism have limited PST activity. She believes that unprocessed phenols and toxic bacteria in the gut act as internal irritants, causing "autistic" and hyperactive behavior.[14] Waring notes that children with low levels of PST also have trouble digesting gluten and casein.[15]

While all foods contain phenolic compounds, some have higher content than others. Phenols occur in foods containing artificial dyes, colors, and flavors, as well as the preservatives Butylated Hydroxyanisole (BHA), Butylated Hydroxytoluene (BHT) and Tertiary Butlyhydroquinone (TBHQ),[16] which inhibit the production of PST and suppress its activity in the gut.[17] Malvin, a phenol present in foods that are naturally red, blue, or purple, is one of the most problematic.[18] High-phenolic foods that children on the autism spectrum eat frequently are apples, grapes, strawberries, bananas, almonds, and vanilla. Consuming high-phenolic foods is not a problem unless PST is low, because then the phenols cannot be properly digested.

The Yeast Connection

The late William Crook, MD, a country pediatrician for over 50 years, wrote extensively about the relationship among childhood ear infections, treatment with antibiotics, and a later autism diagnosis.[19] As early as 1982 he noted a child named Rusty with a history of colic and ear infections in the first year of life. By age two Rusty showed both hyperactivity and autistic symptoms.

Dr. Crook believed that many children on the autism spectrum, like Rusty, have problems with a yeast known as *Candida albicans.* Dr. Bernard Rimland of the Autism Research Institute also suspected a relationship between Candida and autism in 1985.[20] Children who crave sugar from candy, soft drinks, fruit juices, and baked goods are highly suspect of having yeast-based problems, because yeasts feed off of sugar to grow. Dr. Crook commented that eating sugar is like adding kerosene to a fire.[21]

Symptoms of yeast overgrowth are mood swings, headaches, muscle aches, abdominal pain, itching (especially around the genitals or anus), digestive issues, excessive gas, bloating, putrid-smelling stools, irritability, depression, fuzzy thinking, crankiness, brain fog, hyperactivity, and attention problems. In babies, thrush, recurrent and persistent diaper rash, colic, recurrent ear infections with repeated or prolonged antibiotic use, and chronic allergies including rashes, wheezing, and coughing are all red flags for yeast.

William Shaw, PhD, the former Director of Clinical Chemistry and Toxicology at Children's Mercy Hospital and the founder of Great Plains Laboratory (both in Kansas), proved Dr. Crook right in 1995. Shaw, a biochemist, who had no previous experience with autism, identified very high levels of tartaric acid and arabinose, by-products of yeast overgrowth, in the gut flora of brothers who he later learned were autistic.[22]

Arabinose and tartaric acid have drastically negative effects on human metabolism. Tartaric acid inhibits and limits energy production, causing muscle weakness throughout the body. Arabinose impedes the absorption of vitamins essential for the production of digestive enzymes.

Aware that yeast metabolism is a likely source of tartaric acid and arabinose, Shaw concluded that the brothers with autism had yeast in their intestinal tracts. He began seeing a common pattern of ear infections, antibiotics, and yeast overgrowth in children who eventually were diagnosed with autism. Read more about this relationship and immune system dysregulation in chapter 5. Dr. Shaw has become a world authority on yeast-based problems and their role in autism spectrum disorders.

Leaky Gut

A leaky gut occurs as partially digested food particles, proteins, and toxins pass into the bloodstream through tiny holes yeasts produce in the thin mucosal membrane that lines the intestinal wall—a process similar to ivy attaching itself to a brick house and slowly destroying the mortar.[23] Antibiotic overuse, heavy metal toxicity, and destructive enzymes secreted by yeasts further contribute to the breakdown of the gut lining.

The intruders into the bloodstream trigger antibody responses that can then elicit allergic, physical, emotional, or cognitive reactions. As yeasts continue to proliferate, the immune and endocrine systems weaken, the chances of infection and antibiotic usage increase, and the vicious cycle continues.

"Leaky gut syndrome" is the nickname for this condition of increased intestinal permeability. According to veteran nutritionist Elizabeth Lipski, PhD, a leaky gut underlies an enormous variety of illnesses and symptoms, including autism.[24]

The presence of a leaky gut makes elimination diets tricky, as irritants can interact. That is, exposure to a single food may cause few symptoms, but when two mildly reacting foods are present, together they can trip a response by overloading the system. In these "load" reactions, a little bit of a food may be tolerable, but too much of one or a combination of two or more causes trouble. The culprit of this phenomenon is usually a leaky gut.

Constipation and Diarrhea

Parents often report that their children with autism experience chronic constipation accompanied by serious abdominal pain and bloating, frequent diarrhea, or alternating constipation and diarrhea. Some go weeks at a time without a bowel movement; others have five or more a day. Stools are abnormal in color, consistency, and smell, as well as frequency. Others have impacted bowels which lead to alternating diarrhea and constipation. What appears to be diarrhea may in fact be leakage around a hardened stool.[25] Once measures are taken to remove the impaction, bowel and brain function usually improve.

An examination by a gastrointestinal (GI) specialist familiar with autism is essential at this point. The doctor performs a physical exam, which includes listening to the abdomen with a stethoscope and lightly palpating it. A hard, bloated abdomen and discomfort upon palpation may determine a diagnosis.[26]

Gastrointestinal problems in children with autism have generated a great deal of interest among clinicians, researchers, and parents.[27] Two GI experts who have made autism their specialty are Arthur Krigsman, MD, of New York University Medical Center, and Timothy Buie, MD, at Harvard University Medical Center. They have scoped hundreds of children with ASDs.

Gluten and Casein

For at least 30 years, doctors have recognized that problems digesting wheat and/or cow's milk products are related to many chronic health problems, including eczema, asthma, childhood diabetes, constipation, diarrhea, and reflux, as well as behavioral and learning problems.[28] The American Academy of Pediatrics recommends against introducing cow's milk into a baby's diet until after the first birthday for that reason.[29] Cow's milk has seven times as much casein—the protein in dairy products—as human milk, and cows also have four stomachs to our one!

Most children on the autism spectrum have or have had some or all of the above ailments, and frequently eat a very limited diet consisting almost entirely of wheat- and dairy-based food. The intolerance to certain foods, especially those containing gluten and casein, is a common occurrence among children with autism spectrum disorders. Why?

In the late 1990s Karen Seroussi, the mother of a young boy diagnosed with autism at 19 months, began researching treatment options for her son. She discovered that in 1990 biochemist Karl Reichelt and his colleagues found that 90% of a sample of children with autism had abnormally high levels of certain opioid peptides in their urine.[30] The researchers believed that these opioid peptides come from an incomplete breakdown of gluten, the protein in wheat and other cereal grains—including rye, oats, and barley—and casein. One of the approaches that Seroussi tried was eliminating gluten- and casein-containing foods from her son's diet. He made such dramatic improvement that, by age four, he was no longer considered autistic.

When her heart-warming story, *Unraveling the Mystery of Autism and Pervasive Developmental Disorder: A Mother's Story of Research and Recovery* broke in 2000, Seroussi was the first person to publically propose diet as the foremost step to take in treating a child with autism, and the first to use the words "autism" and "recovery" in the same sentence.[31] This book, detailing how Seroussi left no stone unturned in trying to discover what caused her son to regress into autism and then how to return him to normalcy, is still the first book many newly diagnosed families read that offers them hope.

Seroussi's discovery coincidentally was of great interest to her then-husband, Alan Friedman, PhD, a physical chemist at Johnson and Johnson Labs. He and his colleagues compared urine samples of normal children with those of children with autism. The urine of the latter contained undigested food particles, supporting a leaky gut syndrome. Furthermore, they discovered that in children with autism the enzyme Dipeptidyl peptidase IV, responsible for effectively breaking down gluten and casein, was either reduced, inactivated, or absent via a genetic mechanism. Mercury, abundant in the bodies of many kids on the spectrum, has the ability to inhibit or block this enzyme.[32]

Seroussi remains a staunch crusader for dietary intervention, and with her friend Lisa Lewis, PhD, she has written an *Encyclopedia of Dietary Interventions for Autism* to help parents through the gluten elimination journey.[33]

The Opioid Excess Theory

What Seroussi unearthed is called the "opioid excess theory." Many years before she put Reichelt's work into action, he and researcher Jaak Panksepp speculated that people with autism may have elevated levels of opioids because their behavior resembled that of drug addicts.[34]

The main premise of the opioid excess theory is that incomplete digestion of gluten and casein creates small peptides instead of fully broken-down amino acids. These peptides pass through the damaged permeable intestinal membrane and enter the central nervous system, exerting an opioid-like effect.[35]

The brain has receptors for opioids, as well as many other different types of peptides, the role of which is to switch on a neuron's sensitivity to a variety of neurotransmitters. A small amount of opioid peptides is useful; an overload is harmful. Excessive peptides can mimic some of the good hormones and neurotransmitters, thus disturbing perception, behavior, mood, emotions, brain development, and immune function.[36]

Partially digested proteins have odd configurations and mimic other complex molecules such as endorphins. Endorphins are nervous system proteins that act as painkillers. Partially digested gluten or casein proteins may bind to pain-killing (opiate) receptors and cause behavioral symptoms of poor eye contact, irritability, or disconnection.

Parents Speak Out

Since its establishment in the 1960s, the Autism Research Institute (ARI) — under its founder, the late Bernard Rimland, PhD, psychologist and father of son diagnosed with autism — has prioritized the tracking of promising autism treatments. Dr. Rimland, and now director Stephen Edelson, PhD, have to-date collected anecdotal evidence from over 27,000 parents on the results of dietary modification. Over 50% saw positive behavioral changes when removing targeted foods.[37] Here are the results:

PARENT RATINGS OF BEHAVIORAL EFFECTS OF BIOMEDICAL INTERVENTIONS
Autism Research Institute • 4182 Adams Avenue • San Diego, CA 92116

The parents of autistic children represent a vast and important reservoir of information on the benefits—and adverse effects—of the large variety of drugs and other interventions that have been tried with their children. Since 1967 the Autism Research Institute has been collecting parent ratings of the usefulness of the many interventions tried on their autistic children.

The following data have been collected from the more than 27,000 parents who have completed our questionnaires designed to collect such information. For the purposes of the present table, the parents responses on a six-point scale have been combined into three categories: "made worse" (ratings 1 and 2), "no effect" (ratings 3 and 4), and "made better" (ratings 5 and 6). The "Better:Worse" column gives the number of children who "Got Better" for each one who "Got Worse."

BIOMEDICAL/ NON-DRUG/ SUPPLEMENTS	Parent Ratings				
	Got Worse[A]	No Effect	Got Better	Better: Worse	No. of Cases[B]
Calcium[E]	3%	60%	36%	11:1	2832
Cod Liver Oil	4%	41%	55%	14:1	2550
Cod Liver Oil with Bethanecol	11%	53%	36%	3.4:1	203
Colostrum	6%	56%	38%	6.8:1	851
Detox. (Chelation)[C]	3%	23%	74%	24:1	1382
Digestive Enzymes	3%	35%	62%	19:1	2350
DMG	8%	50%	42%	5.3:1	6363
Fatty Acids	2%	39%	59%	31:1	1680
5 HTP	11%	42%	47%	4.2:1	644
Folic Acid	5%	50%	45%	10:1	2505
Food Allergy Trtmnt	2%	31%	67%	27:1	1294
Hyperbaric Oxygen Therapy	5%	30%	65%	12:1	219
Magnesium	6%	65%	29%	4.6:1	301
Melatonin	8%	26%	66%	8.3:1	1687
Methyl B12 (nasal)	10%	45%	44%	4.2:1	240
Methyl B12 (subcut.)	6%	22%	72%	12:1	899
MT Promoter	8%	47%	44%	5.5:1	99
P5P (Vit. B6)	11%	40%	48%	4.3:1	920
Pepcid	11%	57%	32%	2.9:1	220
SAMe	16%	62%	23%	1.4:1	244
St. Johns Wort	19%	64%	18%	0.9:1	217
TMG	16%	43%	41%	2.6:1	1132

BIOMEDICAL/ NON-DRUG/ SUPPLEMENTS	Parent Ratings				
	Got Worse[A]	No Effect	Got Better	Better: Worse	No. of Cases[B]
Transfer Factor	8%	47%	45%	5.9:1	274
Vitamin A	3%	54%	44%	16:1	1535
Vitamin B3	4%	51%	45%	10:1	1192
Vit. B6/Mag.	4%	46%	49%	11:1	7256
Vitamin C	2%	52%	46%	20:1	3077
Zinc	2%	44%	54%	24:1	2738
SPECIAL DIETS					
Candida Diet	3%	39%	58%	21:1	1141
Feingold Diet	2%	40%	58%	26:1	1041
Gluten- /Casein- Free Diet	3%	28%	69%	24:1	3593
Low Oxalate Diet	7%	43%	50%	6.8:1	164
Removed Chocolate	2%	46%	52%	28:1	2264
Removed Eggs	2%	53%	45%	20:1	1658
Removed Milk Products/Dairy	2%	44%	55%	32:1	6950
Removed Sugar	2%	46%	52%	27:1	4589
Removed Wheat	2%	43%	55%	30:1	4340
Rotation Diet	2%	43%	55%	23:1	1097
Specific Carbo-hydrate Diet	7%	22%	71%	10:1	537

A. "Worse" refers only to worse behavior. Drugs, but not nutrients, typically also cause physical problems if used long-term.
B. No. of cases is cumulative over several decades, so does not reflect current usage levels (e.g., Haldol is now seldom used).
C. Antifungal drugs and chelation are used selectively, where evidence indicates they are needed.
D. Seizure drugs: top line behavior effects, bottom line effects on seizures.
E. Calcium effects are not due to dairy-free diet; statistics are similar for milk drinkers and non-milk drinkers.

Table 4.1.

Parent Ratings of Behavioral Effects of Supplements and Special Diets Autism Research Institute March, 2009 (Reprinted with permission)

The impact of food reactions on behavior can be profound. Foods that bother kids' digestion are often the very same ones they crave. After removing offensive foods, parents report seeing remarkable positive changes in target behaviors, such as the understanding and use of language, eye contact, and relatedness. Most important is that unlike using medications, very few children's behavior worsened with dietary elimination.

Recent Research

In the past 10 years, the scientific literature has exploded with well- and not-so-well-designed research on diet and autism. One recent poorly designed study was funded by the National Institutes of Health (NIH) and the National Center for Research Resources, two staunchly conservative groups. The study, conducted on only 14 children for only 4 weeks duration, saw no benefits to sleep, attention, or bowel function by removing gluten and casein-containing foods.[38] This new study ignored (purposefully?) an exhaustive body of research that supports dietary modification.

Outrage emanated from the autism community following the release of these findings because it was counter to the observations of so many parents and clinicians. Many criticized the small sample size, the short time period of the study, the lack of supplementation to address nutritional deficiencies, and the inclusion of sugar-laden products.

Recall that the two foods in this study are only two of many foods to which children with autism react. In Total Load sometimes a little bit of a food is not a problem, but when eaten with other reactive foods, it causes symptoms. In order for children to benefit fully, many potentially reactive foods, such as soy, eggs, and sugar must also be removed for at least three months. The additional time allows opioid peptides to leave the body and for symptoms to improve gradually.

Furthermore, those implementing a gluten-free, casein-free diet always recommend supplementing it with calcium, as well as other deficient nutrients. Finally, nutrient-rich fruits, vegetables, and protein-containing grains are preferable to substituting with gluten- and casein-free junk food, as this study did.

Current dietary research studies are focusing on urinary peptides, gut bacteria, dysbiosis, and reproducing the now-classic findings of Dr. Karl Reichelt and other scientists who have been examining dietary issues in autism for over two decades.

Food Allergy Reactions and Testing

Before adopting an elimination diet, many parents choose to consult an allergist to determine if a restrictive diet is necessary. Surprise! After extensive scratch testing, the child is often found not to be allergic to any foods. Some choose to eliminate gluten and casein proteins anyway, and frequently they report that their youngster responds with improved attention, sleep, or language skills.

How is this improvement possible if the child was not allergic in the first place? The answer lies in understanding the different types of chemical reactions the body can have to food.

"Allergies" are defined as specific immediate reactions such as hives, congestion or swelling involving an antibody called *Immunoglobulin E (IgE)*. Traditional scratch testing identifies IgE triggers, such as pollen, peanuts, or strawberries, that can cause symptoms ranging from annoying to lethal.

A second type of reaction is an *Immunoglobulin G (IgG)* response, which is sometimes called "intolerance" or "sensitivity" rather than "allergy" because it can be delayed and is not usually life-threatening. IgG symptoms are cumulative in nature, and appear as chronic skin problems such as eczema and thrush, gastrointestinal problems such as diarrhea and constipation, and behavioral reactions such as mood swings and hyperactivity.

An extremely helpful test that many health care professionals order for those with autism spectrum disorders is the Enzyme-Linked Immunosorbent Assay, known as ELISA. It screens for both immediate (IgE) and delayed (IgG) reactions in a panel of about 100 food proteins, including gluten and casein. A basic test of the 10 most common allergies is also available. Most labs rate food sensitivities 0–4, where the highest number requires strict avoidance and the lowest is a well-tolerated food. In between, foods can be consumed once in a while, rotated, or avoided except on occasion. The ELISA method is reproducible, reliable, and valid in the detection of food-specific antibodies.[39]

If either IgG or IgE testing shows casein or gluten sensitivity, chemical messages in the body have tripped an allergic response. An IgG casein or gluten reaction is most likely due to poor digestion. The body's immediate response is to clear the incompletely digested particles by producing IgG antibodies.

A third type of reaction is an **Immunoglobulin A (IgA)** response, which is indicative of inflammation, especially of the gastrointestinal lining, and leads to intestinal irritability, stomachache, or diarrhea. Health care professionals are seeing more of this type of immune reaction in children on the autism spectrum. IgA antibodies are often the body's reaction to stress. Prolonged stress changes the immune system's ability to respond quickly. As less blood flows to the intestines, digestion slows and the body heals more slowly.

Bottom line: Many children on the autism spectrum have IgE, IgG, *and* IgA allergic reactions.[40] Semantics permit health care professionals to use the word "allergy" legitimately to describe any symptoms, immediate or delayed, occurring after exposure. Reactions to gluten or casein usually occur more than two hours after eating a food and are most often IgG or IgA reactions, with symptoms such as sleep disturbance, bed wetting, sinus and ear infections, or crankiness. A number of immunological measures are necessary to determine the immune status of an individual with autism.

Special Diets

Once parents understand the havoc existing in their child's gut and that some of the behaviors their child displays could be a result of physiological reactions to foods, they are much more willing to expend the effort necessary to go "cold turkey" on problematic foods. A special diet could help. Remember, each child is unique and one size does not fit all. The ultimate goal is to remove load factors that are taking up a good amount of room, and to free up energy for talking, relating, and learning.

Special diets are the foundation for all children on the autism spectrum. Families of children on special diets must work hard. Daily cooking is mandatory because eating out and relying on pre-prepared foods at home make complying with any diet extremely challenging. When picky eaters with ASDs move to a special diet, of course they choose processed foods over kale and broccoli. All members of the immediate family, including grandparents, aunts, uncles, cousins, and anyone else who spends any time with a child must be "on board" for special diets to work. If just one person feels sorry for a child who cannot eat ice cream and cake at a birthday party, that individual can undermine the program.

Therapists, teachers and their assistants, shadows, and all members of the school family must also comply, including using acceptable substitutes for positive reinforcers. Fortunately, once they see the results, compliance should not be so difficult.

Gluten-Free, Casein-Free (GF/CF) Diet

The basic diet many families start with is the same one Karen Seroussi recommended 15 years ago: the gluten-free, casein-free (GF/CF) diet. Numerous studies since Seroussi's discovery show that removal of gluten and casein from the diet can make a marked and often immediate difference in many children on the autism spectrum.[41]

The best candidates for the GF/CF diet are children who

- already eat a limited diet of mostly gluten- and casein-containing foods;
- get sick easily or have chronically loose stools;
- have a history of ear infections or colic; and/or
- have poor eye contact and are difficult to engage.

According to clinicians I know, approximately one-third of children with autism in their practices improves dramatically and sometimes no longer qualifies for the diagnosis. Another third show improvement in secondary symptoms, such as poor sleep and perseverative behavior, although the diagnosis of autism remains. An unanticipated result is that for some, seizure frequency diminishes with a GF/CF diet. According to ARI (see table 4.1), about 80% of children on the spectrum show some improvement on this diet; thus, many doctors believe that every person with an autism diagnosis should be on a GF/CF diet for at least three months.

Parents must understand that, while full compliance is optimal, 100% is not necessary for a child to improve. Because gluten and casein masquerade under many names, avoiding every food containing gluten or casein may be difficult at first. In most cases avoiding the major offenders will be adequate as a start. Stricter adherence comes with practice and after seeing small gains.

Be sure to include naturally occurring gluten- and dairy-free products, such as vegetables and fruits, in menus, and avoid the trap of switching from empty-calorie wheat and dairy products to empty-calorie GF/CF foods. Use lunch to introduce new food ideas. Take kids shopping to help choose some of the goodies. Let them pack the lunch box themselves. Even the youngest kids can do that! Include:

- *Protein:* Last night's leftovers, a turkey thigh, drumstick, lamb chop, roast beef, tempeh, or tofu salad sandwich on GF/CF bread; a GF/CF tortilla, wrap, or crackers to dip into bean dip or hummus. Eggs for those who can tolerate them—hard boiled is very portable. Mock egg salad made with tofu can be a hit, too. Almond, cashew, pumpkin seed, sunflower seed, and other protein "butters" are great on anything from a rice cake to a celery stick. Small packets of nuts work for those who don't like sandwiches. So do cold hot dogs and even cold GF/CF pizza! Of course, choose organic if possible.

  A once-a-week treat can be an Andibar®, the brainchild of Dr. Lisa Lewis. Available in four delicious flavors, they are gluten- casein-, soy-, corn-, and GMO-free. They also contain no artificial flavors, colors, or preservatives. What they *do* contain are nutritionally balanced vitamins and minerals, flax seeds, and a whopping 10 grams of protein! Start with a 12-bar multi-pack to test your child's tastes.

- *Fruit:* Try to stay in season—apples and pears in fall and winter, berries in the spring, orange sections and grapes any time. Use no-sugar-added pearsauce and applesauce with or without berries. Dried fruits, especially little boxes of raisins and cranberries, and trek mixes work all year round.

- *Vegetable:* Carrots, celery, pea pods, dried green beans (from Trader Joe's), cucumbers, peppers, zucchini sticks, cherry tomatoes. Pair these with GF/CF ketchup, salsa, or a dip like guacamole, GF/CF "ranch" or spinach/artichoke dressing.
- *Something fun or crunchy:* a GF/CF homemade muffin (maybe with some carrot or zucchini hiding in it!), chips, popcorn, a GF/CF cookie, or a few compliant chocolate chips.
  A love note, joke, sticker, or prize like in a Happy Meal.

Some suggestions for cutting down expenses and time when going to a GF/CF diet include:

- *Make your own or buy already-blended flours and bake from scratch.* Buy flours in bulk and keep them in the freezer, then mix them into small blended batches.
- *Plant a garden or fruit trees.* If you're new to gardening or do not have a big plot of land, plant herbs like basil in pots indoors or tomatoes and garlic in a window box or on a patio.
- *Make friends with the local farmers.* Buy eggs directly from them. Pick your own fruits and vegetables. This is fun and encourages eating in-season. Barter with your farmer. Many farmers need help on the farm or would love to trade food or other goods. Find ones that have a Community-Supported Agriculture program, and share your bounty with friends.
- *Dehydrate and can.* Invest in a dehydrator or look for one at a yard sale. You can make turkey and beef jerky, dried fruit, and other foods, particularly when you have bulk or in-season buys. Can extra fruits and vegetables for winter use.

Help going GF/CF is available from many sources. Autism Network for Dietary Intervention (ANDI) at www.AutismNDI.com, founded by Lisa Lewis and Karyn Seroussi, is still educating families about GF/CF. Lewis's *Special Diets for Special Kids*, originally in two volumes, is updated and now available as a single book containing a CD with printable recipes.[42] It outlines the theory behind the diet and has recipes that meet kid standards—such as GF/CF macaroni and cheese, pizza dough, and chicken nugget coating—as well as adult-friendly healthy casseroles and imaginative breakfasts.

Websites detailing gluten- and dairy-free cooking, along with thousands of recipes are available online. Cookbooks abound. Try the following:

- *The Kid-Friendly ADHD and Autism Cookbook: The Ultimate Guide to the Gluten-Free, Casein-Free Diet* by developmental pediatrician Pamela Compart, MD, and nutritionist Dana Laake[43]
- *The Autism Cookbook: 101 Gluten-Free and Dairy-Free Recipes* by Susan Delaine[44]
- *The Autism & ADHD Diet: A Step-by-Step Guide to Hope and Healing by Living Gluten Free and Casein Free (GFCF) and Other Interventions* by Barrie Silberberg[45]
- *Special-Needs Kids Eat Right: Strategies to Help Kids on the Autism Spectrum Focus, Learn, and Thrive* by Judy Converse[46]
- Any of the six great cookbooks published by Connie Sarros, a pioneer in living gluten-free

All of these experts keep good nutrition as well as gluten and casein avoidance in mind.

Subscribe to newsletters and magazines, both online and in print. *Living Without* magazine is a quarterly publication offering tips and recipes in a beautiful format. To subscribe, go to www.livingwithout.com. Connie Sarros, mentioned above, also has a free newsletter at www.gfbooks.homestead.com.

The demand for pre-prepared gluten-free foods is growing at a rapid pace. The market-research firm AC Nielson reports that sales are increasing nearly 25% every year, swelling to $4.2 billion in 2013, and expected to reach $6.6 billion annually by 2017.[47] More and more companies sell products and mixes that make GF/CF cooking a breeze. Go to www.gfcf.com, www.glutenfree.com, www.wellamy.com, and www.enjoylife.com. The Gluten-Free Registry lists over 20,000 restaurants, bakeries, caterers, grocers, and other businesses in every state; all are searchable by location online or as an app for your tablet or phone (www.glutenfreeregistry.com). Still prefer a book to technology? Buy the annually-updated *Gluten/Casein Free Grocery Shopping Guide* from www.CeceliasMarketplace.com. It lists every imaginable product by brand.

Allergy Elimination Diet

If allergy testing showed intolerances to additional foods, such as corn, soy and eggs, a more stringent diet may be necessary, especially for kids with a history of ear infections. A now-classic study showed the elimination of chronic ear infections and fluid in 86% of children when milk, wheat, corn, eggs, soy, and chocolate were removed.[48] Improvement also occurred in other aspects of health and function like respiration and language.

Clinical evidence suggests that soy may also bother some children who react to casein. The chemical structure of the soy protein is similar to casein, and a cross sensitivity may exist in up to 50% of those who react to dairy products. Therefore, it is inadvisable to substitute soy milk for cow's milk during elimination trials. For an extensive treatise on the controversies concerning the use of soy in human diets, read *The Whole Soy Story* by Kayla Daniels.[49]

Feingold Diet

Another doctor who jumped on the food and behavior bandwagon early was Ben F. Feingold, MD, Chief of Allergy of the Kaiser-Permanente Medical Center in San Francisco in the mid-1960s. After seeing that a change in diet made a dramatic difference in the behavior of an adult patient, he began to explore the link between foods and food additives in children's behavior. When he implemented the protocol he dubbed the "K-P Diet" in his clinic, he began receiving reports from parents that not only had their kids' allergies improved, but behavior was more acceptable. Hyperactivity and impulsivity lessened, while attention and focus heightened.

Feingold's K-P diet is now called simply the Feingold diet or Feingold program. It eliminates artificial colors and flavors, synthetic sweeteners, dyes, three preservatives (BHA, BHT, and TBHQ), and salicylates. Feingold removes foods containing salicylates at the start of the diet and reintroduces them one by one after a child manifests a favorable response. Most preservatives and dyes come from petroleum. Obviously, "crude oil" is not listed among a food's ingredients.

Salicylates are a natural ingredient in some fruits, including apples (again!), berries, and oranges; in some vegetables, including tomatoes, peppers, and cucumbers; and in aspirin. The liver breaks down salicylates using drug detoxification pathways. Salicylates in the diet may cause irritability and hyperactivity for youngsters on the autism spectrum because their bodies cannot metabolize them properly. Research supports implementation of the Feingold diet for some children with autism due to their impaired detoxification capacities.[50]

Feingold's legacy is the Feingold Association of the United States (FAUS). For under $100 per year, a family receives

- a **member handbook** with an extensive Foodlist of acceptable and unacceptable food, a two-week menu plan, recipes, a diet diary form, and more;
- a **supplement guide** of acceptable brands;
- a **mail order guide** for hard-to-find products;
- a **fast food guide** based on information provided by popular fast food chains;
- **"Pure Facts" newsletter**, printed 10 times a year with updates to the Foodlist, new research, member issues, etc.;
- access to the password-protected **members' section on the website**;
- access to a free **help line** by both e-mail and phone; and
- **product alert** notifications via e-mail.

FAUS researches the products with the manufacturers and shares this information with their members. Most of the food used on the Feingold diet is readily available in local supermarkets; specialty items can be mail-ordered.

Parents use the Feingold food list to shop and can thus avoid having to read every label. This list is kept up-to-date with monthly addenda as new products come on the market and old ones are modified.

Jane Hersey, a veteran Feingold parent and volunteer, has written a wonderful book, *Why Can't My Child Behave?*, about the advantages of the Feingold program for children with all types of learning and behavioral issues, including autism.[51] To learn more or to join FAUS, go to www.feingold.org and take advantage of the extraordinary materials this organization has to offer. *Every* family that cares about health should belong.

Yeast-Free Diet

Health care practitioners often recommend going yeast-free when on the GF/CF and Feingold diets. Beware that a yeast-free diet rules out many otherwise acceptable additive-, allergy-, gluten-, and dairy-free baked goods and products. A yeast-free diet eliminates baked goods such as breads, crackers, pastries, pretzels, cakes, cookies, and rolls because most contain copious amounts of sugar. It also eliminates fermented foods such as pickles, foods that are naturally moldy like cantaloupe and peanuts, and natural fungi like mushrooms.

Recall the findings of Dr. William Shaw, who found that children with a diagnosis of autism had extremely high levels of toxic yeast by-products in their urine.[52] Restricting yeast minimizes these secondary irritants. Because of Shaw's groundbreaking work, the yeast-free diet has become a staple of biochemical intervention for autism. The yeast-free diet includes the following additional restrictions:

- *Eliminate sugar.* Why? Because sugar feeds yeast. Yeasts ferment sugars into alcohol, leaving a child acting drunk, hung over, unfocused, or hyperactive.[53] When an individual consumes too much sugar or the immune system is weak, the yeast population can grow aggressively.

  More than 100 recognized substances are described as sugars.[54] These include, but are not limited to, sucrose, turbinado, honey, fructose, molasses, barley malt, rice, yinnie and maple syrup, dextrose, sorbitol, aspartame, mannitol, agave nectar, and lactose. Stevia and xylitol are two natural sugars from the rainforest that do not increase yeast.

- *Introduce good bacteria.* An important component to the yeast-free diet is supplementation of good bacteria called "probiotics" to replenish the gut microflora in overcoming the yeast. Probiotics occur naturally in some common fermented foods such as yoghurt and are even being added to some junk foods such as candy to make them "healthy."

You can buy inexpensive probiotics off the shelf or pharmaceutical-grade ones from apothecaries and health food stores. High quality probiotics usually require refrigeration. The number and variety of bacteria determines their power. Look for ones with over one *billion* organisms. Millions of organisms are insufficient to repopulate the guts of those on the spectrum.

A novel way of introducing good bacteria into sick people, especially those with *Clostridium difficile* (*C. diff*), a stubborn bacterium that has become antibiotic-resistant, is through fecal transplants. A 2011 literature review found that 92% of 317 patients with recurrent *C. diff* infection or pseudomembranous colitis had disease resolution upon fecal transplant.[55] The use of fecal transplants for those with autism is just beginning.

A recent innovation, fecal transplant by pill, makes this treatment a little more palatable. Doctors process the donor stool (usually from a relative), taking out food and extracting and cleaning the bacteria, then pack the bacteria into triple-coated gel capsules so they won't dissolve until they reach the intestines. No stool is left—just bugs. Doctors are also testing freezing the stool, which doesn't kill the bacteria, so this "medicine" can be stored and shipped to a needy patient.

• **Use antifungals.** In many cases, removing sugar and adding probiotics is sufficient to rebalance the gut. However, in severe cases, substances to kill the yeast are also required. Natural yeast killers, such as oregano oil, garlic, olive leaf extract, caprylic acid, uva ursi, and other herb combinations might work. Stubborn cases require those available only by prescription, such as Nystatin, Diflucan, and Nizoral. Antifungal therapy is least effective with individuals who have normal or marginally elevated yeast.

The most usual improvements noted with antifungals are increased focus and concentration and diminished bowel symptoms. Other improvements may include increased and clearer vocalization, less spinning, decrease in aggressive or self-abusive behavior like head-banging, better sleep patterns, increased socialization, and improved eye contact.

Even though antifungals remove the yeast from the blood, they may transfer it to the tissues, causing more intensified yeast overgrowth which can demand further intervention sometime in the future. Hyperbaric Oxygen treatment from pressurized oxygen in hard chambers can be an effective way of treating systemic yeast in the tissues.

The easiest way to follow a yeast-free protocol properly is to use a guidebook, such as *Feast Without Yeast: 4 Stages to Better Health*,[56] *The Yeast Connection Handbook*,[57] or *The Yeast Connection Cookbook*.[58] Almost 60% of parents responding to the ARI survey reported that their kids' behavior improved on this diet.

Specific Carbohydrate Diet (SCD)

The Specific Carbohydrate Diet (SCD) takes GF/CF and yeast-free a step further for those kids who still have gut problems. The goal is to stop the vicious cycle of malabsorption and microbe overgrowth by eliminating both the microbes and many more foods upon which the microorganisms feed.

The SCD starts with an introductory plan for about a week or two, consisting of proteins and a limited selection of specific carbohydrates. The introductory plan:

- *Allows* most fresh fruits and vegetables, beans, unprocessed meats, fish and poultry, natural cheeses, olive and coconut oils, and honey. All fruits and vegetables must be peeled, seeded, and cooked in order to make them more digestible.

- *Prohibits* all complex carbohydrates, cereal grains, processed meats, soy products, cow's milk, sugars, and canned fruits and vegetables because partially digested complex carbohydrates sit in the intestines and provide a breeding ground for yeast and bacteria, which thrive on sugar.

- *Includes* a specially fermented homemade goat milk yoghurt as a source of good bacteria; the culturing changes the structure of the casein and renders it harmless. Most children tolerate the goat yoghurt if they start out with a tiny amount and gradually increase it.

Nuts, seeds, raw fruits, and certain vegetables, such as salad greens, carrots, celery, and onions, are not allowed at this stage, but are introduced after diarrhea is under control.

Like so many other treatments and diets for autism, discovery of the SCD's potential for helping autistic families came from a parent. Year after year, Judy Chinitz searched for a way to help her son Alex, who screamed in agony for hours at a time, didn't sleep, couldn't stop moving, bit and scratched himself until he bled, and suffered from endless bouts of diarrhea and vomiting. She tried every medical treatment and special diet that doctors could offer, without success.

Then Chinitz found the SCD, developed by the late biochemist and cell biologist, Elaine Gottschall, for people with diagnosed ulcerative colitis and other bowel diseases. That diet, Chinitz says, "saved our lives." Judy shares her remarkable story in the book she collaborated on with her physician, Sidney Baker, MD: *We Band of Mothers: Autism, My Son, and the Specific Carbohydrate Diet.*[59] Gottschall's pioneering work is detailed in *Breaking the Vicious Cycle: Intestinal Health Through Diet*, published in 1994.[60] Read both of these informative sources to understand thoroughly the progression of allowed foods and to implement the SCD with many delicious recipes.

Online resources include www.breakingtheviciouscycle. info www.pecanbread.com, www.newstarnutrition.com, www. lucyskitchenshop.com www.scdrecipe.com, and www.scdiet.org.

Low Oxalate Diet

Oxalates and oxalic acid are organic acids that come from three sources: foods; fungi such as aspergillus, penicillium, and possibly candida; and normal human metabolism. Oxalic acid is the most acidic organic acid in the body; it is so acidic that car mechanics use it commercially to remove rust from car radiators! Some foods especially high in oxalates are spinach, beets, chocolate, peanuts, wheat bran, tea, cashews, pecans, almonds, and berries. Neither meat nor fish contain significant oxalates.

In children with autism, yeast overgrowth, commonly associated with antibiotic usage, might lead to increased oxalate production. In the presence of mercury, high levels of oxalates slow mercury elimination. Researcher Susan Owens proposed that the use of a diet low in oxalates could reduce symptoms in children with autism. In 2005, she founded the Autism Oxalate Project under the auspices of the Autism Research Institute.

Owens's research shows that those with autism have five to six times the normal amount of oxalates in their urine. None of the children on the autistic spectrum had elevations of the other organic acids associated with genetic diseases of oxalate metabolism, indicating that oxalates are high due to external sources. Reported benefits of the low oxalate diet are more focus and calm; better gross and fine motor skills, sleep, receptive and expressive language, and sociability; and reduced self-abusive behavior and bed wetting.[61] For more information on this diet, go to www.lowoxalate.info.

Body Ecology Diet (BED)

Developed by nutritional consultant Donna Gates, the Body Ecology Diet (BED) is, in my opinion, the best diet of all not only for individuals on the autism spectrum, but for anyone with digestive issues. This diet is compatible with both the GF/CF and Specific Carbohydrate diets. It fights chronic yeast infections by combining the best of Western and Eastern philosophies, with additional guidelines to improve the health of those on these favorite programs. The BED both heals the gut by reestablishing colonies of good gut flora and nourishes it with nutritious foods to allow organ systems to rebuild.

Gates views autism as a combination of disorders — all correctable. She believes that the intestinal-brain infection distances the child from his or her surroundings. The goal of the BED is to "bring the children back into our world and back to their true selves" with dietary intervention. Since 2003, many with autism and related disorders have shown rapid and remarkable improvement on the BED.

The BED removes all of the most problematic edibles: sugars, gluten, casein, soy, and processed foods. It includes the best quality, most nutritionally dense foods from all the food groups:

- *Plentiful, nutritionally dense, dark, leafy green and root vegetables,* such as collard and mustard greens, kale, broccoli, onions, parsnips, winter squash, and potatoes
- *Animal proteins* that are hormone- and antibiotic-free and easy-to-digest, such as fish, chicken, and softly scrambled eggs in small quantities (sometimes amino acid supplements may be needed to aid protein digestion)
- *Four gluten-free grains:* quinoa, millet, amaranth, and buckwheat, all of which are high in vegetable proteins
- *Organic, unrefined, virgin oils and fats,* such as coconut, cod liver, flaxseed, macadamia nut, olive and pumpkinseed oils, ghee, raw butter, and cream, which provide monounsaturated fats, antioxidants, zinc, and omega-3 fats
- *Selected fruits*, including berries, grapefruit, kiwi, green apples, and pineapples, eaten with at least four ounces of coconut kefir (see below) to counteract the negative effect of fruits' natural sugars.

The following seven BED principles encompass all the other diets:

1. *Principle of Uniqueness:* Individual dietary and nutritional needs change daily, with the seasons, and with the number of load factors.

2. *Principle of Blood Type:* Certain food choices might be better for individuals from one blood group than another.[62]

3. *Principle of Balancing Expansion and Contraction:* Based on the macrobiotic principles of yin (expansive) and yang (contracting) in food, this principle helps a person maintain dietary balance by avoiding foods and substances that are too contracting, such

as meat, eggs, and salt, or too expansive, such as sugar. The BED encourages primary food selection from the middle of this continuum, which includes many types of vegetables.

4. *Principle of Acid and Alkaline:* Keeping blood in a slightly alkaline condition is vital to restoring health. Too much acid encourages yeast, viruses, parasites, and other unhealthy critters to thrive. A good reference book for this principle is *Alkalize or Die.*[63] Consult a food chart showing the pH of foods; many are available online. To ensure an alkaline gut, the BED uses Vitality SuperGreen® or other powdered, nutrient-rich green drinks to alkalinize the intestines and restore and maintain a healthy inner ecosystem.

5. *Principle of 80/20:* Every meal should contain 80% alkaline-forming foods and 20% acid-forming foods. 80% of food should be land or ocean vegetables. The remaining 20% is animal protein (fish or poultry), an acceptable grain, and starchy vegetables.

Different nutrients require different conditions in the stomach to be properly digested. Protein requires a high-acid environment; starch requires an alkaline environment. Mixing starch and protein in a single meal does not allow the stomach to digest either properly. Separating starch and protein into separate meals and eating fruit separately increases the efficiency of digestion. Always eat

- protein with non-starchy or ocean vegetables;
- allowable grains and starchy vegetables (acorn and butternut squash, lima beans, peas, corn, water chestnuts, artichokes, and red skin potatoes) with non-starchy or sea vegetables; and
- fruits alone, on an empty stomach.

Eat until your stomach is 80% full, leaving 20% available for digestion. Limit a meal to one portion of grain or starchy vegetables, and, if you're still hungry, eat more alkaline vegetables. Eating until your stomach is 100% full slows digestion and furthers yeast overgrowth; leaving a little room for the digestive juices to do their job is essential for efficient digestion.

6. *Principle of Cleansing:* Humans must continually cleanse to remove the toxins of modern-day living. The BED is unique in recommending regular colon hydrotherapy.

7. *Principle of Step-by-Step:* True healing takes place in small steps, which happen in their own time and their own order. The toxins that have accumulated over years cannot be eliminated in days. The body goes through cycles of progress followed by periods of rest. Each step gets deeper and deeper into the body to pull out toxins and heal. Quick fixes, such as drugs, halt the body's innate wisdom to cleanse, drive sickness deeper into the body, and open the potential for more serious illness later. To assist the body in healing, Gates makes the following suggestions:

- Reduce or eliminate all stressors
- Don't cheat on the diet
- Eat foods that aid in cleansing (see below)
- Eliminate medications that suppress healing
- Rest and sleep
- Use probiotics

The BED also includes signature foods that aid in detoxification and healing: kefir and fermented coconut pudding from young coconuts, cultured and sea vegetables, raw butter, Celtic sea salt, and whey protein. These fermented and other important foods are the real "stars" of the BED protocol that can put a big jumpstart on healing.

- *Young coconut kefir (yck) and coconut pudding* are made from the green or white, unripe baby versions of the mature fuzzy brown coconuts most people recognize. These gems are available in most health food or natural food stores. Their sterile, pale milk and gelatinous meat are full of minerals and enzymes. Gates "kefirs" these parts of the coconut using a special starter that she sells, to make a drink and pudding that most children love. She recommends drinking at least ¼ – ½ cup of the kefir in the morning upon rising, with meals, and at bedtime. The fermented meat, great for breakfast or a snack, provides a raw, easily-digested, vegetarian protein that contains valuable lauric (antimicrobial) and caprylic (antifungal) fatty acids.

• *Cultured vegetables (CVs)* are made by fermenting any vegetables with Gates's special starter. You can buy common CVs like sauerkraut in health food stores; to save money, make your own with any vegetables like carrots, cabbage, beets, or radishes. One pint of store-bought sauerkraut can cost up to $8 a pint, and one bottle of kombucha over $3. You can easily make these at home for about one-tenth the price. Give them a couple weeks on the counter and nature does the rest. Once in the refrigerator they last for months; sauerkraut can last for six months.

CVs aid in digestion, especially when eaten with meals containing animal protein. Ideally everyone should have some CVs or yck with every meal. Puree cultured vegetables for children who do not chew well. They taste tart and sour, and can be made more palatable when combined with olive or pumpkinseed oil, raw cream, homemade mayonnaise, Celtic sea salt, or stevia.

• *Raw Butter* is almost 100% fat, while over 50% of breast milk is raw fat. The goal is to duplicate the raw fat in a healthy mother's breast milk. Raw butter contains vitamins A, D, and E, and butyric acid. It is very healing to the mucosal lining of the gut and helps the microflora adhere there and colonize. All butter is 99% casein-free — that's less casein than in human breast milk. If kids start on raw butter four to seven days after coconut kefir, the small amount of residual casein does not cause a problem for those following a GF/CF regimen. In fact, the butter seems to really jumpstart the healing process. Find a reliable, local source for raw, organic, grass-fed butter.

• *Whey protein*, while a milk product, does not contain casein. Milk is made up of 20% whey protein and 80% casein. Whey protein helps with detoxification. It is also great for muscle development. After being on yck for about two weeks, add one scoop of undenatured whey protein to the Vitality SuperGreen® drink.

BED borrows another food staple from the Weston Price Foundation: bone broths. Make your own stocks and broths: save and store bones from a roasted chicken or turkey carcass (organic and grass-fed, of course!) and freeze your vegetable scraps, such as the ends of carrots or the leafy part of celery, and use them when you have accumulated enough.

The BED can be a very different way of eating for many people, especially those who subsist on a standard American diet replete with wheat and sugar. This description of the BED includes so many details because implementing it can result in some remarkable changes. While some families can quickly make a transition to this healthy way of eating, others may find it very challenging, especially for children who are picky eaters. However, the BED can do no harm, and the whole family is guaranteed to benefit.

Donna Gates has established an online community of those interested in healing their family members with autism using the BED. She calls her group BEDROK for Body Ecology Diet Recovering Our Kids. The goals of the BEDROK program are to:

1. *Nourish* the cells and tissues of the body with high quality, easily-digested foods that contain superior nutrition.
2. *Control* all infections and viruses.
3. *Open* detoxification pathways, thus allowing the body to continually cleanse out toxins that have accumulated since conception.
4. *Create* a strong, vital inner ecosystem in the intestines that ensures the digestion and absorption of foods, and corrects the nutrient deficiencies that accompany autism. This vibrant inner ecosystem also builds a healthy intestinal lining and a strong immune system that protects a child from further infections.

The BED autism support program is available to anyone serious about learning this diet. Gates sells a 12-CD set entitled "The Natural Autism Solution: Dietary Secrets to Help Prevent and Overcome Autism, ADHD, Asperger's and Other Epidemic Childhood Disorders" and teaches seminars on the subject. This product and a list of her trained BED coaches in almost every state are listed on the Body Ecology website at www.bodyecology.com.

Picky Eating

You may be reading this chapter with a huge amount of skepticism. Sure! You want me to get my child to eat what? Right! He'll starve!

You are not alone! Anecdotal evidence from parents of kids with autism continuously confirms that most are picky eaters with extremely limited diets. Amazingly, they are all eating the same things: cereal with milk, macaroni and cheese, noodles with butter and cheese, pizza, bagels and cream cheese, chicken fingers, and french fries (both sprinkled with wheat flour). Not a vegetable (unless you count ketchup or tomato sauce), not a fruit, not a fish in sight!

Don't even consider changing brands—the smallest change in packaging or the slightest shift in color can cause a picky eater to abandon a previously well-loved food choice. Forget sneaking in some crushed up or liquid vitamins; they know instantly! Are these children all in collusion, or is something amiss that is causing their palates to reject what is good for them and beg for wheat and dairy products in every imaginable combination?

One possible cause of eating issues in so many children with autism is that their immature nervous system function can lead to an aversion to certain tastes, textures, or smells. Some youngsters reject foods they have never tasted just by looking at or smelling them. Nobody knows exactly what a child is experiencing when he or she refuses to eat any vegetables or will only eat chicken nuggets from a particular restaurant. The visual system clearly plays a role.

Despite a child's strong need for sameness in foods, getting those with autism to broaden their choices *is* possible. Caregivers must combine a stalwart approach with the utmost patience and perseverance.

Although therapists often interpret picky eating as a behavioral issue and treat it with behavioral modification, frequently other causes are at play. Picky eating, like poor eye contact, is a symptom that something is not right. The adults in a child's life must dig deep to determine what factors might be involved, and by being detectives they can determine which solution is right for an individual child. Here are a few possible causes of picky eating from nutrition guru Kelly Dorfman:[64]

Weak Digestive Function or Nutritional Deficiencies

Children with a history of reflux, colic, frequent antibiotic use, allergies, diarrhea, constipation, and low tone have immature, inflamed, or inefficient digestive systems. These youngsters get a heavy or sinking feeling when eating, and have never experienced how a happy tummy feels. They thus tend to avoid eating, becoming high risk for malnutrition. Refer to the list at the beginning of this chapter to see if your child is well or poorly nourished.

Poor eating creates nutritional imbalances, which further reduce appetite or increase carbohydrate cravings. General malnutrition can contribute to disinterest in food, leading to further malnutrition and reduced appetite over time. Once malnourished, diet alone may not correct the deficiencies, particularly if the child has poor absorption or delivery of nutrients. Children cannot be forced to eat the necessary diet to correct malnutrition. These kids usually need nutrient supplements to correct their deficiencies.

Sensory Misreading in the Mouth or Poor Oral-Motor Skills

A child with tactile defensiveness often exhibits hypersensitivity in the mouth or craves oral stimulation, such as chewing on his clothes. Low muscle tone in the mouth and face often coexists with deeper oral-motor issues. Read more about these issues in chapter 10.

Drug Side Effects

Many medications—including antibiotics and particularly stimulants—decrease appetite. For individuals on medications, parents must reevaluate the side effect/benefit ratio. If the drugs are absolutely necessary, eating a large meal first thing in the morning may be the answer. Then, after school, when the medicine is wearing off, dinner rather than a snack is recommended. Finally, before bedtime, bring out the snacks.

What's for Breakfast?

Breakfast: the most important meal of the day! We've all heard that maxim. What is a good breakfast, and why is it *so* important, especially for kids on the spectrum? It's all about glucose levels. Fasting for 10–12 hours between dinner and awakening in the morning triggers hypoglycemia (low blood sugar) and acidosis. Remember the BED's fourth principle: too much acid encourages yeast overgrowth, viruses, parasites, and other unhealthy cells to thrive.

Research now proves the importance of a good breakfast to prepare children for learning.[65] One British study explored the performance of 19 children ages six to seven years over a four-week period. The children ate meals offering similar calories but different glycemic loads. Two to three hours after breakfast, those who had consumed a low glycemic breakfast performed significantly better on the tests of memory and attention and showed fewer signs of frustration than those who had consumed a high glycemic breakfast.[66]

Follow guidelines from integrative medicine guru Majid Ali, MD, for what to eat in the morning. Breakfast should

- overhydrate the body's cells;
- maintain healthy, even glucose levels;
- tone bowel musculature and stimulate the emptying reflexes;
- provide support for detoxification;
- include restorative oils for brain function;
- offer raw materials for enzymatic action; and
- avoid toxic trans fats, simple sugars, and carbohydrates.[67]

One of the most frequently asked questions from families new to special diets is, "What can we eat for breakfast?" For anyone used to juice, cereal, toast, pancakes, or bagels, breakfast can be a real challenge. Here are some guidelines:

- **_Think protein._** Protein in the morning is the best gift to give your child; any animal or vegetable protein will do. Serve dinner foods for breakfast! Last night's leftovers, a turkey burger, lamb chop, salmon patty, scrambled eggs, lentil soup, bean burrito, or any other meal that gives you at least 10 grams of protein. Children ages three to four require a minimum of 25 grams daily, while those five and up require 30 grams.

• *Think dense nutrition.* Donna Gates suggests a breakfast soup made with fennel, broccoli, garlic, and parsley, cooked in organic vegetable or chicken broth. Delicious!

• *Think quick and easy.* Look in the freezer section for good quality gluten- and dairy-free waffles and pancakes. Up the protein with a nut butter spread. Try GF/CF cereals made with amaranth or quinoa, and added flaxseeds. Make high-protein muffins; if necessary, use premade mixes from excellent suppliers.

• *Think portable.* Try some high-protein GF/CF breakfast bars for a fast breakfast on days when time is a problem. A huge variety is available from good health food stores, Sample several until you find some with a taste you like.

• *Think Essential Fatty Acids (EFAs).* Add flax, hemp, flavored cod liver, pumpkinseed, or other high quality oils to whatever you make. They enhance texture and are close to tasteless.

• *Think drink.* Use nut and grain milks with protein and fruit/vegetable powders to make a quick, nutritious, colorful, drinkable breakfast. Each of the above diets offers online recipes for a multitude of tastes, from chocolate to fruity to nutty. Experiment with ingredients. No two batches will be the same. Here is the flexible recipe naturopathic physician Katie Dahlgren suggests for her patients to drink within an hour of waking to achieve optimal protein and fiber intake and for blood sugar balance.

> 1 cup organic blueberries or mangoes
> 1 cup organic almond, hemp, or coconut milk
> 1 scoop vanilla protein powder
> 1 tbsp organic coconut oil
> 1 tbsp purple or red powder (available as Deep Purple from www.BioPureus.com or as Pro-Red or Pro-Purple from www.nutritionalfrontiers.com or as "Red Powder" from Trader Joes)

1000 mg L-carnitine

1 tbsp freshly ground, organic flax seeds

Rotate four or five of the above breakfasts, never having the same breakfast two days in a row. Once your kids discover several acceptable alternatives, breakfast should be the best meal of the day!

Take-Home Points

Circular thinking might deduce that a child has gastroenterological problems because he has autism, when just the opposite is true: he has autism because his gastroenterological and other bodily systems are dysfunctional. Artificial delineations between digestion and behavior can take parents down diagnostic blind alleys and hinder proper treatment for their children.

After making basic lifestyle changes, learning about digestion and changing the diet are next. At the risk of using a cliché, "A car runs only as well as the gasoline in its tank." The human body, like a car, *must* have excellent fuel to run. Jacqueline McCandless is correct that many children on the autism spectrum have starving brains. Is your child one of them? We must modify what children on the spectrum eat to boost the power of all of the excellent therapies they receive.

Take the second big step in outsmarting autism by committing to one or more of the above diets, and stick to it. Move to a more stringent one if changes do not show up in a couple of months. Get support from family members and the many resources available if you are having trouble. Bon appétit!

---

[1] Dorfman K. Envisioning a Bright Future. Santa Ana, CA: OEPF, 2008, 120.

[2] Pollan M. Food Rules. New York: Penguin Books, 2009.

[3] Carwile JL. Canned Soup Consumption and Urinary Bisphenol A: A Randomized Crossover Trial. JAMA, 2011, 306:20, 2218–20.

[4] Rapp D. Is this your child? New York: Quill Books, 1991.

[5] Dorfman K. Cure Your Child with Food. New York: Workman Press, 2013.

[6] McCandless, J. Children with starving brains, 4th ed. Putney, VT: Bramble Books, 2009.

[7] Lederberg J, McCray AT. 'Ome Sweet 'Omics — a genealogical treasury of words. Scientist, 2001, 15:7, 8.

[8] Mitsuoka T. Bifoidocbacteria and Their Role in Human Health. Jrl of Industrial Microbiology, 1990, 6:264.

[9] Gershon M. The Second Brain. New York: Harper, 1999.

[10] Adams JB, Johansen LJ, Powell LD, Quig D, Rubin RA. Gastrointestinal flora and GI status in children w/ ASD. BMC Gastroenterol, 2011, 11:22.

[11] Williams BL, Hornig M, Buie T, Bauman ML, et al. Impaired Carbohydrate Digestion and Transport and Mucosal Dysbiosis in the Intestines of Children with Autism and Gastrointestinal Disturbances. PLoS ONE, 2011, 6:9.

[12] Finegold SM, Molitoris D, Song Y, Liu C, et al. Gastrointestinal Microflora Studies in Late-Onset Autism. Clin Infect Dis, 2002, 35, S6–S16.

[13] The Autism Enigma. http://cogentbenger.com/autism/. Accessed Oct 24, 2013.

[14] Waring R. Enzyme and sulfur oxidation deficiencies in autistic children with known food/chemical intolerances. Xenobiotica, 1990, 20, 117–22.

[15] Harris RM, Picton R, Singh S, Waring RH. Activity of phenylsulfotransferases in the human gastrointestinal tract. Life science, Sep 2000, 67:17, 2051–57.

[16] Feingold B. Why your child is hyperactive. New York: Random House, 1975.

[17] Brostoff J, Gamlin L. Food allergy and intolerance. London: Bloomsbury Press, 1989.

[18] http://www.desbio.com/database.html?id=P0110&s=Malvin. Accessed Jan 3, 2012.

[19] Crook WG. The yeast connection. New York: Vintage Books, 1986; Crook WG. The yeast connection and the woman. Jackson, TN: Professional Books, 1994.

[20] Rimland B. Candida-caused autism. Autism Res Rev, 1985, 2, 2–3.

[21] Crook, The yeast connection and the woman.

[22] Shaw W, Kassen E, Chaves E. Increased excretion of analogs of Krebs cycle metabolites and arabinose in two brothers with autistic features. Clin Chem, 1995, 41, 1094–104.

[23] D'Eufemia P, Celli M, Finocchiaro R, Pacifico L, et al. Abnormal intestinal permeability in children with autism. Acta Paediatr, Sep 1996, 85:9, 1076–79.

[24] Lipski E. Leaky gut syndrome. A Keats Good Health Guide. Los Angeles, CA: Keats Publishing, 1998, 7.

[25] Chandler S, Carcani-Rathwell I, Charman T, Pickles A, et al. Parent-Reported Gastro-intestinal Symptoms in Children with Autism Spectrum Disorders. Jrl Autism and Developmental Disorders, Dec 2013, 43:12, 2737–47.

[26] Tarasuk D. The Poop on Poop. New Dev, Summer 2005, 10:4, 6.

[27] Mannion A, Leader G. Gastrointestinal Symptoms in Autism Spectrum Disorder: A Literature Review. RevJournal of Autism and Developmental Disorders, Oct 2013.

[28] Oski F. Don't drink your milk. Syracuse, NY: Mollica Press, 1983.

[29] American Academy of Pediatrics. Guide to your child's nutrition. New York: Villard Books, 1999.

[30] Reichelt KL, Ekrem J, Scott H. Gluten, milk proteins and autism: dietary intervention effects on behavior and peptide secretion. J applied nutrition, 1990, 42:1, 1–11.

[31] Seroussi K. Unraveling the Mystery of Autism and Pervasive Developmental Disorder: A Mother's Story of Research & Recovery. New York: Random House, 2000.

[32] http://glutenfreehelp.info/autoimmune-disorders/gluten-enzymes/. Accessed Dec 17, 2011.

[33] Seroussi K and Lewis L. The Encyclopedia of Dietary Interventions for the Treatment of Autism and Related Disorders. Pennington, NJ: Sarpsborg Press, 2008.

[34] Panksepp J. A neurochemical theory of autism. Trends Neurosci, 1979, 2, 174–77; Reichelt KL, Hole H, Hamberger A, Saelid G, Edminson PD, et al. Biologically active peptide containing fractions in schizophrenia and childhood autism. Advances Biochem Psychopharmacol, 1981, 28, 627–43.

[35] Shattock P, Lowdon G. Proteins, peptides and autism, Part 2: Implications for the education and care of people with autism. Brain Dys, 1991, 4:6, 323–34.

[36] McCrone J. Gut reaction: Is food to blame for autism? New Sci, Jun 1998 20, 42–5.

[37] Autism Research Institute. Parent Ratings of Behavioral Effects of Drugs and Nutrients. Mar, 2009.

[38] Hyman S. Autism Diet may not improve symptoms. Presentation at International Meeting for Autism Research, Philadelphia, PA, May 19, 2010.

39 Suen RM, Gordon S. The Clinical Relevance of IgG Food Allergy Testing Through ELISA. Townsend Letter for Doctors & Patients, Jan 2004, 61–66.

[40] Heuer L, Ashwood P, Schauer J, Goines P. Reduced levels of immunoglobulin in children with autism correlates with behavioral symptoms. Autism Res, Oct 2008, 1:5, 275–83; Jyonouchi H, Geng L, Ruby A, Zimmerman-Bier B. Dysregulated innate immune responses in young children with autism spectrum disorders: Their relationship to gastrointestinal symptoms and dietary intervention. Neuropsychobiology, 2005, 51:2, 77–85.

[41] Reichelt KL, Ekrem J, Scott H. Gluten, milk proteins and autism: Dietary intervention effects on behavior and peptide secretion. Journal of Applied Nutrition, 1990, 42:1, 1–11; Knivsberg AM, Reichelt KL, Nodland M. Reports on dietary intervention in autistic disorders. Nutritional Neuroscience, 2001, 4, 25–37; Shattock P, Whiteley P. How dietary intervention could ameliorate the symptoms of autism. The Pharmaceutical Journal, Jul 2001, 267, 7155; Cornish E. Gluten and casein free diets in autism: A study of the effects on food choice and nutrition. J Hum Nutr Diet, Aug 2002, 15:4, 261–69; Whiteley P, Haracopos D, Knivsberg AM, Reichelt KL, et al. The ScanBrit randomised, controlled, single-blind study of a gluten- and casein-free dietary intervention for children with autism spectrum disorders. Nutr Neurosci, 2010 13:2, 87–100.

[42] Lewis L. Special Diets for Special Kids, Vol. 1 and 2 combined. Dallas, TX: Future Horizons, 2011.

[43] Compart P. Laake D. The Kid-Friendly ADHD and Autism Cookbook: The Ultimate Guide to the Gluten-Free, Casein-Free Diet. Gloucester, MA: Quayside Publishing, 2006.

[44] Delaine S. The Autism Cookbook: 101 Gluten-Free and Dairy-Free Recipes. New York: Skyhorse, 2010.

[45] Silberberg B. The Autism & ADHD Diet: A Step-by-Step Guide to Hope and Healing by Living Gluten Free and Casein Free (GFCF) and Other Interventions. Naperville, IL: Sourcebooks, Inc. 2009.

[46] Converse J. Special-Needs Kids Eat Right: Strategies to Help Kids on the Autism Spectrum Focus, Learn, and Thrive. New York: Perigee, 2009.

[47] Gluten-Free Market Estimated at $4.2 Billion. www.specialtyfood.com . Accessed Dec 19, 2013.

[48] Nsouli, et al. The role of food allergy in serious otitis media. Annals of Allergy, 1991, 66, 91.

[49] Daniels, K. The Whole Soy Story. Warsaw, Indiana: Newtrends Publishing, 2005.

[50] James SJ, Cutler P, Melnyk S, Jernigan S, Janak L, et al. Metabolic biomarkers of increased oxidative stress and impaired methylation capacity in children with autism. Am J Clin Nutr, 2004, 80, 1611–17; Haavik S, Altman K, Woelk C. Effects of

the Feingold diet on seizures and hyperactivity: A single-subject analysis. J Behav Med, Dec 1979, 2:4, 365–74.

[51] Hersey J. Why can't my child behave? Why can't she cope? Why can't he learn? Alexandria, VA: Pear Tree Press, 2002.

[52] Shaw W, et al. Increased excretion of analogs of Krebs cycle metabolites and arabinose in two brothers with autistic features. Clin Chem, 1995, 41, 1094–104.

[53] Crook WG. Help for the hyperactive child. Jackson, TN: Professional Books, 1991.

[54] Braly J. Dr. Braly's Food Allergy and Nutrition Revolution. New Canaan, CT: 1992.

[55] Gough E, Shaikh H, Manges AR. Systematic Review of Intestinal Microbiota Transplantation (Fecal Bacteriotherapy) for Recurrent Clostridium difficile Infection. Clin Infect Dis, 2011, 53:10, 994–1002.

[56] Semon B, Kronblum L. Feast without yeast: 4 stages to better health. Glendale, WI: Wisconsin Institute of Nutrition, 1999.

[57] Crook WG. The yeast connection handbook. Jackson, TN: Professional Books, 1996.

[58] Crook WG, Jones MH. The yeast connection cookbook. Jackson, TN: Professional Books, 2001.

[59] Baker SM, Chinitz J. We Band of Mothers: Autism, My Son, and the Specific Carbohydrate Diet. San Diego, CA: Autism Research Institute, 2007.

[60] Gottschall E. Breaking the vicious cycle: Intestinal health through diet. Baltimore, Ontario, Canada: The Kirkton Press, 2004.

[61] http://www.greatplainslaboratory.com/home/eng/oxalates.asp. Accessed Dec 13, 2011.

[62] D'Adamo J. The D'Adamo Diet. Toronto, Ontario, Canada: McGraw-Hill Ryerson, 1989.

[63] Baroody TA. Alkalize or Die. Waynesville, NC: Holographic Health Press, 2002.

[64] devdelay.org/newsletter/articles/html/120-the-picky-eater.html.

[65] Ingwersen J, Defeyter NA, Kennedy DO, Wesnes KA, et al. A low glycaemic index breakfast cereal preferentially prevents children's cognitive performance from declining throughout the morning. Appetite, 2007, 49:10, 240–244.

[66] Benton D, Maconie A, Williams C. The influence of the glycaemic load of breakfast on the behaviour of children in school. Physiol Behav, Nov 2007, 92:4, 717–24.

[67] Dr Ali's Breakfast. http://www.majidalimd.com/breakfast.htm. Accessed Mar 3, 2012.

CHAPTER 5

The Immune System:
What Goes Wrong and How to Fix it

Outsmarting autism by healing the chaos in the gut in this biologically-based disorder is only the beginning. Next is figuring out the complex relationship between the gastrointestinal and immune systems, and their secondary effects on function and behavior. With increasing frequency, medical professionals and parents are recognizing that autism is really an immune disorder. One doctor calls it "an emerging neuro-immune disorder in search of therapy."[1] Because it is *so* crucial that we understand what goes wrong with the immune system and possible ways to strengthen it, this is arguably the most important chapter in the book!

This chapter starts with a basic lesson on the immune system, followed by what goes wrong in autism. Next, it looks at common infections and the possible roles of antibiotics and vaccination in weakening immunity. Finally it introduces a three-pronged approach to healing: strengthening the immune system, fighting infections, and taming inflammation.

Immunology 101

The key to normal immune system function is balancing the different types of immune responses. Humans and infectious microbes have coexisted for as long as humans have walked the earth, and the human immune system has developed a complex and efficient way of dealing with infections caused by viruses, bacteria, and other organisms.

The immune system is divided into two: the *cellular* or "innate" part and the *humoral* or "learned" part. In the presence of an infectious microorganism, the body's first line of defense is an inflammatory response from the cellular immune system, which then signals the humoral part to resolve the inflammation. The learned part produces anti-inflammatory chemicals and antibodies that promote healing and establish resistance to future infection. A healthy, mature immune system requires a delicate balance between cellular and humoral immune responses; an imbalance can lead to allergies and autoimmune disorders.

Receptors for cellular immunity are located in the mucous membranes of the gastrointestinal and respiratory tracts, and in their respective lymph nodes, while humoral immunity resides in the bone marrow, where plasma cells produce antibodies specific to each pathogen. Because microbes naturally enter the body through the mucous membranes of the gut and lungs most of the time, cellular immunity is the primary immune defense system of the body, with humoral immunity playing a secondary role.

The cellular and humoral immune systems are complementary and interdependent, and are governed by thymus (T), helper (H), and lymphocyte cells called TH lymphocytes. Early in development, TH lymphocytes differentiate into either TH1 cells, which monitor cellular immunity, or TH2 cells, which monitor humoral immunity. Differentiation is determined by cytokines, the major cell signaling molecules that TH1 and TH2 cells use to communicate with each other. Once one subset of cytokines dominates, the body's response does not shift easily to the other.

Recall the discussion in the previous chapter about the IgE, IgG, and IgA immune responses. *Immunoglobulin M (IgM)* is another inflammatory immune response. IgM antibodies, found in blood and lymph fluid, make up about 5–10% of the antibodies in the body. A high number of specific IgM antibodies indicates an infection. For example, high levels of IgM antibodies against *Candida* would indicate a yeast infection.

The Role of Antibiotics

Anti-biotic translated literally, means "against life." Just like poisons, such as those that kill roaches, termites, and other undesirable bugs, antibiotics "work," at least in the short term.[2] According to New York microbiologist Martin Blaser, MD, the average child in the developed world has taken 10 to 20 rounds of antibiotics by age 18![3] Blaser is not the only physician who has become concerned about the role of antibiotic overuse in the dysregulation of the immune system.[4]

As bacteria have become resistant to first-generation antibiotics, such as penicillin, doctors have moved to stronger ones, such as Cipro. Today's third-generation antibiotics are "atom bombs" compared to the "water pistols" of the previous generation. No one knows the long-term effects to the digestive, immune, and other systems.

If a baby develops any infection, allowing its immune system to fight the invader appears to strengthen immunity in the long term. When the same invader reappears, the body recognizes it and fights it off. Treating infections with antibiotics further complicates the situation.

If an antibiotic fights the infection, some believe that the antibiotic suppresses the immune system, causing it to fight less vigorously the next time around.[5] By the fourth or fifth infection, the immune system might not even recognize an invader as a threat because it now depends on the antibiotic to do its job.

The antibiotic delivery system is an important factor. External antibiotic creams used to combat skin infections do not typically disturb the gut. However, taken orally, antibiotics kill not only bad bugs that cause infections, but also knock out virtually all of the intestinal bacteria, including beneficial varieties. Many people experience digestive problems after taking an oral antibiotic for this reason.

The gut is a host to hundreds of types of flora that live together cooperatively in the healthy person. Antibiotics usually disrupt this symbiotic environment. The good bacteria, which antibiotics kill along with the bad bacteria, exist to control the growth of yeasts and other fungi in the digestive tract. In their absence, yeasts colonize, and their usually small colonies can then proliferate.[6] Intestinal overgrowth of yeast and bad bacteria is a well-documented outcome of taking broad spectrum antibiotics.[7] Many parents report that their children regressed into autism following antibiotic treatment.

Vaccination

In its attempt to fool the body into believing that it has come in contact with a real infectious microorganism, vaccination does not exactly mimic the natural infection progress. It bypasses cellular immunity and stimulates humoral immunity by injecting viruses and bacteria into the blood instead of letting them enter the body through the gut or lungs, as they would naturally.

After vaccination, the body produces both IgM and IgG antibodies. IgM antibodies are the body's first responders to invaders, with antibody levels typically increasing for several days and then tapering off over the next few weeks, unless a chronic infection persists. IgG antibodies take a bit longer to appear, but once they do, they stay in the bloodstream for months to years, and perhaps for life, providing protection against reinfection.

Newborns do not mount a rapid or strong antibody response to vaccination.[8] "Babies are born with a very immature cellular immune system," says Lawrence Palevsky, MD, a New York pediatrician and cofounder of the Holistic Pediatric Association. "Childhood viral infectious diseases like measles, mumps and chicken-pox initially stimulate the cellular part of the immune system, which leads to the production of the signs of inflammation—fever, redness, swelling, and mucus. This cellular immune response stimulates the humoral part of the immune system to produce anti-inflammatory chemicals and antibodies that assist in recovery from these illnesses. The natural process matures the cellular and humoral immune systems."[9]

Vaccine numbers. Between 1980 and 2006, doctors more than doubled the numbers of vaccines and almost tripled the number of vaccine doses given to children by age 6. In 1980, the CDC and the American Academy of Pediatrics (AAP) recommended that children receive 23 doses of seven vaccines (DPT, polio, MMR) by age 6, with the first vaccinations given at 2 months. Vaccines for the chicken pox, Hib, and hepatitis were added in the 1990s.

Today, the CDC and AAP recommend that children receive 70 doses of 16 vaccines by age 6, with the first dose given at 12 hours old. Half of those 70 doses occur by 15 months. By age 12, children would receive nearly 5-dozen doses of 15 vaccines.[10] Sometimes as many as 7 vaccines are given at a time. The Colorado Immunization Manual includes a line drawing showing a doctor where to administer each shot.[11]

Vaccine additives. Few parents know that in addition to the pathogens, multi-vial vaccines contain preservatives (to keep the vaccine sterile), and all vaccines contain a multitude of potentially toxic additives called "adjuvants." An adjuvant (from the Latin *adjuvare,* to enhance) is a vaccine additive that stimulates the immune system, upping the body's production of antibodies to a pathogen. Adjuvants reduce production costs because the vaccine maker needs less of the expensive antigen; they also increase a vaccine's efficacy.

Vaccine adjuvants include mercury (as the preservative thimerosal), aluminum, formaldehyde, phenooxyethanol, gluteraldehyde, sodium chloride, monosodium glutamate (MSG), yeast, sodium borate, human and bovine albumin, protein, gelatin, and others. These agents are dangerous individually, and the potent toxicity of their interaction is virtually unexplored. The late immunologist Charles Janeway called vaccine adjuvants "the immunologist's dirty little secret."[12]

The preservative thimerosal, which is 49.6% ethyl-mercury by weight, has been used in vaccines and other pharmaceuticals for more than 50 years. Adding thimerosal allows medical personnel to use one vial of vaccine for more than one person, thus reducing the cost. The more expensive single dose vials do not require a preservative to remain sterile.

In 1930, Eli Lilly, the manufacturer, conducted a single study on 22 patients seriously ill with meningitis to prove that thimerosal was safe for injection into humans. All subjects died, but their deaths were attributed solely to meningitis and not to any effects of injected thimerosal. Eli Lily then pronounced thimerosal safe for human use.[13] In 1998 the FDA banned thimerosal from most products, including children's vaccines, because of its toxicity and many adverse reaction reports, but allowed it to remain in multidose vials of killed bacterial vaccines, including those against the flu.

On their own, adjuvants have the potential to cause immune dysfunction and inflammation; when added to a vaccine, they increase the risk of allergies and other adverse effects. Neurosurgeon Russell Blaylock, MD, argues that each successive series of vaccinations containing adjuvants repeatedly stimulates the brain's immune system, resulting in intense inflammatory reactions.[14]

Aluminum (Al), a known neurotoxin,[15] is the only adjuvant licensed to be used in vaccines in the United States. It appears as aluminum gels or aluminum salts such as aluminum hydroxide, aluminum phosphate, and aluminum potassium sulfate in vaccines against hepatitis A and B, diphtheria-tetanus-pertussis (DTaP, Tdap), Haemophilus influenzae type b (Hib), human papillomavirus (HPV), and pneumococcus infection. Symptoms of Al poisoning include personality changes, progressive speech disorder, stuttering, apraxia, tremors, myoclonic jerks, seizures, inflammation, abnormal EEG, psychosis, and dementia.[16]

Peanut oil and peanut allergy. In a groundbreaking 2011 book, *The Peanut Allergy Epidemic: What's Causing it and How to Stop it*, a Canadian mother, Heather Fraser, whose child had an anaphylactic reaction to peanut butter at 13 months of age, convincingly shows the relationship between vaccination and peanut allergies.[17] The following material comes from her extensive research.

In 1964 Merck & Co. announced a new vaccine ingredient promising to extend immunity: Adjuvant 65-4, containing up to 65% peanut oil as well as aluminum stearate. Scientists chose plentiful, inexpensive peanut oil as a replacement for cottonseed oil in vaccines because, from the 1930s through 1950, sensitivity to cottonseed oil in penicillin injections had caused allergies to both products. The inventors of Adjuvant 65-4 knew that allergic sensitization to the peanut oil in the adjuvant was a distinct possibility, and considered toxicity and allergenicity inevitable outcomes of vaccination. Their job was simply to balance potency and safety. Potency won.

Prior to 1941, the literature shows no report of peanut allergies in adults or children. A survey of people showed self-reported peanut allergies in .3% of those born 1944–47, .4% of those born 1948–57, and .6% between 1959–67. Articles published in the late 1950s and early 1960s show a growing awareness of peanut allergy, but the first formal study of peanut allergy in children was not until 1973, and then on only 114 kids.

Between 1997 and 2002, the peanut-allergic pediatric population in the US rose by an average of 58,000 children a year, and doubled between 2002 and 2008. By 2008, more than one million children under 18 and another two million adults were allergic to peanuts in the United States alone. In 2008, over 1% of people born 1944–67, reported allergies to nuts, including peanuts. Doctors watched the mysterious rise in peanut allergies, but few asked "why?"

The answer lies in digestion. French Nobel laureate and immunologist Charles Richet discovered that in all animals, without exception, healthy digestive juices actively transform potentially toxic proteins, rendering them innocuous. Stated alternatively, inadequate digestion is a prerequisite for food allergy. In those with inadequate digestion, the first injection of undigested protein into the bloodstream sensitizes and weakens the person or animal; a second, and subsequent smaller doses then have the potential to produce anaphylaxis, a serious or even fatal reaction.

The possibility that hundreds of thousands of children were sensitized to peanuts by ingredients in one or more routine pediatric vaccinations is just too much to conceive. But it is too obvious to deny. The real clue is the sudden rise in peanut allergy following the escalation of the pediatric vaccine schedule.

Philip Incao, MD, a retired holistic family-care physician in Colorado maintains that "Physically, health is about balancing acute inflammatory responses to infection, which stimulate one arm of the immune system, and chronic inflammatory responses to infection, which stimulate the other part of the immune system. Overuse of vaccines to suppress all acute, externalizing inflammation early in life can set up the immune system to respond to future stresses and infections by developing chronic, internalizing disease later in life."[18]

The elimination of most "natural" experience with infectious "minor" childhood diseases of former times, such as measles and chicken pox, through mass use of multiple vaccines, may be resulting in some unintended consequences. By disrupting the balance of cellular and humoral immunity, mass vaccination may be causing the cellular immune system to atrophy from disuse, instead of becoming stronger.

Two new extremely thorough reviews of the impact of vaccines on the developing immune system are now available: *Vaccine Illusion* by Tetyana Obukhanych, PhD, an impeccably credentialed immunologist,[19] and *A Commentary on Current Childhood Vaccine Programs* by veteran physician, Harold Buttram, MD.[20]

The Immune System in Autism

Immune dysregulation, inflammation, and autoimmune diseases are rampant in the health histories of families with autism, and various symptoms were enumerated in chapter 2. A 2009 Danish study of over 3,000 children showed associations among family history of type 1 diabetes and a maternal history of rheumatoid arthritis, celiac, and autism diagnoses.[21] Genetically vulnerable immune systems eventually become exhausted from continuous efforts to ward off repeated assaults from the environment.

Early studies by Reed Warren, PhD, at Utah State University and others indicate that most children with autism have significant immune system abnormalities.[22] According to longtime autism researcher, Sudhir Gupta, MD, PhD, a professor of neurology, pathology, microbiology, and molecular genetics at the University of California, Irvine, individuals with autism have more TH2 cells than

TH1 cells when compared to neuro-typical children. Gupta believes that the fewer number of TH1 cells explains why these children are more susceptible to viral and fungal infections.[23] The dominance of humoral (TH2) immunity over cellular (TH1) immunity along with persistent inflammation is emerging as one of the hallmarks of ASD.

Further evidence comes from a 2004 Johns Hopkins study in which researchers examined tissue from three different regions of the brain in 11 people with autism, ages 5 to 44, who had died of accidents or injuries. They also compared the number of inflammatory proteins in the cerebrospinal fluid and brains of normal controls, with those of six living patients with autism, ages 5 to 12. Those with autism showed evidence of an ongoing inflammatory process evidenced by abnormally elevated inflammatory proteins called cytokines and chemokines.[24]

A more recent study showed increased cytokines in children with autism compared to those developing typically, when both were exposed to a widespread environmental chemical.[25] Paul Ashwood, an immunologist at the MIND Institute in California and coauthor of the above recent studies, has reviewed over 200 other pieces of research and concluded that autism most probably has an immunological basis.

Vaccination may be instrumental in causing chronic and uncontrolled inflammation in many individuals with and without autism. Remember, a natural stimulation of the immune system can make it stronger and better able to maintain good health. When the immune system does not function normally due to unnatural stimulation, as in many children with ASDs, it can get "stuck" on inflammation and lead to chronic illness.

Inflammation and the role of immune dysfunction are topics of major interest in autism and other disease research today.[26] The comprehensive textbook *Autism, Oxidative Stress, Inflammation and Immune Abnormalities*, with over 400 pages of contributions from experts worldwide, covers this subject in great depth.[27]

Immune system load factors are intimately related to the degree of toxicity and other environmental stressors. Toxins, including mercury and aluminum, disrupt every system of the body, causing them to become inflamed, distressed, and dysfunctional.[28] The bodies of children with autism are in a survival mode, putting all of their energy into just staying alive. Gradually—almost imperceptibly—as the physical body becomes overwhelmed, the brain is affected. Cognitive and/or behavioral problems appear; reactions to foods, pollens, chemicals, and pharmaceuticals accelerate; wheezing, croup, and breathing problems worsen into asthma in some cases. This internal survival state could appear outwardly as distractibility, hyperactivity, or lack of responsiveness.

Allergies and autism go together, as Kenneth Bock, MD, states in his book title, *Healing the New Childhood Epidemics: Autism, ADHD, Asthma, and Allergies.*[29] The exact number of children who have both autism and allergies is unknown, but anyone who works with this population knows it is high. The commonality is immune system dysregulation.

In order to determine how dysfunctional the immune system is for an individual child, an extensive medical and developmental history is necessary. As noted earlier, this must be an exhaustive look at prenatal, natal, environmental, and social factors, such as exposure to medications; vaccine reactions; use of pesticides, chemicals, or tobacco; toxic building materials; pet products; travel; changes in environment; and water.

The history should also include a comprehensive diary of what a child is eating, drinking, and breathing, as well as how much sleep, screen time, and exercise a child is getting. Remember that exposures from air, food, water, dust, and all other sources are cumulative and add incrementally to an individual's Total Load. Although history-taking alone is sometimes adequate to determine an appropriate treatment plan, previously described laboratory testing is frequently necessary to evaluate the body's response to toxic agents, its gut flora, and its nutritional status.

Some environmental assaults may be obvious, such as from an old house with peeling lead paint; others may be subtler, such as toxic lawn treatments tracked into the home. One family became sick when the fertilizer they had been using on their farm was unknowingly "cut" with recycled radioactive material. Extraordinary efforts were necessary to trace the cause of illness and developmental problems in children to this source.

Common Infections in Those with Autism

We now suspect that the many types of early infections in children's health histories are not only risk factors for autism, but are hints that the immune system is overburdened. Many individuals with autism can trace gut, neurological, and behavioral symptoms to exposure to specific infectious agents. Their bodies are teeming with bad bugs to which their immune systems are attempting to respond, resulting in chronic inflammation and neurological reactions. Sometimes these reactions can also be seasonal, such as pollen allergies. Others can be from infections such as the following:

Ear infections. In a 1994 survey of parents by the nonprofit Developmental Delay Resources (DDR), 75% of children later diagnosed with ASDs had five or more ear infections.[30] Later studies confirm this anecdotal evidence.[31] One researcher even targeted early ear infections as a major contributor to autism.[32]

Frequent ear infections are a sign of a weak immune system. A classic 1991 study by Talal Nsouli, MD, an allergist at Georgetown University Hospital, showed that 78% of early childhood ear infections are related to food allergies. By eliminating the offending food from the diet over a 16-week period, he ameliorated the infections in 86% of his subjects. Reintroduction of the food caused a recurrence. By limiting the diet of his patients, Dr. Nsouli avoided the unnecessary use of antibiotics or insertion of ear tubes, often seen as panaceas for such chronic problems.[33] Obviously, less invasive techniques are preferable, especially since current research now shows that ear tube insertion is rarely beneficial.[34]

Maryland nutritionist Kelly Dorfman has coined the term "post traumatic ear infection syndrome" to describe a condition in children who have had continual ear infections, often as result of undiagnosed food allergies.[35] Sequential treatments with stronger antibiotics may increase vulnerability to damage from toxic metals, followed by a gradual behavioral deterioration, including hyperactivity, distractibility, and lessened relatedness.

Boyd Haley, PhD, a world authority on mercury toxicity, found that it takes less mercury to do harm in the presence of the antibiotics ampicillin and tetracycline.[36] Allergies, ear infections, mercury, and antibiotics are a potent cocktail for triggering autism with accompanying auditory processing difficulties, learning disabilities, and attention deficits. Permanent damage to the inner ear could result from complications of immune, toxic, and sensory load factors interacting.

Strep. Some children with autism spectrum disorders, and also those with Tourette syndrome and obsessive-compulsive disorder (OCD), have a history of repeated strep infections. If a strep infection induces tics or OCD, a doctor should suspect Pediatric Acute-onset Neuropsychiatric Syndrome (PANS), the new name for Pediatric Autoimmune Neuropsychiatric Disorder Associated with Streptococcus (PANDAS).[37] The new syndrome covers all cases of abrupt onset or worsening of OCD symptoms triggered not just by a streptococcal infection, but also by a variety of infectious bacteria, viruses, or parasites, followed by a slow, gradual improvement. A subsequent infection might cause symptoms to worsen again.[38]

According to Mady Hornig, MD, at Columbia University's Mailman School of Public Health, what is thought to occur in PANS is that antibodies to strep cross-react with proteins in the basal ganglia of the brain that are responsible for movement and repetitive behavior, thus causing the tics or obsessive-compulsive symptoms.[39]

Lyme. A new bug that is showing up in the bodies of autistics with more frequency is *Borrelia burgdorferi* (Bb), the carrier of Lyme disease. This insidious disease can be passed between sexual partners and from mother to unborn child, and may even be airborne! Bb is very prevalent and underdiagnosed, especially in young children diagnosed with ASDs, according to Dietrich Klinghardt MD, PhD, a practitioner both in the US and Europe.[40]

Because motor delays, speech-language issues, sensory and auditory processing problems, and other developmental problems are so common today, the possibility of Lyme is often overlooked. Even without evidence of the telltale tick bite, Klinghardt tests every child with autistic-like symptoms for Lyme, especially those who are not responding positively to other treatments.

Unfortunately, most lab tests for Lyme disease, including the popular Western blot, are not very reliable; doctors see many false negatives. A more-promising new Lyme test from NeuroSciences (www.neurorelief.com), called "My Lyme Immune ID™," uses memory T cells and cytokine responses to five Bb antigens.

Klinghardt has designed a very complex diagnostic procedure involving muscle testing, called Autonomic Response Testing (ART), which compares the body's energy pathways to those of the pathogen. Using ART, which requires intensive training, Klinghardt finds that seven out of eight of his patients test positive for Bb. (See chapter 7 for more on this technique.)

After evaluating and treating many families with children exhibiting autism, Klinghardt has concluded the following: if the firstborn is male and has autism, mercury is probably at fault, as it has a synergistic effect with testosterone (see more on this in the next chapter). If a mother has a typical child first, however, and one of her other children has autism, mercury is not the sole cause. The culprit is probably Lyme and its coinfections that add to the neurotoxin pool in the mother, potentiate mercury, and pass through the placenta to her unborn baby.

Viruses. Viruses are strands of DNA or RNA that are encased in a protective protein shield and looking for a host. They are parasites that cannot exist outside the body or reproduce on their own, so they get cozy in the cells of their hosts, where they can live for years. Unlike bacteria, viruses do not respond to antibiotics. Most colds and the flu are caused by viruses. Viruses have the ability to mutate and shift within the body, wreaking havoc with function.[41]

The role of viruses in autism is well-documented.[42] Borna disease virus,[43] congenital rubella,[44] Epstein Barr,[45] herpes simplex,[46] and measles virus[47] are all considered to be possible contributors to autism. While Bb is a bacterium and is most often treated with strong antibiotics, it too acts like a virus. That's one reason it is so difficult to diagnose and control. John Martin, MD, PhD, believes that many autistic children have acquired a "stealth virus" that the immune system does not recognize. The immune system thus puts out no antibodies against it, leading to chronic low-grade infection and accompanying inflammation.[48]

The Possible Role of Vaccination in Autism

While the government wants us to believe that there is no relationship between vaccination and autism,[49] strong controversy still exists as parents who believe otherwise make their opinions known.

In *Evidence of Harm*[50] and *The Vaccine Epidemic*,[51] the authors convincingly review evidence for a cover-up by government health officials and vaccine manufacturers of data linking autism and thimerosal. A hot-off-the-press study demonstrated that children who received mercury-containing vaccines were significantly more likely to become autistic.[52]

Proposed biological mechanisms for thimerosal-induced autism have focused on mercury-containing vaccines and genetic factors interacting to create

- oxidative stress leading to impaired methylation and lowered levels of cysteine and glutathione[53]
- DNA damage and death of brain cells[54]
- brain inflammation[55]
- autoimmunity and/or genetic susceptibility[56]

More than 10 years after thimerosal was banned, autism continues to increase because mercury from thimerosal is only one of many contributors to the Total Load. A current study confirms that, although mercury has been removed from many vaccines, other culprits may link vaccines to autism, since many thimerosal-free vaccines have twice the aluminum of those containing thimerosal.[57]

Mercury is not the only problematic adjuvant. The results of a recent Canadian study show that aluminum as an adjuvant is also suspect in the presence of autism. Children from countries with the highest ASD prevalence had the highest exposure to Al from vaccines. The increase in exposure to Al adjuvants significantly correlates with the increase in ASD prevalence in the United States observed over the last two decades, and a significant correlation exists between the amounts of Al administered to preschool children and the current prevalence of ASD in seven Western countries.[58]

Elevating the humoral system to dominance over the cellular system through vaccination and thus reversing the natural immunologic scheme that humans evolved with, is an important overlooked factor in trying to understand immune issues in autism. Furthermore, many of the bacteria and viruses that infect individuals with autism can come only from vaccinations. Since many of these "bugs," including measles, have disappeared from the environment in developing countries, the pathogens must enter the body through the blood.

Vaccine reactions. Every vaccine carries a risk of injury or death, and some individuals can be at higher risk than others for suffering a vaccine reaction. Adverse reactions to a vaccine can begin within hours, days, or weeks after vaccination. Reactions vary from not-so-obvious signs, such as behavioral changes, sleep disturbances, confusion, flapping, loss of relatedness, eye contact, delayed developmental milestones such as speaking, and other signs of physical, mental, and emotional regression, to acute physical symptoms, such as redness at the site of the injection, high-pitched screaming, inconsolable crying, high fever, paralysis, seizures, loss of consciousness, and even death.

Vaccine reactions in infants are often misinterpreted as shaken baby syndrome, as in the famous case of Alan Yurko. His infant son received a hepatitis B shot within hours of birth, as do many babies. This vaccine is known to cause brain hemorrhaging and death in some patients.[59] Yurko was accused of child abuse and jailed for eight years until finally acquitted.

Often what is called "autism regression" is a vaccine reaction, which can be accompanied by symptoms of immune dysfunction such as new food and environmental allergies, asthma, digestive problems, skin disorders, and chronic respiratory and ear infections. Together, these symptoms of vaccine-induced brain and immune system dysfunction may persist. Later, a team of specialists makes a diagnosis of a learning disability, attention deficit, or autism.

Some parents of now-grown vaccine-injured children born during the last two decades of the 20th century, reported the above symptoms of vaccine reactions and regression after the diphtheria-pertussis-tetanus (DPT) vaccination. Witnessing how their children regressed and were left with various kinds of brain and immune system damage, a small group led by Barbara Loe Fisher founded the National Vaccine Information Center (NVIC). They also worked with

Congress on the historic National Childhood Vaccine Injury Act of 1986 (PL99-660), which required the Institute of Medicine to examine the literature for evidence that vaccines can kill and injure.

For the next 15 years additional parents watched in disbelief as their children were regressing into autism after DPT, MMR, and other vaccinations. Empirical evidence for a vaccine-autism connection continued to grow at the same time doctors and scientists inside industry, government, and medical organizations repeatedly denied a vaccine-autism relationship.

Many consider a "one size fits all" vaccination schedule to be inappropriate, especially for premature and immune-compromised babies and toddlers. Before vaccination, doctors are required to inform all parents of the benefits of each vaccine, *and* to discuss the risks, signs, and symptoms of a vaccine reaction. This knowledge allows parents to monitor their children closely for several weeks after vaccination, and recognize and report the sometimes subtle signs that a reaction has occurred to the Vaccine Adverse Event Reporting System (VAERS).

Parents whose children suffer injury or death following vaccination, can receive damages from the federal Vaccine Injury Compensation Program (VICP) created under the 1986 Vaccine Injury Act. Since its inception, this program has awarded over one billion dollars to more than 2,500 families whose children have died or been injured after vaccine reactions.

Mitochondrial Disorder

Mitochondria are the power centers inside cells that are essential to converting food to energy. Well-functioning mitochondria create readily available and sustained energy, resulting in toned and well-formed muscles. When these muscles are exercised, they get stronger steadily and predictably. In mitochondrial disorders, the ability of the mitochondria to generate energy is damaged. Environmental toxins such as heavy metals and pesticides and aggressive antibiotic use can all injure the mitochondria, resulting in loss of muscle tone, stamina, and other functions.

That is what happened in the case of Hannah Poling, the daughter of an MD/PhD neurologist/biophysicist father and a lawyer/nurse mother. In 2000, when she was 19 months old, Hannah received five "catch-up" vaccines in a single day because she had missed some recommended in the vaccine schedule due to a series of chronic ear infections. At the time, Hannah was interactive, playful, and communicative. Two days later, she was lethargic, irritable, and febrile. Ten days after vaccination, she developed a rash; months later she was showing delays in communication, relatedness, and behavior consistent with an autism spectrum disorder. Doctors diagnosed "encephalopathy" caused by a "mitochondrial disorder."

"Encephalopathy" is medicalese for "brain inflammation." Neither Hannah's medical records nor her parents' observations indicated that prior to her catch-up vaccinations she had any symptoms of mitochondrial disorder. Hannah's parents believed that vaccines had triggered her encephalopathy, mitochondrial disorder and autistic-like behavior. They sued the Department of Health and Human Services (DHHS) for compensation under the VICP and won.[60]

A Three-Pronged Approach

So if antibiotics work *against* the body's ability to heal itself, what works in consort *with* the body? A three-pronged program of strengthening the immune system, eliminating the infections, and fighting the inflammation. With this plan "autistic" behavioral symptoms frequently diminish or disappear entirely.

1. Strengthening Immunity

Food. About 400 BC, Hippocrates proclaimed, "Let food be thy medicine and medicine be thy food." Over 2,000 years later, that advice is still sound!

The best way to boost a sluggish immune system is *still* to choose nutrient-dense foods over empty calories. Refer back to the previous chapter which explains why the best choices are *real* food: fresh fruits, vegetables, seeds, nuts, beans, whole grains, spices, plant and animal proteins, and good quality fats. An extremely helpful book on this subject is Lucy Burney's *Boost Your Child's Immune System: A Program and Recipes for Raising Strong, Healthy Kids*.[61] Burney codes each recipe for allergens, showing which are wheat-, gluten-, and dairy-free.

Lately some specialty foods are earning high marks as immune boosters. One of the most interesting is highly nutritious camel milk. No joke! Nomads in the desert have recognized the power of camel milk for centuries.[62] With five times the vitamin C, ten times the iron, and more omega-3 fats and calcium than cow's milk, it may just be the "perfect food," since the type of casein it contains is non-reactive for even the most sensitive kids.

Camel milk targets all three steps: it can not only strengthen the immune system, but also eliminate food allergies and gut problems, fight viruses and bacteria, *and* lessen inflammation![63] Its immune-fighting qualities are truly amazing because of the small size of the immunoglobulins that can penetrate deep into the tissues to fight infection.[64] After a 2005 research study showed that camel milk was like intravenous immunoglobulin therapy (see below) for children with autism,[65] mothers jumped all over it. The latest study shows that one of the reasons camel milk is so beneficial is that it decreases oxidative stress by increasing the antioxidant glutathione.[66] (More about that in the next two chapters!)

Some fruits and vegetables (and juices made from them) are antioxidants, which act like Pac-Man and gobble up the free radicals that cause oxidative stress. Tomatoes, broccoli, garlic, red beans, pecans, walnuts, green tea, blueberries, pomegranates, acai berries, cinnamon, cardamom, turmeric, cumin, mustard seeds, oregano, and parsley are all strong antioxidants.

Bottom line: The best way to strengthen immunity is with a nutrient-rich diet!

Supplements. If a child will not eat nutritious, immune-boosting foods, the second best choice is using immune-boosting supplements. The now-classic book *Superimmunity for Kids*, by physician Leo Galland, is a keeper for a lifetime, as chapters move sequentially from prenatal to adult immunity with both food and supplement options.[67]

Here are some special immune boosters for individuals with autism, and anyone with poor immune function for that matter.

Vitamin D is a fat-soluble vitamin that is produced naturally as D_3 or cholecalciferol when sunlight hits the skin. The body makes what it needs, accumulating and storing significant reserves in the tissues, liver, spleen, bones, and brain; it can then be available during darker months. Vitamin D acts more like a neuro-steroid hormone than a vitamin, directly affecting brain development and regulation of behavior. It is crucial in immune system function.

Recent research suggests that vitamin D offers neuro-protection, anti-epileptic effects, and immuno-modulation of several brain neurotransmitter systems and hormones. It is important in autism because it enhances the body's ability to fight inflammation and destroy dangerous microbes.

Evidence supports a vitamin D deficiency theory of autism.[68] Maybe the high autism incidence among Somalis living in Minnesota[69] is due to the possibility that their bodies are programmed to the extremely high levels of vitamin D from the strong sun in their native land and lacking in their new home. In 2012, Chinese doctors measured vitamin D levels in their patients with autism and found that the lower the levels, the more severe the autistic symptoms.[70] That same year, researchers at the Gillberg Neuropsychiatric Institute in Sweden found the vitamin D-autism connection so strong that they called for "urgent research."[71] Convinced yet?

According to John Cannell, MD, of the Vitamin D Council, blood levels of vitamin D should be at least 50 ng/ml. The most common way to have your vitamin D level tested is to see a doctor. But a new $65 at-home test is available through the Vitamin D Council, which has partnered with ZRT Laboratory. The test measures 25-hydroxyvitamin D or 25 (OH) D, an inactive form of vitamin D. Stick a finger or heel to get a few drops of blood and send the kit back. The results are mailed to you without involving a physician.

Work with a health care practitioner to find a supplementation program that is right. Some bodies absorb drops more easily than tablets or caps. Others require high dosages for a short time to reach acceptable levels. Monitoring is essential to avoid toxicity.

The Mitochondria Cocktail. The mitochondria can be more efficient if they are fed properly. Healthy mitochondria provide the sustained energy necessary for optimal growth and development. Nutritional guru Kelly Dorfman offers a basic cocktail of nutrients critical for mitochondrial function.

- **B-vitamins:** Thiamine (vitamin B-1) and riboflavin (vitamin B-2) are both required cofactors for different parts of energy making. A typical mitochondria formula may contain 50–100mg each of vitamins B-1, B-2, and/or B-3 (as niacinamide). Some children do well with thiamine but get irritated with riboflavin and vice versa. In other cases, both B-vitamins plus are necessary. Because it is hard to know what to support (without a specific diagnosis), the B-vitamins should be added one at a time. Some children will have a clear response to one B-vitamin or may need them all. Keep in close contact with the supervising medical professional and adjust the B-vitamins if the child becomes agitated.

- **Vitamin E (mixed tocopherols):** The mitochondria must be protected against damage from destructive molecules called free radicals, which can damage their fragile cell membranes and disrupt energy production. Vitamin E is an important anti-free radical agent for protecting and healing these membranes. Vitamin E is well-tolerated and it has no known toxicity. Natural vitamin E is usually derived from wheat or soy. In rare cases, it may cause allergic problems.

- **Acetyl-L-Carnitine (ALC):** ALC helps maintain the membranes of the mitochondria and facilitate the transport and utilization of fats so they can be used to make energy. ALC can sometimes cause irritability or stomach distress but is not toxic.

Colostrum, the liquid breast-fed babies get postpartum for the three or four days before a woman's milk supply comes in, is an amazing combination of substances that strengthen and support the immune system, potentiate the development and repair of cells and tissues, and ensure the effective and efficient metabolism of nutrients. It includes cytokines that inhibit inflammation and growth factors that promote maturation of the immune system.[72]

Bovine colostrum has been used successfully to boost immunity in other immune-deficient illnesses,[73] and some health care professionals are now recommending it for patients with autism. To be beneficial, colostrum supplements must be collected from the first milking within six hours after birth of the calf and contain all components, including the fat and not gluten or casein.[74] Some manufacturers offer chewable colostrum in chocolate, orange, cherry and pineapple!

Transfer factors (TFs) are naturally occurring molecules that contain an individual's immune history. They are made by white blood cells that travel to the maturing mammary glands and release the donor's immune history into the maturing mammary tissues. As the newborn nurses, he receives his mother's immune history via her immune factors, hence the name. If one thinks of vitamins and minerals as the bricks and mortar that build immune system cells, TFs are the blueprints that determine where the bricks will be placed.

Transfer factors are now available in capsules, chewables, and powders. They are extracted from cow colostrum and chicken egg yolks and are available alone or combined with other immune-boosting ingredients, including vitamins, minerals, and foods.

Hugh Fudenberg, MD is the researcher usually associated with TFs. In a group of 22 children with autism, 15 of whom had become autistic following an MMR vaccine, all but 1 responded positively to TF, with 10 regaining sufficient skills to enter mainstream schools. After discontinuing treatment, some showed regression, but none returned to their prior baseline levels.[75] In another study, 88 children who used TF at the recommended doses for at least 6 months were compared to a matched sample. The TF group had a 74% reduction in illness and an 86% reduction in antibiotic use.[76]

Kenneth A. Bock, MD, sees the benefit of transfer factors as part of his treatment protocols to boost the immune system in his patients with autism. He believes that TF is an effective immune modulator, especially for those with chronic viral infections and certain autoimmune disorders. A small study of his patients with autism who took polyvalent TF at a dose of three 200-mg capsules three times daily show both behavioral improvements and a marked decrease in incidence of infectious illnesses.

Transfer factors should not be combined with digestive enzymes. For more information, read *Transfer Factor: Natural Immune Booster* by William Hennen.[77]

Intravenous immunoglobulin (IVIG) improves immune function by giving a patient copious antibodies to fight infection and decrease autoimmune reactions. This process, known as "passive immunity," is an expensive and time-consuming therapy.

The pioneer in IVIG therapy for autism is Sudhir Gupta, MD, at the University of California, Irvine. Remember, he is the one who first suspected the imbalance of TH1 and TH2 cells in those with autism. Gupta's first patient in the early 1990s was Garrett Goldenberg, whose mother, Cindy, convinced that the MMR vaccine had triggered her son's autistic behavior, urged him to administer IVIG infusions.

Cindy had eliminated milk and wheat from Garrett's diet and had given him vitamin and nutritional supplements to enhance his immune and gastrointestinal function, with only slight benefit. Within weeks of beginning IVIG injections along with the dietary changes and nutritional supplement therapy, Garrett's behavior improved dramatically. As his rubella antibody levels decreased and his IgG and IgA levels stabilized, Garrett became less and less autistic.

Cindy was the first "Autism Mom" to recover her son from vaccine-induced regressive autism through dietary and immune-modulating therapies. Her voice in the early 1990s pointed doctors toward developing protocols to help heal autism, and gave new hope to a generation of parents who had been told that autism had no cure.

A more current study on this treatment, done on 26 children with autism over a six-month period, showed significant improvement in 37%. However, unlike Garrett, most regressed following discontinuation of the therapy.[78]

Master Mineral Solution (MMS). The new kid on the block is MMS, the acronym for Chlorine Dioxide (CD), which is produced when sodium chlorite is mixed with citric acid. CD is not bleach

(NaOCl), as some are claiming. MMS allegedly kills pathogens through oxidation, is able to neutralize heavy metals, and thus reduces inflammation. Really?

This treatment is *so* "hot" that is being included in this book for completeness. However, because it is also *so* new and *so* controversial, details are not provided. Anyone interested in learning more about it is referred with extreme caution to the only book on the subject, *Healing the Symptoms Known as Autism*, available as an e-book from www.mmsautism.org .[79]

2. Eliminating Allergies and Infections

Practitioners have designed several novel techniques that target the IgE, IgG, and IgA food and environmental reactions that are part of the Total Load of many children with autism. These allergy elimination techniques have limited research; however, they are worthy of mention because they have made such a difference for many on the autism spectrum.

• **Nambudripad's Allergy Elimination Techniques (NAET®)** is a complex, sequential intervention that combines applied kinesiology, chiropractic, acupuncture, and nutrition, the various professional degrees of its developer, Devi S. Nambudripad, DC, LAC, RN, PhD. Using a form of muscle testing, the therapist locates blockages related to a specific allergy, such as milk, on one of the acupuncture meridians. Allergens are "cleared" in a specific sequence, one at a time, and only one item per day. The substance must be completely avoided for 25 hours following treatment and is then permanently neutralized. If an individual has exceptionally high sensitivity, the process is repeated.

When an NAET practitioner eliminates blockages in the presence of the allergens, the brain learns to respond differently. A year-long controlled research study on 60 children with autism diagnoses who were treated for 50 common allergens showed improvement in 30 of 35 symptoms, including communication skills, on a standardized autism checklist. Some were able to function in regular classes following treatment.[80]

Since 1983, Dr. Nambudripod has trained over 9,000 licensed medical practitioners in NAET procedures all over the world. Those wanting to know more about this intervention should read *Say Good-Bye to Allergy Related Autism*[81] or go to www.naetautismtreatmentcenter.com.

• **BioSET™** desensitization, like NAET, is an acupressure technique that utilizes energetics and enzymes to clear or reprogram an individual's immune response. BioSET (for Bio-energetic Sensitivity and Enzyme Therapy) balances meridians blocked by allergens. This natural, noninvasive desensitization was developed over 25 years ago by Ellen Cutler, DC, who has also trained practitioners worldwide. For more information on how this method is being applied to autism, read her book *The Food Allergy Cure: A New Solution to Food Cravings, Obesity, Depression, Headaches, Arthritis, and Fatigue*[82] or go to www.drellencutler.com.

• **Low Dose Allergen (LDA) therapy**, originally called Enzyme Potentiated Desensitization (EPD), was discovered in the early 1960s by Frantisek Popper, MD, and later perfected by British allergist Leonard McKewin, MD, and American Butch Shrader. Doctors mix minute amounts of a specific allergen with an enzyme called Beta glucaronidase, a natural biological response modifier that up-regulates the immune system. The desired result is shifting the immune system from an allergic state (TH2) to a less allergic state (TH1). LDA is prepared at compounding pharmacies, so it does not require FDA approval.[83]

• **Sublingual immunotherapy (SLIT)** is an approach to immune system issues in autism that is novel in the United States but has been practiced abroad for decades. SLIT is a particularly useful method for kids whose "allergies" include needles! After an assessment using a noninvasive, computer-based screening instrument, a doctor prescribes daily sublingual (under the tongue) drops to desensitize allergic reactions to foods and environmental triggers.[84]

Killing the bugs and treating the infections. In their book *The Puzzle of Autism: Putting it All Together,*[85] Garry Gordon, MD, DO, and Amy Yasko, PhD, raise the hypothesis that chronic viral and bacterial infections act as accomplices to the heavy metals, aiding in their retention. From ancient times, healers have prescribed herbs and other natural substances to eliminate all types of pathological organisms living within the human body. Here are some recommendations to fight against specific bugs, mostly from Dr. Dietrich Klinghardt, a master in this arena:

• **Borna virus:** This nasty bug attacks the limbic system and is thus responsible for psychiatric symptoms, especially manic depression. High levels of Borna viruses are apparent in mania. Klinghardt uses herbal antivirals, like olive leaf and mushroom extracts, as well as the drug Amantidine, for at least four months.

• **Giardia, amoebas, and protozoa:** Klinghardt treats these and other bugs with rizoles, a new class of bioactive compounds created by ozonating plant oils, including clove, wormwood, marjoram, cumin, and others, for several weeks. Ozone, a form of oxygen therapy, kills anaerobes — bugs that live without oxygen.

• **Herpes viruses, including Epstein-Barr, varicella (chicken pox), and cytomegalovirus:** Treatment depends upon type. While some doctors choose pharmaceutical medications such as valacyclovir hydrochloride (Valtrex), Klinghardt prefers Heel homeopathics (see chapter 7), chlorella, freeze-dried garlic, and ozonated oils. Others like using turmeric and milk thistle as antivirals.

• **Lyme (*Borrelia burgdorferi*):** Klinghardt has developed a very complex Lyme treatment protocol that emphasizes herbs rather than antibiotics. His latest interventions are available at www.klinghardtacademy.com.The nonprofit

Lyme-Induced Autism Foundation (LIA), a clearinghouse for research, educates the public with periodic conferences and seminars about the latest Lyme treatments. Go to www. lymeinducedautism.org.

• **Measles virus:** Klinghardt treats measles with Vitamin A palmitate in a prescribed regime of 400,000 units in three divided dosages for two consecutive days only. Dosage is repeated every six weeks several times, then once annually. Klinghardt says that using this protocol immediately following a vaccine reaction can possibly prevent future problems.

• **Molds and fungi:** Aspergillus, cladosporium, stachybotrys, and other toxic molds are potentially deadly to the developing immune system. Use propolis, a waxy balsamic resinous substance that forms inside beehives in Somalia, Eritrea, Saudia Arabia, and India, and is a potent antimicrobial. The word "propolis" is made up of two Greek words: *pro* meaning "in front or in defense of," and *polis*, which means "town." Propolis is thus the town of the bees, or a beehive. Rich in flavonoids, hydroxyacids, terpenes, aromatic alcohols, and essential oils, propolis kills molds and has a fantastic long-term anti-inflammatory effect. Its antimicrobial properties were discovered several centuries BC.

Propolis can be taken orally or applied externally. It can also be heated in a vaporizer and released in the home and car to eliminate most bacteria, viruses, fungi, and mold from the air in an all-natural way.

• **Parasites like roundworms, threadworms, tapeworms, and liver flukes** are all very hearty bugs that should never be underestimated. Rizoles are good for treating all worms, cysts, and larvae. Klinghardt also uses Alinia (which crosses the blood-brain barrier), Albendazole, and Biltrocide in high doses to attack these critters.

• **Strep infections including PANS**, Klinghardt believes, often reside in the decaying tonsils of children with autism. The tonsils are a group of five lymphatic tissues found at the back of the throat. Tonsil tissues are arguably the most active parts of the immune system. As lymph tissue, they expand or swell when exposed to germs. Once illness passes, healthy tonsils shrink. In chronic illness, low-grade infections, or allergies, however, sometimes they do not. Because swollen tonsils can interfere with eating, breathing, and sleeping, they are often considered more troublesome than useful.

The standard treatment for chronically inflamed tonsils is to snip them out. This approach does not address why the tonsils became swollen in the first place. While a tonsillectomy may resolve chronic tonsillitis, infections then move and can become pockets of pus around teeth and in sinus cavities.

Instead of removing the tonsils, Klinghardt has established a protocol to heal them. It starts with injecting them and gargling a fermented product to kill the infections, using Heel homeopathic remedies (see chapter 7) to build the immune system, and finally restorative cryotherapy to burn them off. Like flower bulbs they regenerate, good as new. For more information on this treatment, which is available only in Germany, go to www.kryopraxis.de.

In addition to these specific treatments, Klinghardt has pioneered the use of some other unique preventative therapies. As a precautionary measure he suggests spraying a product called "Matrix Microbes" throughout the entire house twice a week. The fulvic acid in Matrix Microbes is death to many viruses, but the spray also includes many "good bugs" that the brain absorbs very quickly.

The best prevention is establishing rules regarding behaviors at home. Return to chapter 3 and review immune-boosting practices such as not wearing street shoes inside the house and washing hands with pure soap (not anti-bacterial soap) and water as you enter. Choose non-toxic products for simply *everything*! Bugs, molds, worms and flukes love toxic environments. Avoid giving them places to set up housekeeping.

Klinghardt has also recorded CDs with the strange vibrations of various bugs in action recorded underground. The patient plays the CD while sleeping, and the bugs respond as if they are being attacked, dying in the process. This is an extremely effective treatment for viruses.

The "bug vibration" CDs come in a 22-disc set or can be purchased individually. Dr. Klinghardt arranged for the recordings under strict, natural, controlled, studio-like conditions which allowed for no interfering sounds. Slides of the damaging viruses, bacteria, fungi, molds and parasites are also available to use with signal enhancers and a polarized filter.

Rizoles, Propolis vaporizers for home and car, Matrix microbes, and CDs are all available from www.klinghardtacademy.com.

3. Taming Inflammation

The third part of boosting and balancing the immune system is to put out the fire of inflammation in various parts of the body. Everyone knows the symptoms of inflammation: swelling, pain, redness, warmth, and discoloration. In autism, most of these symptoms occur internally, especially in the gut and brain,[27] and are invisible. To tackle this dilemma doctors are investigating possible treatment alternatives that bypass the digestive system, because many medicines further compromise the already-disturbed autistic gut.

Bugs and the infections they cause are all part of an inflammatory reaction and cycle that mobilizes the immune system. Because of the variety of pathogens, the immune system in autism over-responds, and the response persists; in other words, inflammation triggers more inflammation.

One of the symptoms stemming from inflammation is the occurrence of seizures in 11–39% of children with autism,[86] with numbers increasing as the more impaired children get older.[87] In one study of 86 patients with childhood-onset seizure disorder, 42% also had ASD.[88] Recent evidence indicates that neuro-inflammation due to allergy, excito-toxicity, environmental, or stress triggers could be contributing to seizures. Treating the inflammation often reduces seizure activity.[89]

- **Low Dose Naltrexone (LDN)**, an opiate blocker, is one of the most-studied anti-inflammatories for treating autism.[90] LDN is administered as a transdermal cream (TD-LDN), which is easy to apply nightly before bed. According to Kurt Woeller, MD, a physician with a mostly autism practice, the result of the opioid block is that the body compensates by producing even more natural endorphins. These feel-good chemicals can stay elevated for up to 18 hours.[91]

LDN appears to correct the imbalance between TH1 and TH2 safely, with few side effects and no known toxicity. Benefits are improved sleep, decreased pain, better digestion, and general resolution or improvement of behavioral symptoms.[92]

- **Actos®** (pioglitazone), a diabetic medication used to control blood sugar, is another anti-inflammatory compounded transdermal cream prescribed off-label for autism by Dr. Woeller and Philip DeMeio, MD. A small study funded by the Autism Research Institute found Actos to be helpful in some children,[93] although some negative side effects such as fevers can occur.

- **Hyperbaric oxygen therapy (HBOT)**, a powerful treatment previously proven efficacious for those who have had drowning accidents, stroke, and other brain injuries, is another popular treatment for neurological inflammation.

Patients of all ages are entirely enclosed in a chamber in which they breathe oxygen at a pressure of 1.3–1.5 atmospheres below sea level. Both the enclosed chamber and the pressure are necessary for HBOT to work. Those electing HBOT must make sure that both of these factors are in place. Treatments last one to two hours. Oftentimes, 40–60 sessions are necessary to see significant benefit.

Pressurized oxygen has tremendous healing capabilities. HBOT increases blood flow to the areas of the brain, and the pressure seems to help decrease some of the inflammatory problems. HBOT delivers oxygen deep into the tissues of the body where it attacks and kills yeasts and anaerobic (oxygen-hating) bacteria, with a short-lived die-off that is not hard on the liver.

Some physicians are very enthusiastic about HBOT as an adjunct therapy for individuals on the spectrum.[94] While the application of this treatment to those with autism shows promise, more research is necessary.

• **Curcumin**, the active ingredient in turmeric, an Indian spice, is known to have an anti-inflammatory effect.[95] It is showing good success in reducing both gut and neurological inflammation. Two products especially formulated for kids on the spectrum are Meriva-SR a patented time-release curcumin product from Thorne Research and Enhansa Curcumin, compounded by Lee-Silsby Pharmacy. Curcumin is high in phenols and should be used cautiously with children who are phenol intolerant.

Take-Home Points

Autistic symptoms appear almost certainly to be related in large part not only to gastrointestinal problems, but also to immune system dysfunction in genetically vulnerable children. Inflammation and lessened immunity are huge load factors, caused and exacerbated by environmental toxins and medical treatments, such as antibiotics.

Lyme and other bacteria and viruses contribute to the inflammatory process and further compromise immunity. Vaccines and their additives add to the Total Load by artificially tricking the body into an unnatural state of humoral system dominance over the cellular system. For over 200 years the medical literature has shown that neurological and immune system dysfunction can be caused by both infectious diseases and vaccines created with those same viruses and bacteria. A host/disease or host/vaccine interaction causes inflammation, which is acute at first, and becomes chronic rather than resolving and leaving the host with good health. In both cases, the end result is unresolved inflammation leading to brain dysfunction of varying degrees of severity, which is the same profile many have observed in children with ASDs. The vaccine-autism relationship goes far beyond the pathogens in the shots.

Treatment involves a three-step plan of boosting the immune system, fighting the infections, and taming the inflammation naturally. In the past decade protocols that combine these essential components using special foods, supplements such as colostrum and anti-viral herbs and oils, and natural anti-inflammatories that bypass the disturbed gut are showing promise. Allergy elimination and desensitization is a lengthy and often worthwhile process for those with severe reactions.

Families striving to outsmart autism must become knowledgeable about available options and work with experienced health care practitioners who are sharing their understanding through webinars and conferences on respecting and supporting the body's ability to heal itself.

---

[1] Theoharides TC, Kempuraj D, Redwood L. Autism: An emerging 'neuroimmune disorder' in search of therapy. Expert Opin. Pharmacother, 2009, 10:13, 2127–43.

[2] Pollan M. Cooked: A Natural history of Transformation. New York: Penguin Press, 2013, 331.

[3] Blaser M. Antibiotic Overuse: Stop the Killing of Beneficial bacteria. Nature, 2011, 476, 393–94.

[4] Levy SB. The antibiotic paradox: How the misuse of antibiotics destroys their curative power. Cambridge, MA: Perseus Books, 2002.

[5] Schmidt M. Beyond Antibiotics: Strategies for Living in a World of Emerging Infections and Antibiotic-Resistant Bacteria. Berkeley, CA: North Atlantic Books, 2009.

[6] Crook WG. The yeast connection handbook. Jackson, TN: Professional Books, 1996.

[7] Samonis G, Gikas A, Anaissie E. Prospective evaluation of the impact of broad-spectrum antibiotics on gastrointestinal yeast colonization of humans. Antimicrobial Agents and Chemotherapy, 1993, 37, 51–53.

[8] Siegrist CA. Neonatal and early life vaccinology. Vaccine, 2001, 19:25–26, 3331–46.

[9] Fisher BL. In the Wake of Vaccines. Mothering Magazine, Sep/Oct 2004, 44.

[10] Recommended Immunization Schedule for Persons Aged 0 Through 6 Years. www.healthychildren.org. Accessed Jan 19, 2012.

[11] Giving all the Doses. www.dcphe.state.co.us/dc/Immunization/immunmanual/sec09.pdf, 9–17. From Habakus LK, Holland M. Vaccine Epidemic. New York: Skyhorse Pub., 2011.

[12] Adjuvants, Once Immunologist's 'Dirty Little Secret.' www.emoryhealthsciblog.com/?p=3307. Accessed Mar 3, 2012.

[13] Jamieson WA, Powell HM. Merthiolate as a preservative for biological products. Am J Hyg, 1931, 14, 218–24.

[14] Blaylock, RI. The danger of excessive vaccination during brain development. Med Veritas, 2008, 5:1, 1727–41.

[15] Yokel RA. The toxicology of aluminum in the brain: A review. Neurotoxicology, 2000, 21:5, 813–28.

[16] Johnson VJ, Sharma RP. Aluminum disrupts the pro-inflammatory cytokine/neurotrophin balance in primary brain rotation-mediated aggregate cultures: Possible role in neurodegeneration. Neurotoxicology, 2002, 24:2, 261–68.

[17] Fraser H. The Peanut Allergy Epidemic: What's causing it and How to Stop it. New York: Skyhorse Publishing, 2011.

[18] Fisher BL. Shots in the Dark. The Next City, Summer 1999, 4, 4.

[19] Obukhanych T. Vaccine Illusion. www.amazon.com: Kindle book, 2012.

[20] Butram HE. A commentary on current childhood vaccine programs. Quakertown, PA: Philosophical Publishing Company, 2010.

[21] Atladóttir HO, Pedersen MG, Thorsen P, Mortensen PB, Deleuran B, Eaton WW, Parner ET. Association of family history of autoimmune diseases and autism spectrum disorders. Pediatrics, Aug 2009, 124:2, 687–94.

[22] Warren RP, Margaretten N, Pace N, Foster A. Immune abnormalities in patients with autism. J. Autism Develop Dis, 1986, 16, 189–97; Warren RP, Singh VK, Averett RE, et al. Immunogenetic studies in autism and related disorders. Molec Clin Neuropathol, 1996, 28, 77–81; Jyonouchi H, Sun S, Itokazu N. Inate immunity associated with inflammatory responses and cytokine production against common dietary proteins in patients with autism spectrum disorders. Neuropsychobiol, 2002, 46:2, 76–84.

[23] Gupta S, Aggarwal S, Heads C. Dysregulated immune system in children with autism: Beneficial effects of intravenous immune globulin on autistic characteristics. J Autism Dev Dis, 1996, 26:4, 439–52.

[24] Vargas DL, Nascimbene C, Krishnan C, Zimmerman AW, Pardo CA. Neuroglial activation and neuroinflammation in the brain of patients with autism. Annals Neurol, Jan 2005, 57:1, 67–81.

[25] Ashwood P, Schauer J, Pessah IN, Van de Water J. "Preliminary evidence of the in vitro effects of BDE-47 on innate immune responses in children with autism spectrum disorders." J Neuroimmunol. 2009 Mar 31; 208 (1– 2): 130–5.

[26] Ashwood P, Corbett BA, Kantor A, Schulman H, Van de Water J, Amaral DG. In search of cellular immunophenotypes in the blood of children with autism. PLoS One, May 2011, 6:5, e19299; Jyonouchi H, Geng L, Streck DL, Toruner GA. Children with ASD who exhibit chronic GI symptoms and marked fluctuation of behavioral

symptoms exhibit distinct innate immune abnormalities. Jrl Neuroimmunology, Jul 29, 2011.

[27] Chauhan A, Chahan V, Brown WT, ed. Autism, Oxidative Stress, Inflammation and Immune Abnormalities. Boca Raton, FL: CRC Press, 2010.

[28] Bernard S. Autism: A novel form of mercury poisoning. Medical Hypothesis, 2001, 56:4, 462–71.

[29] Bock K. Healing the New Childhood Epidemics: Autism, ADHD, Asthma, and Allergies: The Groundbreaking Program for the 4-A Disorders. New York: Ballantine Books, 2008.

[30] Dorfman K, Lemer PS, Nadler J. What puts a child at risk for developmental delays? Unpublished survey of Developmental Delay Resources (DDR), Pittsburgh, PA, 1995.

[31] Niehaus R, Lord C. Early medical history of children with autism spectrum disorders in a large group-model helath plan. Pediatrics, Oct 2006, 118:4, e1203–11.

[32] Konstantareas M, Homatidis S. Ear infections in autistic and normal children. J Autism Dev Dis, 1987, 17, 585.

[33] Nsouli TM. The role of food allergy in serious otitis media. Ann Allergy, 1991, 66, 91.

[34] Paradise JL, Feldman HM, Campbell TF, Dollaghan CA, Rockette HE, Pitcairn DL, et al. Tympanostomy tubes and developmental outcomes at 9 to 11 years of age. N Engl J Med, Jan 2007, 356:3, 248–61.

[35] Dorfman K. Post-traumatic ear infection syndrome. New Dev, Spring 2004, 9:3, 7.

[36] Haley BE. Toxic overload: Assessing the role of mercury in autism. Mothering, Nov/Dec 2002, 115, 44–6.

[37] Schrock K. Could an Infection Cause Tourette's-Like Symptoms in Teenage Girls? Scientific American, Feb 2, 2012.

[38] The official PANDAS webpage. http://intramural.nimh.nih.gov/pdn/web.htm. Accessed Jan 5, 2012.

[39] Antibodies to Strep Throat Bacteria Connected to Obsessive Compulsive Disorder In Mice. Red Orbit, Aug 11, 2009.

[40] Greenburg E. Treating Lyme Disease. EXPLORE for the Professional, May 2006, 15:3.

[41] Rountree R and Colman C. Immunoitics: Your Personal Immune-boosting program. New York: Perigee, 2000, 37.

[42] Libbey JE, Sweeten TL, McMahon WM, Fujinami RS. Autistic disorder and viral infections. J Neurovirol, Feb 2005, 11:1, 1–10.

[43] Pletnikov MV, Jones ML, Rubin SA, Moran TH, Carbone KM. Rat model of autism spectrum disorders: Genetic background effects on Borna disease virus-induced developmental brain damage. Ann NY Acad Sci, Jun 2001, 939, 318–19.

[44] Swisher CN, Swisher L. Letter: Congenital rubella and autistic behavior. N Engl J Med, Jul 1975, 293:4, 198.

[45] Caruso JM, et al. Persistent preceding focal neurologic deficits in children with chronic Epstein-Barr virus encephalitis. J Child Neurol, Dec 2000, 15:12, 791–96.

[46] Ghaziuddin M, Tsai LY, Eilers L, Ghaziuddin N. Brief Report: Autism and Herpes Simplex Encephalitis. Jrl Autism and Developmental Disorders, 1992, 22:1, 107–113.

[47] Bradstreet JJ, El Dahr J, Anthony A. Detection of measles virus genomic RNA in cerebrospinal fluid of children with regressive autism, a report of three cases. Jrl Amer. physicians and surgeons, Summer 2004, 9:2, 38–45; Singh VK, Lin SX, Yang VC. Serological association of measles virus and human herpes virus-6 with brain auto-antibodies in autism. Clin Immunol and Immunopath, Oct 1998, 89:1, 105–8.

[48] Martin WJ. Complex intracellular inclusions in the brain of a child with a stealth virus encephalopathy. Experimental and Molecular Pathology, 2003, 74, 197–209.

[49] Institute of Medicine. Adverse effects of vaccines: Evidence and causality. Washington, DC: National Academies Press, 2011.

[50] Kirby D. Evidence of Harm: Mercury in vaccines and the autism epidemic, a medical controversy. New York: St. Martin's Press, 2005.

[51] Habakus L, Holland M. Vaccine Epidemic: How corporate greed, biased science, and coercive government threaten our human rights, our health, and our children. New York: Skyhorse Publishing, 2011.

[52] Geier DA, Hooker BS, Kern JK, King PG, Sykes LK, Geier MR. A two-phase study evaluating the relationship between Thimerosal-containing vaccine administration and the risk for an autism spectrum disorder diagnosis in the United States. Transl Neurodegener, Dec 2013, 2:1, 25.

[53] James SJ, Slikker W, Melnyk S, New E, et al. Thimerosal neurotoxicity is associated with glutathione depletion: Protection with glutathione precursors. Neurotoxicity, 2005, 26, 1–8.

[54] Parran DK, Barker A, M Ehrich. Effects of Thimerosal on NGF signal transduction and cell death in neuroblastoma cells. Toxicol Sci, 2005, 86:1, 132–140.

[55] Herbert MR. Autism: A brain disorder, or a disorder that affects the brain? Clinical Neuropsychiatry, 2005, 2:6, 354–79.

[56] Haley BE. Mercury toxicity: Genetic susceptibility and synergistic effects. Medical Veritas, 2005, 2, 535–42.

[57] DeLong G. A positive association found between autism prevalence and childhood vaccination uptake across the US population. J Toxicol Environ Health, 2001, Part A, 74, 903–16.

[58] Tomljenovic L, Shaw CA. Do aluminum vaccine adjuvants contribute to the rising prevalence of autism? J Inorg Biochem, Nov 2011, 105:11, 1489–99.

[59] Grotto I, Mandel Y, Ephros M, Ashkenazi I, Shemer J. Major adverse reactions to yeast-derived hepatitis B vaccines—a review. Vaccine, 1998, 16, 329–34.

[60] Young A. Georgia girl helps link autism to childhood vaccines. http://www.ajc.com/health/content/health/stories/2008/03/06/autism_0306.html. Accessed Jan 19, 2012.

[61] Burney L. Boost Your Child's Immune System: A Program and Recipes for Raising Strong, Healthy Kids. New York: Newmarket Press, 2005.

[62] Price WA. Nutrition and Physical Degeneration. La Mesa, CA: The Price-Pottenger Nutrition Found, 1997, 157.

[63] Shabo Y, Barzel R, Margoulis M, Yagil R. Camel milk for food allergies in children. IMAJ, 2005, 7, 796–98.

[64] Yagil R. Camel Milk and Autoimmune Diseases. Historical Medicine, 2004.

[65] Shabo Y, Yagil R. Etiology of autism and camel milk as therapy. International Journal on Disability and Human Development, 2005, 4:2, 67–70.

[66] Al-Ayadhi LY, Elamin NE. Camel Milk as a Potential Therapy as an Antioxidant in Autism Spectrum Disorder (ASD). Evid Based Complement Alternat Med, 2013, 602834.

[67] Galland L. Superimmunity for kids: What to Feed Your Children to Keep Them Healthy Now, and Prevent Disease in Their Future. New York: Dell, 1989.

[68] Glaser G. What if Vitamin D Deficiency is a Cause of Autism. Scientific American, Apr 29, 2009.

[69] Minneapolis Somali Autism Spectrum Disorder Prevalence Project. http://rtc. umn.edu/autism/. Accessed Dec 23, 2013.

[70] Gong ZL, Luo CM, Wang L, Shen L, et al. Serum 25-hydroxyvitamin D levels in Chinese children with autism spectrum disorders. Neuroreport, Oct 1, 2013.

[71] Koaovska E, Fernell E, Billstedt E, Minnis H, et al. Vitamin D and autism: Clinical review. Res. Dev Disabil, Sep–Oct 2012, 33:5, 1541–50.

[72] Jepson B. Changing the course of autism. Boulder, CO: Sentient Publications, 2007, 235.

[73] Kelly GS. Bovine colostrums: A review of clinical uses. Altern Med Rev, Nov 2003, 8:4, 378–94.

[74] Kleinsmith A. Colostrum for Autism. http://EzineArticles.com/3955895, Accessed Jan 10, 2012.

[75] Fudenberg HH. Dialyzable lymphocyte extract (DLyE) in infantile onset autism: A pilot study. Biother, 1996, 9:1–2, 143–7.

[76] Markowitz DM. Quiet victories: A journey towards health and wellness: A quarterly newsletter. www.shirleys-wellness-cafe.com. Accessed Jan 10, 2012.

[77] Hennen W. Transfer factor: Natural immune booster. Orem, UT: Woodland Publishing, 1998.

[78] Boris M, Goldblatt A, Edelson S. Improvement in children treated with intravenous gamma globulin. J Nutr Environmental Med, Dec 2006, 15:4, 1–8.

[79] Rivera K. Healing the Symptoms Known as Autism, 2nd ed. E-book, 2014.

[80] Teitelbaum J, Nambudripad JS, Tyson Y, Chen M, et al. Improving Communication Skills in Children With Allergy-related Autism Using Nambudripad's Allergy Elimination Techniques: A Pilot Study. Integrative Medicine, Oct/Nov 2001, 10:5, 36–43.

[81] Nambutripad D. Say Good-Bye to Allergy Related Autism. Los Angeles, CA: Delta Publishers, 1999.

[82] Cutler EW. The Food Allergy Cure: A New Solution to Food Cravings, Obesity, Depression, Headaches, Arthritis, and Fatigue. New York: Three Rivers Press, 2003.

[83] Shrader WA. Enzyme Potentiated Desensitzation: American EPD Society Patient Instruction Booklet. Santa Fe, NM: American EPD Society, 1997.

[84] Ingels D. Allergy Desensitization: An Effective Alternative Treatment for Autism. In Lyons T, Siri K, McIlwain, Arranga T. Cutting Edge therapies for Autism. New York: Skyhorse Publishing, 2012.

[85] Gordon G, Yasko A. The Puzzle of Autism: Putting it All Together. Matrix Development Pub., 2004.

[86] Trevathan E. Seizures and epilepsy among children with language regression and autistic spectrum disorders. J Child Neurol, Aug 2004, 19 Suppl 1, S49–57.

[87] Tuchman R, Rapin I. Epilepsy in autism. Lancet Neurol, Oct 2002, 6, 352–58.

[88] Matsuo M, Maeda T, Ishii K, Tajima D, Koga M, Hamasaki Y. Characterization of childhood-onset complex partial seizures associated with autism spectrum disorder. Epilepsy Behav, Mar 2011, 3, 524–27.

[89] Theoharides TC, Zhang B. Neuro-Inflammation, Blood-Brain Barrier, Seizures and Autism. J Neuro-inflammation, Nov 2011, 8:1, 68.

[90] Elchaar GM, Maisch NM, Augusto LM, Wehring HJ. Efficacy and safety of naltrexone use in pediatric patients with autistic disorder. Ann Pharmacother, Jun 2006, 40:6, 1086–95.

[91] Woeller K. Autism: The benefits of low dose naltrexone. http://drkurtwoeller. blogspot.com/2009/01/autism-benefits-of-low-dose-naltrexone.html. Accessed Jan 12, 2012.

[92] www.lowdosenaltrexone.org. Accessed Dec 23, 2013.

[93] Boris M, Kaiser CC, Goldblatt A, Elice MW, et al. Effect of pioglitazone treatment on behavioral symptoms in autistic children. Journal of Neuroinflammation, 2007, 4:3.

[94] Granpeesheh D, Tarbox J, Dixon DR, Wilke AE, et al. Randomized trial of hyperbaric oxygen therapy for children with autism. Research in Autism Spectrum Disorders, Nov 2009; Rossignol DA, Rossignol LW, James SJ, Melnyk S, Mumper E. The effects of hyperbaric oxygen therapy on oxidative stress, inflammation, and symptoms in children with autism: An open-label pilot study. BMC Pediatrics, 2007, 7:36.

[95] Curcumin (Turmeric) Suppresses Inflammation and Pain. http://curcumin-turmeric.net/inflammation.html. Accessed Jan 12, 2012.

CHAPTER 6

The Endocrine System:
Hormones and Autism

Outsmarting autism is *so* complicated! The gut is healing, inflammation is lessening, and behaviors are gradually changing. Maybe a child is a little more responsive, speaking more frequently. Grandma, who doesn't see him every day, notices that he seems happier. What else could be going on?

After boosting immunity and lowering inflammation, the next step is dealing with endocrine and hormone disruption. Chapter 2 enumerated the frightening number of chemicals that can set off a cascade of unnatural reactions that interfere with the synthesis, transport, binding, and action of hormones. Disruption in any aspect of hormonal function during any stage of life, especially during the first two years, can impair normal brain development. Cheer up! Ongoing research is making it more and more possible to know what to do. First, a short course on the endocrine system.

Endocrine System 101

The endocrine system is a convoluted network of glands that regulate many of the body's organs and functions such as growth, development, mood, metabolism, immunity, and reproduction. (What else is there?) The hypothalamus, pituitary, thyroid, adrenals, ovaries, testes, pancreas, and thymus are the endocrine glands that release minute amounts of molecules called hormones.

Human hormones are too numerous to list. Some, like estrogen, testosterone, and insulin, are well-known; others, such as melatonin and oxytocin, are becoming more familiar as scientists gain knowledge about their roles in sleep and feelings of well-being. Appropriate hormone levels are critical for controlling and regulating all of the above functions throughout the lifespan. Hormones flow into the bloodstream and fluid surrounding the cells along with chemicals from the environment and nutrients from foods.

"Neurotransmitters" are what scientists call the chemical messengers that do their jobs at nerve endings and synapses. The names of some neurotransmitters, such as serotonin, dopamine, norepinephrine, and epinephrine (adrenaline), are also entering the lay vocabulary with increasing frequency as medical professionals check their levels in patients presenting with mood swings, learning problems, disrupted sleep, and autistic symptoms. Unremitting biological and environmental stress from toxic heavy metals, chemicals, viruses, and other immune aggravators can produce a chronic state of neurotransmitter imbalance.

Let's look at some of the endocrine organs and the hormones they secrete. Further in the chapter we will examine their role in autism spectrum disorders. The importance of these organs and glands varies among individuals, so the order presented here is random. What is significant, though, is that the relationship among organs and hormones is **so** complex that over-simplification is necessary in this short introduction.

The *hypothalamus* and its companion, *the pituitary*, sit side-by-side in the middle of the brain. This team has many important functions: they stimulate the thyroid gland, produce the hormones oxytocin and vasopressin, and regulate several others. When the hypothalamus and the pituitary detect low levels of thyroid hormones in the blood, they tell the thyroid to produce more thyroid hormone.

The hypothalamus and pituitary are also responsible for controlling body temperature, hunger, thirst, appetite, circadian rhythms (day/ night cycling), and emotions. Pretty important, wouldn't you say? If toxins alter their ability to produce hormones, any or all of those functions can be "off."

Oxytocin (Oxt) is a hormone that signals, modulates, synchronizes, and sensitizes the body's cells to communicate and work with each other. Oxt bridges communication between the physical body, its energetic fields, and emotions.[1] It plays a major role in childbirth, when the hypothalamus and pituitary work together to produce and release large amounts during labor to facilitate birth, and afterwards in letdown, when milk is released into the breasts. Scientists are now investigating oxytocin's role in many behaviors and emotions.

Vasopressin (VP) is a hormone that enhances muscle tone, peer bonding and memory. It is also known as the "antidiuretic hormone" (ADH) because it increases water permeability and absorption in the collecting ducts of the kidneys. Like Oxt, most of ADH is stored in the pituitary, where its release plays an important role in social behavior and bonding.

The *thyroid* is a butterfly-shaped gland that lives in the front of the neck, attached to the lower part of the larynx (voice box) and to the upper part of the windpipe. Its name comes from the Greek word for "shield" because its main role is protecting the body from toxins, especially radiation. In today's toxic world, thyroid cancers have more than doubled since the early 1970s, making it the fastest-growing cancer in the United States.[2]

The thyroid receives chemical messages from the pituitary and hypothalamus, signaling when to produce its own hormones. The thyroid must have sufficient iodine to do its job properly; too little iodine disrupts thyroid function. Any iodine will do—if it is unable to get adequate supplies from food or water, it takes it from the air. Families living adjacent to nuclear reactors or power plant disaster sites are given iodine supplements to supercharge their thyroids so that this gland does not absorb radioactive iodine from the reactors.

Research is extremely strong confirming that a pregnant mother's thyroid function is a factor in the health of her unborn baby. See the next section on what is thought to happen to the thyroid in babies later diagnosed with autism.

The *adrenal glands*, vital to our body's response to stress, are a pair of endocrine glands that are located on top of the kidneys. Their name denotes their location: *ad* is Latin for "near," and *renes* for "kidneys." The adrenals produce the hormones cortisol, epinephrine, and norepinephrine in response to stress.

Cortisol is classified as a glucocorticoid because its primary job is to raise blood sugar and to turn down immune activity. Proper regulation of glucocorticoids is essential for normal brain development, especially affecting an individual's vigilance and cognition. Cortisol also prevents the release of substances that cause inflammation. Cortisol levels vary during a 24-hour cycle: they peak in the early morning, double after waking, fall during the day, and bottom out three to five hours after falling asleep, or midnight to four a.m.

Epinephrine, *norepinephrine*, and *dopamine* are catecholamines, another category of neurotransmitters. The adrenal glands manufacture epinephrine and norepinephrine in response to fight-or-flight; both are critical for attention and focus. Dopamine acts in concert with other neurotransmitters to enhance many functions, including motor control, arousal, and motivation. Dopamine inhibits norepinephrine release.

In addition, the adrenal glands produce most of the body's **dehydroepiandrosterone, (DHEA)**, which is also made in the brain and skin. Low DHEA levels are a sign of chronic stress. DHEA is a steroid hormone that boosts immunity by preventing the destruction of tryptophan, thus increasing the production of serotonin. Low DHEA, low immunity. Low DHEA, low tryptophan. Low DHEA, low serotonin.

Tryptophan is one of the amino acids that the body uses to synthesize proteins. It is well-known as the ingredient in turkey that makes everyone drowsy after a traditional Thanksgiving meal. Another food source of tryptophan is quinoa, a gluten-free grain that can raise melatonin production and thus improve sleep quality.

Serotonin is a neurotransmitter that affects many basic psychological functions, such as mood and anxiety in interaction with many other neurotransmitters, including tryptophan and dopamine. It is not produced by an endocrine gland, but rather by the brain and in the gut. Thus, dysbiosis and gut inflammation can disrupt its production. The link is a TH2 cell called Interleukin 13, a mediator of allergic inflammation that is implicated in bowel disease.[3]

Estrogens are hormones, secreted mostly by the ovaries, that stimulate and control female characteristics. Some foods, including soy, are estrogenic, which means they can raise the body's supply of estrogen, resulting in more female features and traits.[4]

Testosterone, mainly from the testes, is an androgen—a hormone that stimulates and controls the development and maintenance of male characteristics. Mercury is androgenic and raises the body's testosterone levels, resulting in more masculine features and traits.

Melatonin, a hormone that is produced in every cell of the body and secreted by the pineal gland, is an antioxidant for the brain. Remember the vital importance of antioxidants in health. Melatonin is essential in the sleep cycle because it monitors circadian rhythms by inducing drowsiness, lowering body temperature, and calming the nervous system. Its supplementation for insomnia is well documented.[5]

The pineal gland needs darkness to secrete melatonin. Klinghardt believes that many individuals with sleep disorders have melatonin deficiency because the pineal gland is not getting the darkness it requires. In addition, excessive exposure to electromagnetic fields (EMFs) disturbs the pineal gland's production of melatonin.

The interaction between the endocrine glands and the hormones they excrete, as well as interaction among the body's organ systems, the foods we eat, and the chemicals in the environment, is extremely complex. Some believe that what we call "autism" is perhaps the outcome of very confused hormones.[6]

Endocrine and Hormone Disruption in Autism

According to naturopathic physician Jared Skowron, endocrine disruption probably begins prenatally as babies are conceived, carried by, and born to parents whose egg and sperm cohabit with endocrine-disrupting toxins.[7] When a pregnant woman's body detects the presence of toxins such as pesticides, plastics, and metals, it acts to remove the offenders. The deeper the toxins are in the tissues, the stronger it tries, putting additional stress on the mother's body.

As stress increases, cortisol levels rise, other endocrine production must adjust, and a cascade of hormonal reactions begins. In children later diagnosed with ASD, a mother's melatonin production decreases, altering her circadian rhythms. Serotonin—melatonin's precursor—diminishes, contributing to this dysregulation. Hypothalamic-pituitary dysfunction is next, leading eventually to low production of thyroid hormones.[8]

Weak thyroid function is very common among mothers of children later diagnosed with autism.[9] Raphael Kellman, MD is a New York internist specializing in autism who believes that many children with ASDs have inherited thyroid dysfunction that health care professionals can miss by running only routine blood testing. After treatment for their low thyroid, these children experienced significant improvement in focus, speech, eye contact, interaction, attention, cognition, and mood.[10]

Following a baby's birth, early infant vaccinations, as we learned in the last chapter, alter immune response. Resulting gut problems, inflammation in other organ systems, and further endocrine disruption put additional stress on the developing nervous system, adding to the developing child's Total Load.

Almost imperceptibly, an initially "perfect" baby begins to experience minor illnesses. If vaccination proceeds according to schedule, the baby begins drinking cow's milk, and toxic exposure continues, soon sleep becomes disrupted and the child gets "sicker." Gastrointestinal problems followed by significant respiratory distress are the next stages as overall health deteriorates. Antibiotics for ear or other infections, sometimes administered prophylactically, add further stress to the immune system. As stressors on all systems increase, an autism diagnosis is inevitable.

Puberty can be a stage of significant endocrine dysfunction in autism. Precocious puberty is common in males with autism because high testosterone levels and mercury exposure traceable to thimerosal in vaccines are an unhealthy combination.[11] High testosterone levels may be the answer to why so many more individuals with autism are male than female. The potentially volatile combination of testosterone and mercury might also explain why so many children with autism develop seizures in adolescence.

High testosterone is a little-known cause of precocious puberty.[12] Mark Geier, MD, a geneticist, and his son David found that approximately 80% of boys and girls with autism experienced precocious puberty. Females with autism are affected by hormone disruption at puberty as well. Curiously, affected girls seem to have even higher testosterone levels than the affected boys, leading the Geiers to conclude that high testosterone was necessary to overcome the naturally protective effects of estrogen.[13] One study showed both testosterone-related medical conditions and delayed puberty in women with high-functioning autism and their mothers.[14]

Paralleling thyroid imbalance in autism is extreme adrenal dysregulation. Cortisol production becomes deficient, and adrenocorticotropin hormone (ACTH) production rises significantly due to imbalanced melatonin and ACTH.[15] Two common symptoms of ASD, hypersensitivity and insomnia, have a strong connection to this imbalance in the adrenal system.

British researchers have found that some individuals with high-functioning autism do not experience expected morning cortisol peaks.[16] In fact, their cycles are quite atypical, sometimes reaching peak levels in the middle of the night. This could account for their sleeping difficulties. Theoharis Theoharides, MD, at Tufts University is emerging as the researcher in this area, and he is just beginning to unravel the complexities of how some glucocorticoids are affecting those with autism.[17]

Balancing Hormones

Review the chart of medications that doctors prescribe for those with ASD in the first chapter (table 1.1). Antidepressants like Abilify, Luvox, Paxil, Prozac, Tofranil, and Zoloft are "serotonin-uptake inhibitors," which means they allow the body to recycle (rather than use up) its precious supplies of serotonin to fight depression. Stimulants like Adderall, Cylert, and Ritalin increase levels of the fight-or-flight neurotransmitters norepinephrine and dopamine. Instead of relying on drugs, which can have deleterious side effects, many health care practitioners are prescribing hormones and their precursors for those with ASD.

Melatonin

High on the list of prescribed hormones is melatonin because it addresses both the devastating sleep problems rampant in this population and the toll it takes on both the child and the family. In a study of over one hundred children with autism, melatonin was beneficial in improving sleep in over half. Dosages range from one to six milligrams, starting low and working up if needed, given a half-hour before bedtime. Melatonin was found to be safe, with only one child showing worsening of sleep.[18] Melatonin is available as a liquid, so it is easy for children to take.

SAMe, Tryptophan, and 5HTP

Dr. Amy Yasko, an autism specialist in Maine, has delved deeply into neurotransmitter anomalies in autism. Her testing often shows results of excessive norepinephrine, for which she suggests S-adenosyl methionine (SAMe, pronounced "sammy"). SAMe assists in changing neurotransmitters into other substances. It helps convert serotonin into melatonin, and norepinephrine into epinephrine (adrenaline).[19]

Another option is supplementing tryptophan and 5-hydroxytryptophan (**5HTP**), which combine and convert to serotonin. Dr. Skowron, cited above, combines melatonin with zinc and the above serotonin precursors to rebalance circadian cortisol rhythms. He also recommends the herb holy basil (ocinum sanctae) to even out cortisol spikes.

Oxytocin Supplementation

A review of the literature shows more than one hundred articles on oxytocin supplementation for autism in the past two years, many of them positive. Oxytocin, sometimes called the "anti-stress hormone" is, in fact, one of the hottest topics in autism research right now.[20]

Psychiatrist Martha Welch, MD, a specialist in bonding relationships, believes that autism results from the dysregulation of oxytocin combined with oxidative stress in the gut, which disrupts the whole gut-brain network.[21] Supplementing oxytocin in those with autism decreases their social anxiety and increases social behaviors, including trust, empathy, eye contact, generosity, facial recognition, and bonding. At the end of 2013, a hot-off-the-press, multi-national study in the Proceedings of the National Academy of Sciences confirmed the role of OXTR, the gene that encodes the receptor for oxytocin, not only in social interactions such as mother-infant bonding, but also in the ability to recognize faces.[22]

A deficiency of oxytocin could explain many of the symptoms and behaviors of those on the spectrum. However, the big, important question is, why would individuals with autism have too little?

The oxytocin-Pitocin connection. The answer appears to stem from something that happened at birth: OXTR has been turned off.[23] By what? Pitocin, the synthetic oxytocin often administered to induce and accelerate labor.

Veteran autism researcher Eric Hollander, MD, of New York's Mount Sinai School of Medicine discovered that while only about 20% of all births are assisted by Pitocin, 60% of the patients with autism in his clinic had been exposed to Pitocin in the womb. Significant or just a coincidence? You decide. Is Pitocin during childbirth a load factor in autism?

Hollander has tracked 58,000 children whose mothers' procedures were monitored during pregnancy. The oxytocin/Pitocin connection could be a perfect example of epigenetics in action: In genetically vulnerable infants, administering Pitocin at a critical time when the brain is still developing could down-regulate the oxytocin system, leading to developmental problems. To test this hypothesis, Hollander and his colleagues supplemented oxytocin and found that it consistently reduced repetitive behaviors in his patients with autism.[24]

Another theory is that Pitocin interferes with the natural rhythms of birth and can cause enormous pressure on the baby's brain and cranial nerves during the birthing process, compromising the developing nervous system[25]. If that is true, any baby enduring a Pitocin-assisted delivery would benefit from the therapies for structural impediments and birth trauma described in chapter 8.

One more problem with Pitocin: a 2009 study shows that administering Pitocin during labor decreases glutathione (GSH) levels in newborns.[26] Read more about the essential role of GSH in detoxification in the next chapter.

Recall that oxytocin appears to stimulate receptors in the regions of the brain that involve social memory and social affiliation. More recent work with intranasal oxytocin by the Hollander team and others in Australia showed additional positive effects, including heightened ability to recognize emotions and show empathy.[27] Dr. Angela Sirigu, an Italian neuroscientist, and her team at the Centre de Neuroscience Cognitive in Lyon, France, further confirmed that inhalation of oxytocin holds significant therapeutic potential for autistic and other individuals with impaired social skills to interact more effectively.[28]

A large-scale study called SOARs-B, for "**S**tudy of **O**xytocin in **A**utism to Improve **R**eciprocal **S**ocial **B**ehaviors," is using nasal oxytocin versus a placebo on children and adolescents age 3 to 17. Funded by Autism Speaks, it is a joint project of University of North Carolina School of Medicine, Massachusetts General Hospital, Vanderbilt University, and Seattle Children's Hospital. Results should be interesting.

Oxytocin is delivered as either sublingual drops or in a nasal spray. The spray is absorbed into the bloodstream more rapidly. Both deliveries last for two to three hours. For longer, more lasting effects, some practitioners are prescribing homeopathic oxytocin after a couple of months on the medical product. Stay tuned!

Oxytocin and secretin. In her research mentioned above, psychiatrist Martha Welch, MD, has studied oxytocin and its interaction with yet another hormone, secretin. This hormone, a neuropeptide produced by the stomach that aids in regulating gastric function, is also intimately involved in many activities of the brain, including the production and utilization of the neurotransmitter serotonin.

Secretin supplementation was hyped in the late 1990s when Victoria Beck, the mother of a boy with autism, requested an upper-GI procedure to find the cause of her son's severe diarrhea and gut pain. Immediately following the procedure, which included an infusion of secretin, her son, who had not spoken in months, startled everyone by speaking coherently. Many were hopeful that by replenishing secretin in those with autism, language delays and difficulties with relatedness could be reversed.

Secretin, as a supplement, went out of favor after a negative research report by its manufacturer, but still the demand for natural secretin was great. However, the FDA banned its use, shut down the lab that produced it, and created secretin as a prescription drug in a transdermal form that required approval by the US Department of Agriculture. The drug never seemed to have the same effect as the original natural secretin. Today secretin is available in a homeopathic form.

Recently, Turkish investigators have shown that oxytocin could possibly be helpful in ameliorating gut inflammation.[29] Oxytocin and secretin taken together may be the magic combination for resolving both the chronic gastrointestinal and social-emotional issues in some children with autism. Another area worth following.

Estrogen and Testosterone

In the body DHEA breaks down into the more well-known hormones estrogen and testosterone. It should therefore be no surprise that some individuals with autism have low DHEA levels. Increasing DHEA levels can actually reduce high cortisol levels and, thus, chronic stress.

Several scientists have concluded that high testosterone levels are a load factor in both males and females with autism. Neuroscientist C. Sue Carter, PhD, from The Brain-Body Center at the University of Illinois at Chicago has studied the implications of depressed oxytocin and vasopressin (VP) in autism spectrum disorders.[30] VP levels are dependent on testosterone and are thus of particular importance to male behavior. Carter believes that disruptions in the VP system, which result from epigenetic modifications during early development, could contribute to the vulnerability of males for ASD.

British researcher Simon Baron-Cohen studied 235 mother-child pairs over eight years, periodically giving the children questionnaires designed to measure autistic traits. None of the children in the study received an autism diagnosis, but Baron-Cohen found that those who had been exposed to higher testosterone levels in the womb — measured via amniocentesis during pregnancy — had a greater chance of displaying autistic traits.[31]

A study headed by George Washington University researcher Valerie Hu, PhD, revealed that the excess testosterone in individuals with autism suppresses a gene called RORA, which hinders aromatase, an enzyme it produces from converting testosterone to estrogen. The excess levels of testosterone both stifle the presence of the gene and increase the likelihood of autism.[32] These findings were duplicated by Chinese investigators.[33]

Now the controversy begins. The Geiers believe that mercury also raises testosterone levels, and that the high levels of testosterone block the body's ability to make glutathione, which is necessary for detoxification (see the next chapter). Furthermore, mercury binds to glutathione, thus inactivating whatever stores the body may already have.

The Geiers prescribed the drug Lupron "off-label" to lower testosterone levels in autism patients like Wesley, the son of the Reverend Lisa Sykes. Lupron is approved by the FDA for treating precocious puberty. Tests showed that Wesley's already-high testosterone levels were pushed from "the stratosphere into orbit" by additional testosterone production in puberty.[34] To many parents, including Wesley's mother, it made sense that adolescent seizures and aggressive behavior were related to the high testosterone. They were ecstatic as their son's testosterone levels dropped, and his seizures and aggressive behavior lessened.[35]

However, authorities were not amused by the Geiers' off-label use of Lupron, and they accused them of "chemically castrating" their young patients. In 2011, authorities suspended Mark Geier's license to practice medicine in several states.[36] Dr. Geier is fighting the suspension of his medical license and believes that his practice should be judged on the very positive results parents report. Without Lupron, many of the adolescents and young adults who showed extreme aggression would probably have required psychotropic drug intervention and even institutionalization.

Endocrine and Hormone Testing

Thyroid and cortisol testing are essential for both treatment and monitoring. Testing of other hormones such as melatonin can be helpful. If an individual with autism is showing aggression, testing for the total catecholamines, including dopamine, epinephrine, and norepinephrine, is also strongly recommended. This is because a subset of children with autism possess an aberrant enzyme that affects catecholamine neurotransmitters, causing neurotransmitter imbalances altering mood, attention, and activity.[37] Different labs offer different panels; one that specializes in this type of testing is NeuroSciences at www.neurorelief.com.

Take-Home Points

The more researchers explore dysfunction in and interaction among the nervous, immune, digestive, and endocrine systems in those with autism, the more they are convinced that autism is a biologically-based disorder. Identifying which hormones are disrupted and balancing them requires careful testing, history-taking, and observation. As endocrine dysregulation lessens, so do gut problems, inflammation, and day-to-day issues such as sleep, eating, and behavioral concerns.

The neuro-endocrine issues in autism are far-reaching and include not only estrogen and testosterone, but also lesser-known hormones such as oxytocin and cortisol, as well as neurotransmitters including melatonin, serotonin, dopamine, norepinephrine, and epinephrine. As doctors begin to understand interactions, new protocols are emerging for treatment.

The next chapter focuses on detoxification. Understanding why children with autism are so sick is not just about what they are exposed to, but also why their bodies are unable to rid themselves of the toxins and deleterious bugs. Onto methylation and sulfation: getting the bad stuff out!

---

[1] Klinghardt D. Medicine 2012: New Symptoms, New Causes, New Treatments. Warren, NJ: Klinghardt Academy, 2012.

[2] Davies L, Welch HG. Increasing incidence of thyroid cancer in the United States, 1973–2002.
JAMA. May 2006, 295:18, 2164–67.

[3] Shajib MS, Wang H, Kim JJ, Sunjic I, Ghia JE, et al. Interleukin 13 and Serotonin: Linking the Immune and Endocrine Systems in Murine Models of Intestinal Inflammation. PLoS One, Aug 2013, 8, 8.

[4] Daniels KT. The Whole Soy Story: The dark side of America's favorite health food. Washington, DC: New Trends Pub, 2007.

[5] Buscemi N. Melatonin for treatment of sleep disorders. Evidence Report #108. Prepared for the Agency for Healthcare Research and Quality, US Department of Health and Human Services, 2004.

[6] Tareen RS, Kamboj MK. Role of endocrine factors in autistic spectrum disorders. Pediatr Clin North Am, Feb 2012, 59:1, 75–88.

[7] Skowron JM. Autism and the Endocrine Response. http://www.naturopathydigest.com/archives/2006/oct/skowron.php. Accessed Dec 24, 2013.

[8] Spratt EG, Nicholas JS, Brady KT, Carpenter LA, et al. Enhanced Cortisol Response to Stress in Children in Autism. J Autism Dev Disord, Jan 2012, 42:1, 75–81.

[9] Molloy CA, Morrow AL, Meinzen-Derr J, Dawson G, Bernier R, Dunn M. Familial autoimmune thyroid disease as a risk factor for regression in children with Autism Spectrum Disorder: a CPEA Study. J Autism Dev Disord, Apr 2006, 36:3, 317–24; Roman GC, Ghassabian A, Bongers-Schokking JJ, Jaddoe VW, et al. Association of gestational maternal hypothyroxinemia and increased autism risk. Annals of Neurology, Nov 2013, 74:5, 733–42.

[10] Kellman R. Thyroid Deficiency: Preventing a Metabolic Meltdown. Life Extension Magazine, Sep 2004.

[11] Geier DA, Young HA, Geier MR. Thimerosal Exposure & Increasing Trends of Premature Puberty in the Vaccine Safety Datalink. Indian Journal of Medical Research, 2010, 131, 500–507.

[12] Williams KL. High testosterone in children, Oct 29, 2010. www.livestrong.com. Accessed Mar 18, 2012.

[13] Heckenlively K. Mercury, Testosterone and Autism, a really big idea! Age of Autism, Apr 21, 2008. http://www.ageofautism.com/. Accessed Mar 18, 2012.

[14] Ingudomnukul E, Baron-Cohen S, Wheelwright S, Knickmeyer R. Elevated rates of testosterone-related disorders in women with autism spectrum conditions. Hormones and Behavior, May 2007, 51:5, 597–604.

[15] Curin JM, Terzic J, Petkovic ZB, Zekan L, Terzic IM, Susnjara IM. Lower cortisol and higher ACTH levels in individuals with autism. J Autism Dev Disord, Aug 2003, 33:4, 443–8.

[16] Brosnan M, Turner-Cobb J, Munro-Naan Z, Jessop D. Absence of a normal cortisol awakening response (CAR) in adolescent males with Asperger syndrome (AS). Psychoneuroendocrinology, Aug 2009, 34:7, 1095–100.

[17] Theoharides TC, Doyle R, Francis K, Conti P, Kalogeromitros D. Novel therapeutic targets for autism.Trends Pharmacol Sci, Aug 2008, 29:8, 375–82.

[18] Andersen IM, Kaczmarska J, McGrew SG, Malow BA. Melatonin for insomnia in children with autism spectrum disorders. J Child Neurol, May 2008, 23:5, 482–5.

[19] Yasko A. Autism: Pathways to Recovery. http://www.dramyyasko.com/resources/autism-pathways-to-recovery/chapter-2/.

[20] Gurrieri F, Neri G. Defective oxytocin function: A clue to understanding the cause of autism? BMC Med, Oct 2009, 7:63, 22.

[21] Welch MG, Welch-Horan TB, Anwar M, Anwar N, Ludwig RJ, Ruggiero DA. Brain effects of chronic IBD in areas abnormal in autism and treatment by single neuropeptides secretin and oxytocin. J Mol Neurosci, 2005, 25:3, 259–74.

[22] Skuse DH, Lori A, Cubells JF, Lee I. Common polymorphism in the oxytocin receptor gene (OXTR) is associated with human social recognition skills. Proceedings of the National Academy of Sciences. Pub online Dec 23, 2013; doi: 10.1073/pnas.1302985111.

[23] Gregory SG, Connelly JJ, Towers A, Johnson J, et al. Genomic and epigenetic evidence for OXTR deficiency in autism. BMC Medicine, 2009, 7:62.

[24] Hollander E, Novotny S, Hanratty M, Yaffe R, et al. Oxytocin infusion reduces repetitive behaviors in adults with autistic and Asperger's disorders. Neuro-psychopharmacology, Jan 2003, 28:1, 193–98.

[25] Tsimis M. "Study_Finds_Adverse_Effects_of_Pitocin_in_Newborns" Paper delivered at The American College of Obstetricians and Gynecologists , May 7, 2013. https://www.acog.org/About_ACOG/News_Room/News_Releases/2013/. Accessed March 16, 2014.

[26] Schneid-Kofman N, Silberstein T, Saphier O, Shai I, et al. Labor Augmentation with Oxytocin Decreases Glutathione Level. Obstetrics and Gynecology International, 2009, Article #807659.

[27] Hollander E, Bartz J, Chaplin W, Phillips W, et al. Oxytocin increases retention of social cognition in autism. Biol Psychiatry, Feb 2007, 61:4, 498–503; Guastella AJ, Einfeld SL, Gray KM, Rinehart NJ, et al. Intranasal oxytocin improves emotion

recognition for youth with autism spectrum disorders. Biol Psychiatry, Apr 2010, 67:7, 692–94.

[28] Andari E, Duhamel JA, Zalla T, Herbrecht E, Leboyer M, Sirigu A. Promoting social behavior with oxytocin in high-functioning autism spectrum disorders. Proceedings of the National Academy of Sciences, 2010.

[29] Iseri SO, Sener G, Saglam B, Gedik N, et al. Oxytocin ameliorates oxidative colonic inflammation by a neutrophil-dependent mechanism. Peptides, Mar 2005, 26:3, 483–91.

[30] Carter CS. Sex differences in oxytocin and vasopressin: Implications for autism spectrum disorders?
Behav Brain Res, Jan 2007, 176:1, 170–86.

[31] Auyeung B, Taylor K, Hackett G, Baron-Cohen S. Foetal testosterone and autistic traits in 18 to 24-month-old children. Mol Autism, 2010, 1:1, 11.

[32] Sarachana T, Xu M, Wu RC, Hu VW. Sex hormones in autism: Androgens and estrogens differentially and reciprocally regulate RORA, a novel candidate gene for autism. PLoS ONE, Feb 2011, 6:2.

[33] Xu X, Shou X, Li J, Jia M, et al. Mothers of Autistic Children: Lower Plasma Levels of Oxytocin and Arg-Vasopressin and a Higher Level of Testosterone. PLoS One, Sep 2013, 8:9.

[34] Cohn M. Lupron therapy for autism at center of embattled doctor's case: Some parents embrace alternative treatment for autism that scientists don't support. The Baltimore Sun, Jun 16, 2011.

[35] Sykes L. Sacred Spark. Fourth Lloyd Productions, 2009.

[36] Gorski D. Chemical castration of autistic children leads to the downfall of Dr. Mark Geier. Science-based medicine, May 9, 2011.

37 http://www.springboard4health.com/notebook/health_autism2.html. Accessed Jan 9, 2014.

CHAPTER 7

Detoxification:
Getting the Bad Stuff Out

"Detoxification" is a household term today. At last check, a half dozen popular magazines on the newsstand featured this topic, searching Google yielded 15,400,000 hits, and Amazon carried over 1,500 titles including this word. You can detoxify "naturally," "herbally," "quickly," "slowly," "sensibly," "safely," or "organically." It can be a "relief," a "miracle," or even a "transformation."

While mainstream in the public sector, the topic of detoxification as related to healing autism and related disorders is controversial. In fact, it is *so* controversial that even the idea that kids with ASD diagnoses who flap their arms, avoid eye contact, and do not speak are "toxic" has been rejected by many doctors. I have seen parents show the "proof" to their physicians, with before and after lab tests, and still their doctors attribute positive changes to ancillary therapies. We will rarely change the minds of these providers. The best we can do is thank them for their interest and move on to those who are more collaborative.

For parents and professionals who are "believers," focusing on the process of clearing out the bad stuff must wait until the gut is stable. That is why the subject of detoxification does not appear until nearly halfway through this book.

In this chapter, after a simplified explanation of the detoxification process, including the essential role of the antioxidant glutathione, the focus is primarily on detoxification for individuals with autism through a variety of natural methods. First comes a review of the role of important foods, vitamins, and minerals, followed by external methods, such as Epsom salt baths and a sauna. Precautionary detoxification guidelines follow. Next we look at homeopathy and its 200-year-old history of helping the body heal itself. Lastly are some novel energetic detoxification strategies that can rid the body of tangible toxins as well as psychological trauma and past-generational pain.

Detoxification 101

Detoxification is the human body's way of neutralizing, processing, and eliminating poisonous substances. Efficient detoxification is crucial to good health for everyone. It is a natural process occurring regularly in the body. The liver, an extremely complex organ involved in over 300 different functions, does most of the work. The body has several major routes of detoxification: the digestive system through bowel movements and urine, the skin through sweating, and the hair and nails as they grow out. We now know many ways to assist the body's natural detoxification pathways through a variety of means and methods such as foods, herbs, heat, baths, cleansers, and oils.

Detoxification and Microorganisms

The presence of microorganisms such as fungi, molds, bacteria, and viruses complicates the detoxification picture. As a patient detoxifies, microorganisms may proliferate. Poisons such as insecticides and mercury-based thimerosal that we use to terminate these bugs' growth in the outside world have the same effect on our internal ecosystem—but at a price. These poisons harm not just the microorganisms, but also the environment in which they live: the cells of our body. In our body's attempts to maintain homeostasis, it keeps the load of stored toxins equal to the load of pathogenic microorganisms.

Paradoxically, it is the toxin-induced impairment of our immune system that enables the microorganisms to enter our system in the first place. Once established, they are difficult to eradicate, and simply removing the causative toxin is not sufficient; each individual body also needs help with the elimination of the infectious agents.

Historically, this fact is known as the "Milieu theory of Bechamp." It was discovered in the late 1800s by Antoine Bechamp, one of France's most prominent scientists, teachers, and researchers, with degrees in biology, chemistry, physics, pharmacy, and medicine. He hypothesized that viruses and bacteria do not cause disease, but rather the body's condition or "terrain," according to levels of nourishment contamination, is what determines all diseased states.

Today, Dietrich Klinghardt, MD, PhD, who was introduced in earlier chapters, is one of the few doctors in the United States who understands the complex relationship between toxins and microorganisms and why flare-ups of previously hidden infections occur regularly during detoxification. Listen to interviews in which he eloquently describes the process and his treatments on his website at www.klinghardtacademy.com .

Phases of Detoxification

Detoxification takes place in two phases. In their book, *7-Day Detox Miracle*, Bennett and Barrie compare detoxification to a two-phase wash cycle.[1] In **Phase One**, nutrients in the body convert toxins into less-harmful constituents and prepare them for elimination. First, cells must be cajoled into breaking down stored toxins into intermediate forms. Scavengers called antioxidants facilitate by gobbling up free radicals or oxidants produced during this process. A few toxins are ready for removal at this stage, but others need a second wash cycle. If the process stops after phase one, sickness and even death can occur because bad toxins are floating around impeding function in all systems of the body.

Phase Two is the actual elimination phase, during which the body attempts to excrete toxins safely, usually in partnership with an "escort" nutrient. Six steps—methylation, sulfation, acetylation, glutathione conjugation, amino acid conjugation, and glucuronidation—make up phase two detoxification. Five of the six pathways are dependent upon sulfur chemistry. Since this process is so very complicated, it will not be completely covered here. Here are the highlights.

Methylation and Sulfation

A body's strong ability to methylate is the key to detoxification. During methylation, the sulfur amino acid methionine (considered "the queen of amino acids" by Dr. Baker) gives away a methyl group and becomes "horrible homosysteine," a potentially toxic molecule. Homosysteine is then converted to cysteine, a process dependent upon an ample supply of methyl B-12, which many of those with autism lack. Cysteine is one of the raw ingredients for making the body's most powerful antioxidant, glutathione. Read more about this powerhouse of detoxification below.

Proper sulfation requires the pathway to the production of sulfates to be functioning optimally. This pathway takes the amino acid cysteine through numerous steps to make sulfite, which is then processed into sulfate through an enzyme called sulfite oxidase. Many nutrient interactions must take place for this pathway to function properly. Efficient processing of sulfur, deficient in many on the spectrum, is essential for sulfation.

Sulfur molecules are "sticky," allowing cells to adhere to one another.[2] In other words, cells containing sulfur can grab onto heavy metals and other toxins and escort them out of the body. When sulfur metabolism or sulfation is lacking, cells "leak." Leakiness, or excessive permeability creates different problems in different parts of the body. Leakiness in the gut lining, or "leaky gut" is described in chapter 4. Leaky skin creates eczema; leakiness in the joints leads to arthritis; leakiness in mucus membranes creates otitis, sinusitis, and rhinitis.

Efficient sulfation pathways are necessary for the body to break down and remove chemicals called phenols (remember them from chapter 4?) If sulfation pathways are inefficient, phenols build up.[3]

Many of the body's own chemicals are also phenolic, and need the sulfation process to metabolize properly. Hormones, including testosterone, estrogen, DHEA, and others, all require efficient sulfation to maintain proper function.

Defective sulfation results from the combination of an overload of phenolics from foods, an imbalance of both hormones and neurotransmitters, and decreased levels of the enzyme phenol sulfur-transferase (PST). Dr. Rosemary Waring's now-classic findings of low levels of PST in autism are also described in chapter 4.

Glutathione: The Body's Most Powerful Antioxidant

Glutathione (GSH) is created by every cell of the body from three amino acids: cysteine, glycine, and glutamic acid. The body makes about half the GSH it needs. N-Acetyl-Cysteine (NAC), methyl B-12, folinic acid, trimethylglycine (TMG), and vitamin C are all important nutrients for increasing and maintaining healthy glutathione levels in the body by giving it the raw materials to build from.

Glutathione and its cofactors bind with hundreds of environmental toxins, including the metals cadmium, lead, and mercury, dragging them out of the blood to the liver, gall bladder, and gut, through which the body excretes them. When levels of toxins are high, the body's natural store of GSH becomes depleted. As GSH levels fall, the body accepts more heavy metals. Each molecule of a toxin uses up a molecule of glutathione.[4]

A body's glutathione level determines how many toxins it absorbs. Adequate levels of GSH are also necessary for many aspects of immune function. Low levels impair immunity, which leads to frequent infection. The body's poor response to infection causes inflammation and oxidative stress, which, in turn, lowers GSH. A vicious cycle perpetuates when there is inadequate GSH to offset oxidative stress, further reducing immunity and allowing opportunistic infections like yeasts and parasites to proliferate. As GSH levels rise, the body is better able to excrete poisons.[5]

Detoxification and Autism

For those with autism, the detoxification process can be life-changing because many individual load factors fall into the category of "toxicity." Chemicals, metals, food additives, radiation, and non-tangibles, such as abuse, neglect, abandonment, poverty, and other psychological and sociological burdens all require detoxification for healing to take place.

A Perfect Storm: Exposure + Poor Detoxification Pathways = Autism

The main issue for individuals with autism is that the rate at which toxins increase is more rapid than the rate at which the body is able to rid itself of them. Limiting exposures is only half the battle; having efficient detoxification pathways is the other half. Continuous toxic exposure requires continuous detoxification.

Only semipermeable membranes — our skin and mucosal surfaces — separate us from our toxic environment. Staying "clean" requires our inherent detox systems to work overtime against the osmotic pressure of the incoming toxins. As the toxicity of our environment increases, so does the osmotic pressure that pushes poisons into our body.[6]

S. Jill James, PhD, and her colleagues at the University of Arkansas have carried out some game-changing research that has increased our understanding of the genetic and chemical relationships that impair detoxification pathways in autism. James shows that many of those with autism have deficiencies in both cysteine and methyl B-12, thus impeding phase two detoxification without supplementation.

Her team studied blood samples from 95 children with autism and 75 healthy controls, and found that the affected children had significantly lower blood levels of GSH. They believe that the stores of GSH in the children with autism were depleted by their overexposure to mercury, specifically from thimerosal-containing vaccines.

Furthermore, because high levels of oxidative stress are due primarily to low GSH levels, low GSH is an important contributor to the neurological, gastrointestinal, and immune system problems seen in these children. Coupled with high production levels of homocysteine, this combination produces the perfect storm for autism.[7]

Knowing where to start and how to get the bad stuff out is a complicated project that is both an art and a science. Most doctors rely upon copious laboratory testing using some of the blood, stool, hair, and urine tests listed in chapter 2. A couple of additions and alternatives to these tests can also be quite revealing.

Two Unique Methods of Testing

Nutrigenomic testing. Amy Yasko, PhD, ND, is the pioneer of nutrigenomic testing analysis for autism. The name is derived from the fact that once this blood test identifies an individual's genetic mutations or polymorphisms called SNPs (single nucleotide polymorphisms), a nutritional supplementation program can be prescribed.

Some SNPs can impair detoxification and deplete the body of glutathione.[8] One, MTHFR damages methylation, while another, SUOX, damages sulfation. Return to chapter 1 for a review of these genetic mutations. Yasko's individualized protocol bypasses and corrects those SNPs affecting an individual's detoxification pathways, allowing the body's natural detoxification systems to operate properly. This option is one of the most exciting new therapies of the last century!

Frequent retesting is necessary (and expensive!) because the body constantly shifts during the healing process. Results are shared through a large online forum of parents, not with the doctor directly.

Some of the nutrigenomic tests pioneered by Yasko are now being offered by other laboratories. Spectracell, which requires a blood draw, offers MTHFR genotyping at www.spectracell.com, and www.23andme.com offers a unique saliva test. There are five SNPs included in Yasko's testing that are not included in the 23andme results. However, you can enter your 23andme results at www.geneticgenie.org and get a methylation and detox analysis for free.

Autonomic Response Testing (ART). Dietrich Klinghardt, MD, PhD, has co-developed Autonomic Response Testing (ART), a form of muscle testing, or kinesiology, that measures autonomic nervous system stress responses in the body. Unlike most "muscle testing," ART is an extremely accurate, elegant, sophisticated, quick, and comprehensive diagnostic system that is the leading bioenergetic technique in Europe today.

Klinghardt sometimes delays expensive laboratory testing, preferring ART to simply start his patients on a safe, gentle detoxification program of all natural, mild, over-the-counter agents like cilantro and chlorella (see below), and adds stronger agents later if testing indicates. Every couple of months, he might use hair analysis to monitor which metals the body is excreting. Interestingly, he prefers pubic hair (if the patient is old enough) to hair from the head, as it grows more slowly and thus delivers a longer excretion history. His experience is that toxic mineral levels register low at first, and then begin rising, with lead and nickel showing up before mercury.

During ART an examiner pushes on an individual's outstretched arm while touching him in a variety of locations and placing possible antidotes to various toxins near the patient, using special tools that enhance the power of the energetic signal to the outstretched arm. Simultaneously, the body reveals what toxic metals, microorganisms, traumas, or other toxins are stressing the patient, the site of the stress, and which products or procedures are beneficial in relieving the stress. Order all tools and instructional DVDs from www. KlinghardtAcademy.com.

If several antidotes are successful, ART has techniques to determine which one works best. The sum of all the antidotes is the patient's "prescription." For young children, an adult surrogate can act as a circuit between the examiner and the child by touching the child's body while the examiner tests his or her outstretched arm. ART is the only type of muscle testing that can establish a diagnosis and prescribe treatment simultaneously.

Klinghardt recommends using ART to fine-tune the results of laboratory testing or as a stand-alone diagnostic tool to further evaluate toxicity. With proper training, professionals from any discipline can learn to use ART as an adjunct to standard in-office laboratory and diagnostic testing. Like any technique, skillful autonomic response testing requires continuous study, practice, and discipline.

Foods and Supplements for Detoxification

As in healing the gut, the first-choice weapons for detoxification are foods. Some fruits and vegetables are natural detoxifiers because they are highly antioxidant and support the body's detoxification pathways. Some highly detoxifying foods are blueberries, acai berries, and pomegranates; dark leafy green vegetables such as kale, collards, dandelion greens, Swiss chard, and broccoli sprouts; walnuts, hazelnuts, and almonds; green tea and red wine; cloves, cinnamon, and turmeric; and everyone's favorite, dark chocolate. Some of these are contra-indicated on the special diets in chapter 4, so cross-check carefully.

Yasko's patients thrive on vitamin- and mineral-rich foods, including nutrient-dense broths made from organic vegetables and bones of grass-fed animals, raw and fermented dairy products, nut milks, and supplements like vitamin B-12, DMG/TMG, magnesium, zinc, and others. For more specifics about the Yasko protocol, go to www.holisticheal.com or read *Autism Pathways to Recovery*, available on her personal website at www.dramyyasko.com.

Children who are vaccine-injured and who eat only foods such as toast, french fries, and noodles are at an increased risk for gut problems during detoxification. Attempting to rid the body of the toxins that wreaked havoc there in the first place without a healthy gut only wreaks more havoc, especially without therapeutic doses of antioxidants. For successful detox, a child must be eating sufficient protein and a fairly wide variety of foods including a minimum of three to four servings per day of fruits and vegetables, not including juice. Heavy metals are not excreted well when the diet is low in protein.

For children who are progressing well with their therapy programs and whose laboratory tests show high metal levels, ingesting detoxifying foods and supplements may be all that is needed for slow, steady progress. Few have negative reactions to this method, although progress may not be noticeable on a day-to-day basis. Over time, youngsters often become better regulated and more responsive to therapy; language often improves more rapidly. An occasional child shows dramatic developmental gains.

Complementing food are important vitamins, minerals, and natural over-the-counter agents made up of either large quantities of food substances or vitamins and minerals derived from antioxidant foods, which can assist in the mobilization of metals. Even gentle nutritional detoxification using foods and supplements requires strict supervision, and should take place only under the guidance of a health care practitioner.

Supporting Detox with Vitamins and Minerals

All safe heavy metal removal programs should include extra vitamins and minerals. According to nutritionist Kelly Dorfman, adding extra nutrients during detoxification, even with a balanced diet, only makes sense. The poorer the diet, the more nutrients a child needs, even with mild detoxification techniques. A good nutrient program alone naturally encourages detoxification and gentle heavy metal displacement. Antioxidant supplementation alone often jump-starts the body's natural methylation and sulfation mechanisms.[9]

Heavy metal excretion depletes minerals and antioxidants; thus, safe detoxification requires extra nutrients. During the detox process, Klinghardt protects the brain and gut with electrolyte-enhanced drinking water, since many detox agents deplete minerals.

A sample base nutrient program for a child over three includes:

• *Vitamin C* is an extremely safe water-soluble antioxidant that immensely benefits the brain and body in a multitude of ways. Doctors are using it extensively as a detoxification tool. Diarrhea occurs before the body can absorb too much, so there is little concern about toxicity.

• *Vitamin E* is an important fat-soluble antioxidant that many health care professionals are adding to nutritional programs for autism to aid in detoxification. Since cell membranes are basically a layer of fat, vitamin E is important for protecting membrane integrity. It also helps the mitochondria clean up debris for more efficient energy production.

• *Calcium* enhances detoxification as it neutralizes excess aluminum. Individuals with calcium deficiency, perhaps due to a casein-free diet, may be irritable, hyperactive, sleep-disturbed, or inattentive, and may have stomach and muscle cramps and tingling in arms and legs. Though dark green vegetables and almonds are calcium-rich, in practice children rarely eat enough of these foods to cover their calcium needs without supplementation. Calcium must be properly balanced with magnesium, which improves absorption, and can cause loose stools. Dorfman recommends 800–1000 mg per day for children ages one to ten.

• *Magnesium (Mg)*, the eighth most plentiful element on the planet and the fourth most abundant mineral in the body, is essential for over 300 biochemical bodily reactions, including digestion and kidney function. Two major functions of Mg are stabilizing cell membranes and maintaining proper electrical balance. Signs of magnesium deficiency include constipation, hypersensitivity to loud and high-pitched sounds, irritability, muscle cramps and twitches, cold hands and feet, insomnia, and carbohydrate cravings. Mg deficiency is most likely in those who eat many processed foods, overcook foods, and drink soft water. Deficiencies can develop when Mg elimination is increased by taking many medications, like antipsychotics, because these products—as well as alcohol, caffeine, and sugar—leach Mg. Foods high in Mg are avocados, beans, molasses, almonds, Brazil nuts, cashews, pumpkin and sunflower seeds, whole grains, fish, kiwis, and leafy greens, especially spinach.

• *Molybdenum (Mo)* is an essential element in human nutrition whose role was little understood until recently. If a person has the SUOX mutation, then Mo is an especially important supplement because it is vital for the processing of sulfur. Low Mo, poor sulfation. How does one get molybedenum? Some foods contain it. Your best bets are barley, yams, beef kidneys and liver, buckwheat, eggs, leafy ɪs, spinach, sunflower seeds, oats, and potatoes. If that ...'t help, supplementation is necessary. Work closely with a licensed health care professional on this one!

• *Copper (Cu) and Zinc (Zn)* must be balanced carefully. With too much copper and too little zinc, psychiatric symptoms occur. Molybdenum is also important in maintaining the proper Cu/Zn ratio. Research on Cu/Zn imbalances is the work of William Walsh, PhD, an innovative biochemist who reports that 85% of his sample of 603 patients with autism showed a highly statistically significant Cu overload and Zn depletion when compared to typicals matched for age and gender. Imbalanced Cu/Zn impairs the hippocampus and amygdala, which monitor social-emotional function. Patients thus have a biochemical tendency for emotional meltdowns and attentional deficits.[10]

• A comprehensive mineral supplement containing 30 mg of zinc, 100–200 mcg of the strong antioxidant *selenium*, and 2–5 mg of *manganese* is essential. Adequate zinc protects against adverse effects from heavy metals, including lead, cadmium, and copper. To minimize the number of pills try a mineral combination such as Minerall from Kirkman (www.kirkmanlabs.com) or Basic Nutrients Plus from New Beginnings Nutritionals (www.nbnus.com).

• *Essential Fatty Acids (EFAs)* are a crucial part of the structure of the nervous system, which is 60–70% fat. Grandma was correct: take cod liver oil! It is no longer a stinky job because fats now are available in flavored capsules, liquids, and gummies. EFAs must be ingested because the body cannot produce them. The pattern in children with autism is usually a deficiency of omega-3 fatty acids, with elevations of arachidonic acid (an omega-6 fat) and transfatty acids. Symptoms of EFA-deficiency are hair loss, dry or peeling skin, eczema, fatigue, aggression, dry brittle hair, eating disorders, excessive or diminished thirst, gallstones, growth impairment, immune deficiency, hyperactivity, and impaired wound healing.

Essential fats are fragile, and when over-processed or exposed to air, they can become rancid. Old fish oil is worse than no fish oil, as the body must deal with the results of the fish's oxidative stress! Refrigeration can slow deterioration. Quality in fish oils is of utmost importance; make sure they come from mercury-free fish and are soy oil free!

• *Dimethylglycine (DMG) and Trimethylglycine (TMG).* Before his death in 2006, Bernie Rimland, founder of the ARI, followed the use of DMG (Vitamin B-15) in autism for over 25 years and found it to be nontoxic and potentially helpful. TMG, a related substance, has been added recently to the autism vitamin arsenal to improve detoxification pathways.

• *Folinic acid* is often added to antidote to the irritability sometimes caused by DMG or TMG.

• *Vitamin B-12*, also called *cobalamin*, is one of the most important B vitamins for detoxification. Cobalamin comes in several forms; methylcobalamin, the active form of B-12, is the preferred type for detoxification over the less-expensive, more-available cynocobalamin. James Neubrander, MD, in Edison, New Jersey, pioneered injections of pure concentrated methylcobalamin for children with ASDs. He recommends up to 55 mcg/kg twice a week. Injections, unlike oral B-12, bypass the impaired gut and directly feed the nervous system. Klinghardt's preferred method is to deliver methyl B-12 as a nasal spray with or without folinic acid.

Jacqueline McCandless, MD, believes (and Klinghardt agrees) that combining folinic acid with methylcobalamin and sometimes TMG is probably one of the best formulas for kids on the spectrum. This treatment is especially suited to those with a history of thimerosal-containing vaccines and chronically loose stools. When combined with folinic acid, B-12 facilitates the complicated methylation processes important for creating optimum metabolic balance, which eventually allows the body to detoxify itself.

A novel new product is RevitaPOPs — methylcobalamin lollipops developed by autism Dad, Stan Kurtz. Each contains approximately 3.6 mg of methylcobalamin suspended in five grams of organic evaporated cane juice, which is a natural and wholly unrefined sweetener. Find them at www.revitapop. com.

• *Alpha lipoic acid (ALA)* is an antioxidant that neutralizes free radicals and has the unique characteristic of being able to function in both water and fat.[11] It is thus able to replenish antioxidants such as vitamin C and glutathione after they have been depleted. ALA also aids in the formation of glutathione.[12] It is plentiful in spinach, broccoli, peas, brewer's yeast, brussel sprouts, rice bran, and organic meats.

Dorfman suggests starting nutrients one at a time, three days apart, and carefully monitoring reactions, the most common of which is irritability. Sometimes parents must design creative ways to get supplements into picky kids. Oils mix well into puddings and apple- or pearsauce. Sometimes just holding the nose and biting the bullet, with a great reward for compliance, is the easiest method!

Andrew Cutler, PhD, an expert in mercury toxicity related to dental amalgams, has a detoxification protocol of nutrients that is becoming increasingly popular for those with autism. He recommends dividing supplements into four doses a day because the body can only absorb water-soluble vitamins and minerals in limited doses; giving them all at once could be both wasteful and harmful. In addition to the above nutrients, Cutler also suggests in some cases supplementing with glycine, taurine, lecithin, carotenes, and lypocenes.[13]

Glutathione Supplementation

Dr. Jill James is one of the major proponents of glutathione (GSH) supplementation along with methyl B-12. In James's study, those on this combination showed both improved speech and levels of cognition.[14]

Supplementing GSH in combination with TMG, folinic acid, methionine, methyl B-12, and the essential nutrients like zinc, magnesium, taurine, and others, can assist in breaking down and releasing stored toxins. Infants and toddlers with colic, diarrhea, or constipation and children with suspected vaccine damage and heavy metal exposure are prime candidates for this treatment.

Essential Glutathione™, a liquid that surrounds the GSH with fat droplets called liposomes, is the delivery method of choice by many physicians today. Preliminary studies suggest that liposomes optimize absorption by protecting the GSH from oxidation. Essential Glutathione™ is available without prescription from Wellness Pharmacy (www.wellnesshealth.com; 800–227–2627). Give ¼ tsp. twice daily per 30 pounds of body weight, always starting with a smaller dose in sensitive children. Ongoing feedback from parents is available at the Wellness Pharmacy website.

Intravenous (IV) GSH is also quite popular, although using needles with children who have sensory problems can be challenging. GSH is also available nebulized, as a nasal spray, and a transdermal cream.

Specialty Supplements with Good Safety Records

Doctors and other health care practitioners are using varied and creative methods for ridding the body of unwanted substances and helping it heal from the inside out. Many considerations, such as age, cost, and convenience, are necessary in choosing detox agents. Here are some additional alternatives:

- *Coriandrum sativum,* also known as *cilantro* and *Chinese parsley*, is one of Klinghardt's favorites because it is capable of mobilizing mercury, cadmium, lead, and aluminum from the bones, central nervous system, and the cells.[15] Cilantro is so effective that it may flood the connective tissue with metals, causing "re-toxification," necessitating the simultaneous administration of an intestinal toxin-absorbing agent, such as chlorella (see below). It also can cause the gallbladder to dump bile containing the excreted neurotoxins into the small intestine. The bile-release occurs naturally as we are eating, and is much enhanced by cilantro. Without chlorella, neurotoxins can be reabsorbed on the way down the small intestine by the abundant nerve endings of the enteric nervous system located in the gut.

Cilantro is available in a number of forms: (1) as a **tincture** dosed initially at two drops twice per day in hot water just before a meal. Gradually increase dose to 10 drops three times per day for full benefit. During the initial phase of the detox, cilantro should be given one week on, two to three weeks off; (2) as **chopped, fresh, organic cilantro** placed in hot miso soup; (3) **transdermally**, by rubbing five drops of homemade or commercial cilantro oil twice per day into ankles or wrists; and (4) as a **tea** made from 10 to 20 drops of oil or chopped fresh leaves in a cup of hot water, and sipped slowly.

• *Sodium alginate* and *chlorella* are both extracted from algae. Sodium alginate is an excellent detox agent for barium, cadmium, lead, strontium, and mercury, as well as for detoxing environmental fumes.[16] Chlorella, as can be surmised by its name, contains vast amounts of chlorophyll, nature's own detoxification agent.

Chlorella is another product in the Klinghardt detoxification arsenal because it has multiple health-inducing effects.[17] It is available as capsules, a powder, and chewable tablets. It is not just for autism, but is a staple for anyone interested in maintaining good health.

Chlorella growth factor (CGF) is a heated extract from chlorella that concentrates specific peptides, proteins, and other ingredients for detoxifying every existing toxic metal in a profound way. The research shows that children taking CGF develop no tooth decay and have near-perfect maxillary-facial development. They experience fewer illnesses, grow better, have higher IQs, and are socially more skilled.[18] Klinghardt believes that CGF makes the detox experience much easier, shorter, and more effective.

Some chlorella products are purer than others; try BioPure brand, which is treated with ultrasound, is oxidized, and is guaranteed to be free of metals and other toxins.

• *Heavy Metal Detox (HMD)* is a patent-pending, proprietary all-natural synergistic blend of organic cilantro leaf tincture, CGF, and homaccord cell-decimated chlorella that is taken orally. HMD is proven to eliminate lead, antimony, arsenic, cadmium, mercury, uranium, and other toxic metals successfully without leaching essential minerals, and without negative side effects.[19]

• *METAL-FREE™* is a complex agent containing chlorella, as well as glycine, algae, hyaluronic acid, alpha lipoic acid, and other nutrients, in a liquid base that can be sprayed into the mouth or taken as drops. Start with one spray (or 4 drops) under the tongue for one week, and then two sprays the second week, up to a dose of 4 sprays (16 drops). Take an hour before or after eating, such as before bed. If a child becomes cranky or agitated, decrease the dose. METAL-FREE™ is available from www.bodyhealth.com .

• The healing power of *garlic* has been known to herbalists for over 200 years. Garlic (allium sativum) and Bear's garlic (allium ursinum) protect the white and red blood cells from oxidative damage caused by metals in the blood stream on their way out. Garlic also has its own valid detoxification functions. It contains numerous sulphur components, including alliin, which oxidize mercury, cadmium, and lead and make them water-soluble. Garlic's alliin is enzymatically transformed into allicin, nature's most potent antimicrobial agent.[20]

The half-life of allicin from crushed garlic is fewer than 14 days, so most commercial garlic products have little allicin-releasing potential. Freeze-dried garlic still contains allicin and is available in capsules.

Metal-toxic patients almost always suffer from secondary infections, which are often responsible in part for symptoms. Garlic also contains the most important protective mineral against mercury toxicity: bioactive selenium. Most selenium products are poorly absorbable and do not reach the proper sites. Selenium from garlic is a natural bioavailable source.

Dosage: 1–3 capsules freeze-dried (not fresh) garlic after each meal. Using high-quality freeze-dried garlic ensures purity. Start with 1 capsule after the main meal per day and slowly increase to the higher dosage. Initially the patient may experience die-off reactions, such as diarrhea from dying pathogenic fungal or bacterial organisms.

Detoxification Guidelines and Precautions

Invest in quality supplements. Supplement quality is equally as important as the quality of the food that children with autism eat. Buy vitamins and minerals only from pharmacies, health care providers, and manufacturers who take pride in their products and know this population of kids. The good ones say "pharmaceutical grade." Look at the origin of the supplement and watch for fillers. Many instances of "the supplement did not work" are due to poor-quality products off the shelves of grocery and health food and big-box stores. Supplements are one instance where you get what you pay for.

Use the proper form of a vitamin or mineral to ensure it is absorbable and appropriate for a particular child. Ask your health care practitioner to recommend the form and delivery system.

Start slowly, and gradually increase dosages to make sure that the initial dosage is not too powerful. Err on the side of caution by starting with a small amount and moving gradually to a target dosage. Drop back the dosage or stop the supplement if negative symptoms occur, such as irritability, diarrhea, or constipation. Decrease dosages until symptoms disappear.

Watch for possible detox reactions. Patients are as unique in their responses to detox methods as they are to other interventions. Detoxification is one area where vigilance is essential in the outsmarting process! Some people go through the process without incident. For others, detox reactions occur if agents remove poisons too quickly. Reactions may be as benign as muscle aches that indicate the redistribution of toxins into the connective tissue and an insufficient nutritional support program. Other responses can be serious, such as rage, extreme hyperactivity, depression, headaches, seizures, and increased pain, indicating the redistribution of metals into the central nervous system, again the result of a support program that is too weak. Eye and ear problems that occur during detox indicate redistribution of toxins into these organs.

During a detox program, a patient may also become temporarily "allergic" to a substance that carries out the toxins. Every time a patient receives a detoxifying substance, toxins emerge from their hiding places into the more superficial tissues of the body, where the immune system detects them. The immune system sometimes believes that the detoxifying substance itself is the enemy, and reacts to it. This reaction typically resolves spontaneously six weeks after detoxing.

Look for reappearance of signs of candida. Using probiotics and digestive enzymes can be helpful in avoiding this side effect.

Remove only one toxin at a time, first clearing lead, then mercury, and finally other toxins like pesticides. Each agent has a primary place of action, which determines when, how much, and for how long it is used. In choosing individual detox agents, Klinghardt considers the part(s) of the body where metals are stored, relying upon ART. For example, he finds that chlorella is ideal for removing virtually all toxic metals from the gut, but has too little effect on mercury stored in the brain. Intravenous glutathione may reach the intracellular environment, even in the brain, but is fairly ineffective in removing mercury from the gut.

Pulling multiple toxic compounds simultaneously increases the opportunity for a synergistic effect from which a patient may have difficulty recovering. Using multiple detox agents sequentially (rather than simultaneously) can address various forms of mercury in the body because mercury is bound in the tissues, cells, and organs in virtually hundreds of ways, and no single agent can clear all forms of mercury.

Homeopathy

Homeopathy is a 250-year-old approach to healing used by a small number of medical and osteopathic doctors, by many naturopathic physicians, and by a growing number of lay professionals without medical licenses. It has recently emerged as an extremely efficacious treatment for people on the autism spectrum. Founded by Dr. Samuel Hahnemann, a German physician searching for a safe, effective alternative to conventional medicine, the word "homeopathy" comes from combining the Greek words *homoios*, meaning "similar" with *pathos*, meaning "suffering" or "disease."

Homeopathy is a complete system of healing targeted at achieving homeostasis: the optimal healthy functioning of the entire body. Double-blind, placebo-controlled clinical research studies during the past decade prove its safety and effectiveness.[21] Of course detoxification is a part of the process.

Classical Homeopathy

Many health care professionals practice "classical homeopathy," which focuses on determining the right homeopathic medicine or constitutional remedy for a patient. Remedies are plant, mineral, or animal substances that stimulate the body's "vital force," thus enhancing its ability to heal itself. Remedies come as pellets, tablets, creams, ointments, salves, or liquids, in varying potencies. They are prepared through a process of dilution, which results in a potentized medicine. The higher the number of dilutions, the greater the potency and the more powerful the remedy. Remedies produce symptoms of a specific disease in a healthy person.[22]

Like other treatments in this book, homeopathy focuses on the whole person, not on the diagnosis. The classical homeopath evaluates physical, mental, and emotional symptoms before prescribing.[23] An individual's symptoms and history, as well as the practitioner's interview with the patient and family provide the most important information. Two children with autism may be given different remedies, depending on what symptoms cluster together. The beauty of homeopathy is that a single homeopathic medicine addresses all concerns at the same time. Most homeopathic practitioners are open-minded about combining their treatments with other therapies, especially nutritional supplementation and dietary modification.

The possible relationship between autism and vaccines is of particular concern to homeopaths. Some use homeopathics as alternatives to vaccines for those who are skittish about vaccinating their children, and as a way to mitigate possible adverse vaccine reactions.

Many classical homeopaths believe that homeopathy can help children from the mild to severe end of the autism spectrum. Read *A Drug-Free Approach to Asperger's and Autism: Homeopathic Medicine for Exceptional Kids*[24] and *The Impossible Cure*[25] from "autism mom" Amy Lanksy to learn more.

CEASE Therapy

The late Dutch physician, Tinus Smits, MD, treated more than 300 cases of autism until his death in 2010. His conclusion was that 70% of autism was due to vaccines, 25% to toxic substances, and 5% to physical disease. Today his work continues through a program called CEASE, for Complete Elimination of the Autistic Spectrum Expression.

Smits coined the term "post-vaccination syndrome" to describe the relationship between vaccination and the physical, cognitive, and behavioral problems in children on the autism spectrum. He believed that "vaccination damage can take months to express itself, sometimes starting very insidiously, almost imperceptibly."[26]

Smits thought that homeopathic nosodes are a perfect tool to treat post-vaccination damage. While homeopathic medicines are derivatives of substances that occur in nature, nosodes are derived from the pathogens which cause a disease. The therapeutic administration of homeopathic nosodes is another way to practice homeopathy. Neither nosodes nor homeopathic medicines contain any biochemical trace of the substance from which they are derived, but rather are energetic imprints of those substances.

CEASE addresses all possible causative factors—not just vaccines. Step-by-step, it detoxifies medications, environmental exposures, and other poisons with the homeopathically prepared, diluted, and potentized substances, which clear their energetic imprint out of a patient's field. CEASE also uses supplements, especially Vitamin C, fish oil, and zinc in the detoxification and healing process.

Practitioners trained in Smits' approach offer services around the world. To learn more about this method, read *Autism Beyond Despair*[27] and go to www.cease-therapy.com.

Heel Remedies

In the Klinghardt model, practitioners use products from a German company called Heel. These products are combinations of single homeopathic remedies; they can wake up cells and help them regain their ability to communicate, thus mobilizing toxins from their hiding places. Regulating, balancing, and strengthening patients' lymphatic, endocrine, and organ systems results in increasing the body's ability to dump mercury and other toxins.

Heel remedies come in a saline solution, which holds the energy very strongly — for hundreds of years if stored in glass, not plastic. The remedies can be ingested or squirted up the nose or into the mouth using a syringe. Klinghardt has developed combinations of Heel products for each step of detoxification, always individualizing for unique issues with each patient.

These medicines require little training to use correctly. They are inexpensive and have many years of support behind them, proving their effectiveness and safety. However, classical homeopaths, who use single remedies, are generally not in favor of these products. Heel remedies are available from www.biopureus.com, and instructions on how to use them are available through the Klinghardt Academy at www.klinghardtacademy.com.

Homotoxicology

Homotoxicology is a form of sequential detoxification that evolved from the basic homeopathic concept that the body heals from the inside outward. It addresses an individual's physical and emotional traumas in reverse order from occurrence, going from the most recent to the oldest. It was originally developed by Jean Elmiger, MD, and is detailed in his book *Rediscovering Real Medicine: The New Horizons of Homeopathy.*[28] German physician Hans Henrich Reckeweg, MD, studied the influences of toxic substances in humans, and developed combination formulas of homeopathic remedies to remove them.

Using special equipment, a homeopathic practitioner determines in what order to detoxify the body using combination and low potency remedies that support and stimulate the body's own detoxification pathways. This energetic treatment first opens the detox channels to ensure that the toxins are not reabsorbed, and then sequentially uses substances to rid the body of viruses, bacteria, parasites, metals, plastics, radiation, and other toxins. The body releases the substances naturally via sweat, urine, hair, and stool. If done properly, the patient experiences no discomfort. Sometimes slight diarrhea or skin eruptions occur as substances pass out of the body.

Homotoxicology is fast becoming one of the most popular ways of detoxification for those with autism because it is one of the least invasive, least costly, safest, and most efficient methods we have today. Newly trained practitioners are entering this field weekly. To learn more about homotoxicology and its use with autism spectrum disorders, go to www.realchildcenter.com.

Neural Therapy

Neural therapy, a German form of acupuncture, is a powerful invention that involves the injection of the anesthetic procaine, diluted medications, and homeopathics into scars and specific acupuncture points. Scars from surgeries such as cutting the umbilical cord, performing circumcision, and removing tonsils can create abnormal electrical signals that cause them to become magnets for heavy metals. These traumatized body parts can develop into toxic storage sites.

Injecting the scars with healing substances helps to mobilize the toxins so excretory organs can eliminate them. The injections are superficial, safe, easy to learn, and effective for alleviating a wide variety of medical problems associated with toxicity.[29]

Laser Energetic Detoxification (LED)

Another technique developed in Germany and perfected in the United States by W. Lee Cowden, MD, is laser energetic detoxification (LED). A practitioner can use ART or other testing techniques to determine components of an individual's protocol. Cowden retrofits a device to hold homeopathic preparations of toxins and heavy metals along with detoxification support, and lasers them into the body in a process called photonphoresis. He beams the light through the vial onto targeted acupuncture points on the ears, soles of the feet, and palms of the hands. This procedure allows the body to receive the energetic information from the homeopathic remedy immediately, and can elicit rapid and deep effects.[30]

LED can speed up and amplify detoxification because the power of the laser light affects the body's biophoton field, stimulating it to specifically dump a toxin out of the cells and extracellular spaces. Coupling LED with oral chelating agents such as chlorella binds the toxins and shuttles them out of the body at a much quicker rate than with chelation alone. The beauty of LED is that it is very safe, and side effects are greatly minimized because detoxification support is built into the protocol.

Additional Methods of Detoxification

Epsom Salt Baths

A soothing support for detoxification is magnesium sulfate, also known as Epsom salts, which have long been used for baths. Susan Owens has shown the benefits of Epsom salt baths for autism.[31] Their efficacy is linked to the phenol sulfur-transferase (PST) enzyme, which causes a change inside the cells by adding the molecules adenosine and phosphate to sulfate before any sulfur-transferase enzyme can use it. The molecular additions turn sulfate into its "activated" form.

Pour one cup of Epsom salts into a tub of warm water, and soak for approximately 30 minutes per day. Epsom salts can help with both magnesium supplementation and sulfur levels in the blood.

Sweating in a Sauna

Sweating is one of the oldest, safest, most natural, and least expensive ways to detoxify heavy metals and balance the body's pH. Saunas are finding their way into the lives of many health-conscious people so they can sweat all year around.

A far infrared sauna duplicates the same frequencies as normal body heat. Far infrared heat rays penetrate the body to a depth of 1.5–2 inches. The body's tissues selectively absorb these rays as water in the cells reacts in a process called "resonant absorption," which causes toxins to be released into the blood stream. These toxins are then excreted in sweat, feces, and urine. Because no chemicals are added and the heat forces the use of sweat as the major mode of toxin elimination, this method puts less stress on the kidneys and liver.

Saunas are available for two, three, or four persons; the best are made of poplar, which unlike cedar, redwood, spruce, or pine, does not outgas any chemicals. Some are equipped with stereo speakers. Find one that is totally natural, with no off-gassing or toxic glues. Two great sources are High Tech Health at www.hightechhealth.com and Heavenly Heat at www.heavenlyheatsaunas.com.

Chelation

Chelation is a more aggressive and powerful last resort for those whose testing shows the presence of toxic agents, and who are not making progress either with over-the-counter metal-removal agents or with therapies. Doctors have used chelation for many years to remove lead. Available only by prescription, it involves medical procedures that are *very, very, very* controversial, require special training, and can be costly.

The word "chelation" is derived from the Greek word for "claw," which describes the chemical binding of metal ions that occurs as a pharmaceutical agent attaches itself to toxic metals, allowing the body to expel them. Every mineral taken into the body, whether essential or toxic, binds to a substance called a chelating agent to stabilize it. The heaviest and generally most toxic metals such as lead, mercury, nickel, and cadmium bond to chelating agents first. The resulting chelated minerals are stabilized minerals.

All chelation protocols must be supported by a diet rich in antioxidants and a strong nutritional program designed to alleviate oxidative stress and to replenish minerals that chelators remove along with the metals. Balancing the bowels is a must before starting chelation because heavy metals are partially excreted through the stool. Use dietary modification and nutritional supplementation to get the bowels functioning properly, heal the gut, and to strengthen immunity.

Doctors are continually looking for safe and effective chelation protocols. Here are some chelators they are using:

- *Dimercaptosuccinic acid (DMSA)* has a long safety record and is an effective chelator for many metals.[32] It is delivered orally, through rectal suppositories, or in a transdermal cream, and it can be combined safely with cilantro and/or chlorella. Common negative effects include gastrointestinal disruption and the leaching of essential minerals, especially zinc.

- *Thiamine tetrahydrofurfuryl disulfide (TTFD) cream* is a synthetic version of vitamin B-1 derived from garlic. Dr. Derrick Lonsdale believes that TTFD has three sulfur-related mechanisms that benefit children with autism spectrum disorders.[33]

- *Ethylenediamine tetra-acetic acid (EDTA)* is a synthetic amino acid with a strong binding affinity to calcium and lead, and an effective chelator for aluminum and nickel. Traditionally, it has been used orally for lead poisoning; however, it can remove many metallic ions.[34] Doctors are using EDTA experimentally both orally and by IV. Each requires a different form of the chelator. A tragic medical error occurred in 2005, when the wrong type was administered IV and caused cardiac arrest in a young boy with autism. Although charges were dropped against the family's physician, this incident caused quite an uproar in the medical community about using chelation in autism.[35]

- *Dimercaptopropane sulfonate (DMPS)* is a sulphuric compound that binds to heavy metals, especially mercury. DMPS is used off-label on children, as it is not FDA-approved. Some experience severe detox reactions and zinc loss. DMPS can be delivered transdermally (TD-DMPS), as a highly-stable, oxidation-resistant lotion that is rubbed into the skin, and as suppositories. To avoid mineral depletion, many physicians start an aggressive two-week mineral repletion program prior to initiating treatment with TD-DMPS. Check availability from compounding pharmacies specializing in autism products.

Recently, oral chelation for those with autism has lost favor due to chronic, pesky gut symptoms and reports of developmental regression following treatment. Those practicing chelation often prefer transdermal and intravenous delivery systems because they bypass the gut.

Because methods are rapidly changing and evolving, details of all the different programs are not included here. A 2005 review of chelation for heavy metals describes the options in general.[36] Contact a health care practitioner with years of chelation experience to help sort the possibilities and choose the best program for an individual child.

Chelation and Chronic Cerebro-Spinal Venous Insufficiency

Chronic cerebro-spinal venous insufficiency (CCSVI) is a condition where blood from the brain and spine has trouble getting back to the heart. Klinghardt and others are beginning to look at CCSVI in those with autism because they believe that many chelating products work on the vascular system, reducing CCSVI. In simple English, many detoxifying agents clean out the veins and arteries, especially in the neck area, thus allowing more blood flow to the brain.

Blood that remains in the brain too long creates a delay in deoxygenated blood leaving the head, which in turn can cause hypoxia, a lack of oxygen in the brain. Plasma and iron from blood deposited in the brain tissue can also be very damaging, allowing iron and other unwelcome cells to cross the crucial brain-blood barrier.

The CCSVI hypothesis originates from the treatment of multiple sclerosis (MS) by Italian vascular surgeon Paolo Zamboni, MD, who applied his knowledge and skills to his wife, who was diagnosed with MS. After he dilated vascular restrictions that showed up on a special imaging device, she made dramatic improvement:[37] the perfect example of "when you are a hammer, everything looks like a nail!"

After using a combination of microbe killers and detoxifying agents for a lengthy period of time, which may take two to three years, Klinghardt follows with a balloon treatment of the neck veins. At a talk in New York in February 2012, he reported remarkable benefits of this novel technique—which he calls "one of the biggest breakthroughs in autism to date"—for some of his patients with autism and other neurological diseases. Obviously, this approach needs further study. For more information on CCSVI, go to www. ccsvi.org.

Detoxification and Psychological Issues

A similar strange and often-overlooked association exists between metal toxicity and psychological issues. The degree of physical toxicity is also equal to the number of unresolved psychological issues, according to the Klinghardt model.

Often, as physical detoxification takes effect, repressed emotional material moves out of the unconscious to the subconscious, causing the patient to experience symptoms such as anxiety and anger. Health care professionals can mistakenly interpret these emotions as side effects of detoxification, or "detox reactions." An important component of detoxification thus must also include ridding the body of "toxic" emotions to retain the balance of physical and psychological toxicity.

When detoxification programs do not include the simultaneous elimination of harmful infectious agents and harmful unresolved trauma and emotions, the body stops releasing further toxins because the discrepancy between the infections and/or unresolved psycho-emotional material and the already-released physical toxins is too large. Both are out of balance – the toxin container is less full than the containers of bugs and emotions. Effective detoxification cannot progress without appropriately addressing these needs. The axiom that "for each unresolved psycho-emotional conflict or trauma, there is an equivalent of stored toxins and an equivalent of pathogenic microorganisms" is known as the "Klinghardt Triad of Detoxification." To successfully detoxify the body, Klinghardt addresses all three issues simultaneously.

The Origins and Resolution of Psychological Issues

Unresolved psychological issues and trauma may not have taken place during the lifetime of the patient. They can be epigenetic imprints from previous generations, passed down energetically in the same way physical characteristics are passed down genetically. They can be unhealthy or estranged relationships with another family member in the past or present.

Each unresolved case from the past causes the body to lose some of its ability to recognize and successfully excrete toxic substances. In fact, using ART, Klinghardt has shown that where specific infectious agents and metals reside in the body can be predicted with a high degree of certainty by knowing what type of unresolved psycho-emotional conflict a client has and at what age the associated event occurred!

The proper kind of psychological intervention can lead to a release of deeply stored toxins. Klinghardt utilizes some elegant interventions, including a form of muscle-biofeedback-assisted counseling called applied psycho-neurobiology (APN), to resolve deep-seated emotional issues.

Family Constellations

Another tool for healing multi-generational psychological wounds is family constellations, which is one of the most popular therapeutic approaches in Europe today and just beginning to make headway in the United States. Growing out of the family systems movement of the 1950s, this approach begins with the idea that dysfunction and suffering often relate to painful events in the family's past instead of simply originating in an individual's life history from birth to the present.

While parents' deepest wishes are that their children thrive and their relationships work, Dr. Bert Hellinger, a renowned German psychoanalyst, believes that sometimes an individual's future may be out of his or her control. An entanglement with a deceased relative from a past generation may be at play, sealing an unhappy fate, with a child as the victim.

Nothing is more important to a child than belonging. Sometimes a child's way of being connected, though, is to suffer like those who came before him. A child may become "entangled" in the difficult fate of a past family member and unconsciously draw unhappiness, failure, addiction, or illness into his own life.

Klinghardt believes that the large energetic fields of individuals on the spectrum makes them particularly vulnerable to disturbances in the energy field of the extended family, including unhealed transgenerational issues. Because of their extraordinary energetic sensitivities, they become the recipients of unhealed transgenerational family issues. Stored toxins prevent the physical body from receiving and processing perceptions and communications. Together these factors further perpetuate their illness.

Unresolved transgenerational trauma in the family system, as a psychological stressor, is by far the most common determining factor. Klinghardt believes that the impact of this stressor is grossly underestimated. Family constellations can serve to reverse illness, failure, and conflict by revealing hidden dynamics and pointing the way toward resolution. For a family whose child or children have autism, a constellation can break an energetic bond of pain and suffering, allowing a child to heal. Often therapy and biomedical intervention do not progress until a healing family constellation is done by an experienced facilitator.

Family constellations usually take place in groups. An individual chooses representatives for members of his or her family from the circle of participants and positions them in a way that seems right. In a short time the representatives begin to experience physical sensations, emotions, or urges belonging not to themselves but to the family members they represent. It is as though they have become antennae, receiving information from a family soul mysteriously present in the room. Facilitators refer to this as the "knowing field."

Through observations, questions, trial statements, and movements, the facilitator and client come to see the issue in a new way and create a resolution that enables the client to break his or her connection with difficulties in the family's past. As the hidden dynamic becomes clear and movements of peace and reconciliation arise, the genuine love and strength in a family begin to flow in a healthy way. Klinghardt recommends two or three sessions of family constellation work to free up the system to release more toxins, so other interventions suddenly become more effective.

An example. The family history of one boy with autism was full of turmoil and pain on both sides: the father was excessively involved with his own mother; the boy's mother, an immigrant, had been unable to establish roots in her husband's country; and a decision to abort a child from a former relationship had been made with little respect and seriousness to bring the event to a healthy closure.

As the constellation unfolded, the body language of the boy's representative showed how he was tied to those issues. To lighten the burden on their son, the father needed to free himself from his attachment to his own mother and become more available to his current family. The mother needed to develop a sense of rootedness in and respect for her new country. Together they needed to honor the soul of the aborted child by creating a place for it in their hearts.

Klinghardt suggests that families of children with autism put prodigious effort into healing their own families. The family includes children who have died early, aborted children, husbands excluded after a divorce, mothers who died at childbirth, and men who died in wars. Healing involves relating and communicating to everybody who is alive, as well as holding a loving memory of those who are gone. Don't rest until love and respect flows among everybody in the present and at least two generations prior.

Hellinger Institutes and independent groups offer family constellations across the United States. Hellinger's work, available in many books published by Zeig Tucker & Theisen, continues to evolve from a lifetime of rich experiences, including his years as a priest and living with the Zulu tribe in Africa. To learn more about family constellations, read Ulsamer's *Healing the Power of the Past*[38] and visit www.hellinger.com.

Take-Home Points

Toxins make people sick. When a body's Total Load of toxins exceeds its ability to detoxify, the poisons eventually affect the nervous system, including the brain. Unresolved psycho-emotional issues and traumatic family issues from the past further undermine function, creating the perfect storm and resulting in the undesirable behaviors and symptoms called autism.

For individuals with autism, a comprehensive detoxification program must deal with all of the above "toxins," not just the physical ones, but the energetic and epigenetic ones as well. Using a variety of techniques and tools, practitioners can gradually chip away at the stored aggravators and outsmart autism in patients of all ages. Each healer has his or her favorite methods with which to approach this phase of intervention. Mild, natural herbs and foods can help a body detox slowly. Homeopathic detoxification, which can take a variety of forms, is also a safe, effective method that takes time and patience. Chelation is a more controversial and faster way of removing toxins from the body and is being practiced with less frequency than in the past.

Every child with autism who is undergoing detoxification should be monitored by a professional; a home-based program is not a substitute for appropriate individual medical care. Detoxification is a continual, lifelong process. It can be an elegant, direct route through the maze of treatment options or a frustrating sequence of blind alleys and dead ends. Supervision by an experienced and qualified practitioner is absolutely essential for success. For help in finding an expert to guide you in this still-controversial arena, go to www.epidemicanswers.org or www.devdelay.org.

---

[1] Bennet S, Barrie S. 7-Day Detox Miracle. New York: Three Rivers Press, 2001.

[2] Owens SC. Understanding the Sulfur System. Defeat Autism Now! Conference Proceedings, Philadelphia, PA, May 16, 2003, 65–76.

[3] Defelice K. Enzymes for autism and other neurological conditions: A practical guide for digestive enzymes and better behavior. Johnston, IA: ThunderSnow Interactive, 2002, 241–43.

[4] Rogers SA. Detoxify or Die. Sarasota, FL: Sand Key Company, 2002, 48–49.

[5] McCandless J. Children with Starving Brains. 4th ed. Putney, VT: Bramble Books, 2009.

[6] Klinghardt D. A Comprehensive Review of Heavy Metal Detoxification and Clinical Pearls from 30 Years of Medical Practice. www.healingcancernaturally.com. Accessed Apr 1, 2012.

[7] James SJ, Melnyk S, Jernigan S, Hubanks A, Rose S, Gaylor DW. Abnormal transmethylation/transsulfuration metabolism and DNA hypomethylation among parents of children with autism. J Autism Dev Disord, Nov 2008 38:10, 1966–75.

[8] Gadow KD, Roohi J, DeVincent CJ, Kirsch S, Hatchwell E. Gene polymorphisms associated with anxiety, ADHD and tics in children with autism spectrum disorder. J Autism Dev Disord, Nov 2009, 39:11, 1542–51; Melnyk S, Fuchs GJ, Schulz E, Lopez M, et al. Metabolic imbalance associated with methylation dysregulation and oxidative damage in children with autism. J Autism Dev Disord, Mar 2012, 42:3, 367–77.

[9] Dorfman K. Using Nutritional Supplements with Children. http://devdelay.org/newsletter/articles/html/26-nutritional-supplements.html.

[10] Walsh, W. Nutrient Power: Heal Your Biochemistry & Heal Your Brain. New York: Skyhorse Publishing, 2012.

[11] Packer L, Witt EH, Tritschler HJ. Alpha-Lipoic acid as a biological antioxidant. Free Radic Biol Med, Aug 1995, 19:2, 227–50.

[12] Patrick L. Mercury toxicity and antioxidants: Part 1: Role of glutathione and alpha-lipoic acid in the treatment of mercury toxicity. Alternative Medicine Review, Dec 2002, 7:6, 456–71.

[13] Cutler AH. Amalgam Illness: Diagnosis and Treatment. Sammamish, WA: Andrew Cutler, 2005.

[14] James SJ, Cutler P, Melnyk S, Hernigan S, Janak L, Gaylor DW, Neubrander JA. Metabolic biomarkers of increased oxidative stress and methylation capacity in children with autism. American Journal of Clinical Nutrition, 2004, 80:6, 1611–17.

[15] Chithra V, Leelamma S. Coriandrum sativum changes the levels of lipid peroxides and activity of antioxidant enzymes in experimental animals. Indian J Biochem Biophys, Feb 1999, 36:1, 59–61.

[16] Skoryna SC, Paul TM, Edward DW. Studies on Inhibition of Intestinal Absorption of Radioactive Strontium, Can Med Assoc J, Aug 1964, 91:6, 285–88.

[17] Georgiou GJ. The Discovery of a Unique Natural Heavy Metal Chelator. Explore!, 2005, 14:4, 1–7.

[18] Tokuyasu, M. Examples of diets for infant's and children's nutritional guidance, and their effects of adding chlorella and CGF to food schedule. Totori City, Japan: Conference proceedings at the Nutritional Illness Counseling Clinic, 1983 (Jpn J Nutr, 41:5, 275–283).

[19] Georgiou GJ. The Discovery of a Unique Natural Heavy Metal Chelator. Explore!, 2005, 14:4, 1–7.

[20] Bergner P. The Healing Power of Garlic. New York: Prima Publishing, 1996.

[21] Jonas WB, Ernst E. The safety of homeopathy. In Jonas WB, Levin JS, eds. Essentials of Complementary and Alternative Medicine. Philadelphia: Lippincott Williams & Wilkins, 1999, 167–71.

[22] Marohn S. The Natural Medicine Guide to Autism. Charlottesville, VA: Hampton Roads, 2002, 137.

[23] Zand J, Walton R, Rountree B. Smart medicine for a healthier child. Garden City, NY: Avery Publishing Group, 1994, 33.

[24] Reichenberg-Ullman J, Ullman R, Luepker I. A Drug-Free Approach to Asperger's and Autism: Homeopathic Medicine for Exceptional Kids.Edmonds, WA: Picnic Point Press, 2005.

[25] Lansky, A. The Impossible Cure: The Promise of Homeopathy. R.L. Portola Valley, CA: Ranch Press, 2003.

[26] www.tinussmits.com. Accessed Apr 9, 2012.

[27] Smits T. Autism Beyond Despair. Haarlem, Netherlands: Emryss Publishers, 2010.

[28] Elmiger J. Rediscovering Real Medicine: New Horizons of Homeopathy. Boston, MA: Element Books, 1998.

[29] Klinghardt D. Neural Therapy. Townsend Letter for Doctors and Patients, Jul 1995, 96–98.

[30] Cowden WL. LED in Autism. http://www.youtube.com/watch?v=jKcy2q6xlCk, Accessed Apr 15, 2012.

[31] Owens SC. Understanding the Sulfur System, DAN! Conf Proc, Philadelphia, PA, May 2003, 65–76.

[32] Miller AL. Dimercaptosuccinic acid (DMSA), a non-toxic, water soluble treatment for heavy metal toxicity. Alternative Medical Review, Jun 1998, 3:3, 199–207.

[33] Lonsdale D, Shamberger RJ, Audhya T. Treatment of autism spectrum children with thiamine tetrahydrofurfuryl disulfide: A pilot study. Neuroendocrinology Letters, Aug 2002, 23:4.

[34] Cranton EM, Frackelton JP. Scientific rationale for EDTA chelation therapy: Mechanism of action. A textbook on Chelation Therapy, 2nd ed. Newburyport, MA: Hampton Roads Publishing, 2001.

[35] Autistic boy dies during chelation therapy. Looking Up, 3:12, 2005. http://www.lookingupautism.org/Back-Issues/vol03.12.html. Accessed Apr 5, 2012.

[36] Blanusa M, Varnai VM, Piasek M, Kostial K. Chelators as antidotes of heavy metal toxicity: Therapeutic and experimental aspects. Current Medical Chemistry, 2005, 12:23, 2771–94.

[37] Zamboni P, Galeotti R, Menegatti E, Malagoni AM, et al. Chronic cerebrospinal venous insufficiency in patients with multiple sclerosis. J Neurol Neurosurg Psychiatry, Apr 2009, 80:4, 392–99.

[38] Ulsamer, B. The healing the power of the past: The systemic therapy of Bert Hellinger. Nevada City, CA: Underwood Books, 2005.

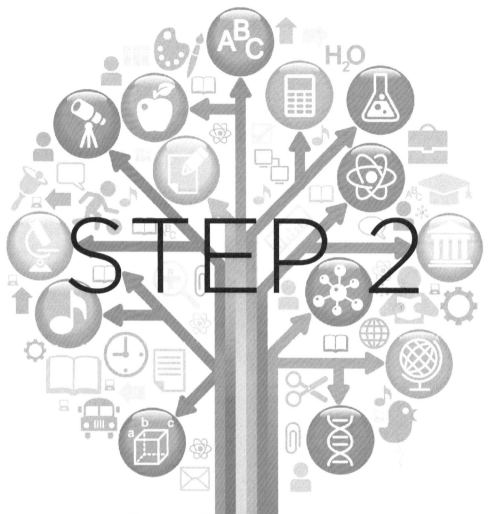

STEP 2

Correct Foundation Issues

CHAPTER 8

Structural and Brain Integration Therapies

A number of treatment modalities take into account the structural and skeletal systems of the body and their relationship to each other. These include chiropractic, chiropractic neurology, osteopathy, craniosacral therapy, and others that cluster under the umbrella of "bodyworks." Included in this chapter are also some unique movement therapies that integrate the body and the brain.

Only a perfectly aligned spinal cord and nervous system allow normal development to proceed along a pre-programmed, prescribed, sequential path without difficulty. Structure and function work hand-in-hand: structure determines function, and function determines structure. Changes in the body's structure changes its function.

Any imbalance among the organs, fluids, bones, and connective tissues disrupts the overall health of the growing organism. When structure is compromised, the body must utilize much of its energy to stay structurally intact, sucking whatever energy it can out of the immune system and elsewhere.

According to Dr. Viola Frymann, a world-renowned osteopathic physician in California, birth trauma is the most common cause of developmental problems.[1] A 2006 British study of children with an ASD diagnosis showed that they are 12 times more likely to have experienced birth trauma or complications than their non-autistic siblings.[2] A premature birth, long labor, problems in delivery (including a breech presentation), a Cesarean section, the temporary compression of the head and body passing through the birth canal, use of forceps, and vacuum aspiration, can all disrupt the structural integrity of the brain, spinal column, and the fluids in and around these organs. The birth histories of children with autism spectrum disorders often include one or more of these possible contributors, from which their skulls and sacra may not fully recover.[3]

For instance, the structural organization of the bones of the skull anchors the brain in place and determines the tension of the membranes that suspend the pituitary gland and the hypothalamus. The ability of the hypothalamus to release and transport its hormones is extremely vulnerable to the positional changes of the pituitary that may occur during a traumatic birth.

Many of the underlying health issues experienced by children on the autism spectrum cluster into specific organ and muscular systems. The nervous and digestive systems are particularly vulnerable. Some children have seizure disorders and gross or fine motor delays, which often originate from birth trauma. Unless health care professionals address structural impediments early in life, they can interfere with health and development, especially the absorption of vitamins and minerals and the detoxification of metals, pesticides, and other poisons.

Structural problems can cause symptoms immediately or take years to be evident; the larger the load of stressors, the sooner and more serious the symptoms. Obvious early signs of underlying structural issues are a delay in sucking; frequent reflux, vomiting, or spitting; a crossed eye (strabismus); "wiggly eyes" (nystagmus); and reduced visual or auditory acuity.

Subtle signals, such as fluctuating visual focus, an asymmetry between the two sides of the body, or missing stages in motor development, are easy to overlook. Both obvious and subtle issues can have profound effects on overall growth and development, especially on behavior and learning.

Structural Therapies

Structural therapies aid in realigning the body's internal parts. They can restore the body's structural integrity by

- releasing blockages in flow of internal fluids and energy,
- balancing the relationships among organs, and
- preparing the body to absorb essential nutrients.

Therapists who deliver structural therapies provide precise, gentle, restorative manipulative treatment by applying pressure — sometimes deep, sometimes light. Each type of pressure and manipulation addresses each dysfunctional system with procedures designed to reactivate that system and bring its function back into balance.

When an osteopath, chiropractor, or other structural therapist corrects structural dysfunction early on, neurological development can progress satisfactorily. Structural treatment facilitates the firing of nerves so they have quicker and more efficient responses to other therapies. Motor, sensory-motor, language, social-emotional, cognitive, and behavioral issues then resolve because optimal anatomic-physiologic integrity is established or restored.

Since practitioners from many disciplines are trained in manipulative techniques, families can sometimes find it difficult to determine which type of structural therapy might be beneficial for a particular child. Because the underlying cause of the problem, rather than the diagnosis, is what is important, knowing a patient's in-depth developmental history is essential before making a referral. Structural therapy procedures address structural and functional abnormalities simultaneously.

Chiropractic

Chiropractors are educated in a four-year graduate program at a chiropractic college. They are considered physicians and called "doctors of chiropractic," using the initials DC. Chiropractors call interferences and abnormalities with the body's structure "subluxations," which can occur in any vertebral or bony area of the body, including the neck and face. A chiropractor first identifies misalignments or subluxations in a patient's structure, then uses a variety of techniques to gently tap a segment back into place, thus restoring the structure and function of that area.

Structural abnormalities in facial development (involving the head, neck, and jaw) can cause defective dentition, such as an overbite, as well as problems with the temporal mandibular joint—both of which are serious stressors on the growing nervous system. Even slight misalignments can compromise the circulatory and lymphatic systems profoundly and impede blood flow and lymphatic drainage in affected areas through low pressure vessels called lymphatics, which are easily compressed. That is why Dr. Klinghardt strongly recommends a whole body evaluation by a well-trained chiropractor, as well a bite assessment of possible dental occlusion by a cranial osteopath or a very experienced orthodontist, for anybody with an autism diagnosis.

Elizabeth Sheehan, DC, CCN, who trained with Dr. Klinghardt, routinely evaluates the spine globally, including all 12 of the cranial nerves, in children with ASDs. The inability of any of the cranial nerves to process sensory stimuli efficiently could cause fatigue and stress. Identifying whether these nerves have the structural capacity to receive and integrate information, and treating them if they do not, ensures their capacity to handle appropriate therapeutic sensory interventions functionally.

Dr. Sheehan believes that cranio, upper cervical, and pelvic misalignments are always present in autism. These stressors on the nervous system, derived from birth and other trauma, can weaken the brain's defenses, making the body susceptible to ear and other infections, as well as invasion by lead, aluminum, mercury, and the micro-organisms that feed on them.

One of the main subluxations Sheehan sees in patients with autism spectrum disorders is a combination of misalignments called the "sphenoid pattern," which includes the sphenoid and occipital bones deep in the cranium. This subluxation pattern can occur from subtle or frank birth injury or head trauma, as well as from swelling and inflammation in the brain and lymph system from a variety of toxins. Misalignments in this joint complex negatively affect pumping of the cerebrospinal fluid and can disturb temperature regulation, increase intracranial pressure, upset balance of neurotransmitters and hormones, and impair taste, smell, hearing, and speech.

To remove subluxations in her patients with autism, Dr. Sheehan often uses an FDA-approved adjusting instrument called an ArthroStim™, which has been refined and perfected over the past 20 years. It provides a fast, accurate, low-force, controlled adjustment, and introduces energetic information into the body to realign segments and remove nerve pressure at a speed of 12 "taps" per second (12 hertz). The ArthroStim™ gives patients a very specific adjustment by addressing only the segment that is out of position, without any twisting, turning, or "cracking" of joints. This technique permits adjusting in many different postures, such as sitting, standing, or lying down.

Chiropractic Neurology. This "hybrid" field marries the biomechanical aspect of chiropractic care with the latest techniques of assessment and rehabilitation of the central nervous system. The result is a brilliant model of diagnosis and care that focuses on the two-way interaction between all of the sensory systems and the central nervous system. To find a chiropractic neurologist, go to www.acnb.org.

Additional Chiropractic Approaches. Some chiropractors and chiropractic neurologists have studied additional techniques that are of great benefit to those on the autism spectrum.

- The *Koren Specific Technique (KST)*, developed by chiropractor Tedd Koren, enables the practitioner to evaluate and treat the position of every joint in the body, including the spine, extremities, cranial and facial bones, and sutures. KST is particularly helpful for the sphenoid pattern of misalignments mentioned above.

KST is an especially quick and effective way of evaluating and treating cranial bone issues, especially for children with autism who are unable to tolerate craniosacral therapy (see below). Dr. Sheehan has observed drastic improvements in children with autism by adjusting them using KST. For more information on this technique, go to www.teddkorenseminars. com.

• *Gonzalez Rehabilitation Technique (GRT)* is a revolutionary "new neurology" system of diagnosis and treatment of the nervous system developed by George Gonzalez, DC. This unique technique closely evaluates and treats the entire nervous system, including the spinal cord as well as motor, sensory, and cranial nerves. Of all the nerves in the body, 20% are motor nerves that supply muscles for motor control and movement, while 80% are sensory nerves, which affect the ability to process sensory information.[4] GRT is crucial in autism because treating the sensory nerves often results in fewer incidences and lessened severity of self-stimulatory behavior.

GRT also evaluates and corrects functional cranial nerve deficits. The 12 cranial nerves originate in the brain and control functions such as sight, smell, eye movements, hearing, balance, motor and sensory control to the face, swallowing, and vocalization. After discovering a functional weakness in a nerve, a practitioner uses a powerful infrared device called a GRT light. Treatment with this instrument rapidly up-regulates (strengthens) the nerve and nerve impulses, reduces inflammation, increases intracellular ATP production, and effectively retrains the body to better multitask and integrate information. For more information about GRT, go to www. grtseminars.com.

In summary, chiropractors and chiropractic neurologists can be valuable members of a multidisciplinary team treating individuals with autism. If the birth history shows any signs of distress, or if any symptoms of structural issues are apparent upon examination, a consultation with a chiropractic professional is strongly recommended.

Osteopathy

Osteopathic medicine, or osteopathy (from the Greek *osteo*, meaning "bone," and *pathos*, meaning "suffering"), is a form of medical practice founded in the late 1800s. Doctors practicing osteopathy or osteopathic medicine are called osteopathic physicians, osteopaths, or DOs, and after four years of post-graduate education they are licensed to practice fully in all 50 states. They prefer to work in fields that enhance wellness, always considering the impact that lifestyle and environment have on health.

Three fundamental principles of osteopathic medicine are

1. structure and function are reciprocally interrelated;
2. the body is one integrated unit of function; and
3. the body has an innate self-healing or vital force within, which can be harnessed to reduce all types of stressors.

A unique component of osteopathic education is training in hands-on techniques that influence the body's structure and enhance the body's innate ability to heal itself and thus function more efficiently. This treatment is called osteopathic manipulative therapy (OMT).

Like chiropractors, DOs view all patients, regardless of diagnosis, as individuals who deserve to be helped to achieve their maximum structural, physiological, and emotional potential. Drawing on the three fundamental principles, DOs determine the most effective combination of treatments for each individual. Treatments often include dietary modification, nutritional supplementation, and detoxification techniques in addition to osteopathic manipulation.

Osteopaths find structural commonalities in children with symptoms of autism. Many show injury (likely from birth) to the back of the skull where the first cervical vertebra attaches to the skull, which results in the neck being jammed up against the skull base or occiput. This condition, in turn, injures three groups of muscles that make up the suboccipital triangle. When these muscles and their fascia become contracted, they compress a space called the jugular foramen (literally a hole in the skull). Several nerves and the jugular vein, which drains 95% of all blood coming from the brain, pass through this area. When the hole is compressed, the amount of blood that can flow through the vein is decreased. OMT can result in marked and quantifiable changes in cerebral blood flow, thus improving brain function.[5]

Several osteopathic physicians have devoted some of their careers to working with patients on the autism spectrum. Two are Sherry Tenpenny, DO, whose primary interest is in vaccine education, and Mary Ann Block, DO, who attended medical school at the age of 39 to help her daughter heal. Dr. Tenpenny runs a multidisciplinary health center located in Middleburg Heights, Ohio. Her website is www.tenpennyimc.com.

Dr. Block believes that structural therapies, when combined with other interventions, are particularly beneficial for treating those who have chronic ear infections. She uses osteopathic manipulation to drain the fluid in the ears, along with dietary modification and nutritional supplementation to enhance the immune system.[6] Her website is www.blockcenter.com.

Additional Bodyworks Interventions

Craniosacral Therapy (CST)

Craniosacral therapy (CST) is a form of treatment developed by John Upledger, DO. It is a gentle, relaxing, hands-on intervention that can help children and their families deal with some of the physical and emotional issues common to autism. Chiropractors, osteopathic physicians, occupational therapists, physical therapists, speech-language therapists, and even some massage therapists use craniosacral techniques.

The brain and the spinal cord make up the body's craniosacral system. The bones of the skull and spinal column are encased in a three-layer membrane system called the meninges. Symptoms appear when the meningeal membranes cannot glide freely over one another or when their capacity for motion is restricted or compromised — even slightly — by physical, emotional, behavioral, or other stressors.

The membranes hold and protect the entire nervous system in nutrient-rich cerebrospinal fluid, as well as house the pituitary and pineal glands, which were discussed in chapter 6. The endocrine system can thus be disrupted if the cerebrospinal fluid does not flow freely.

The outermost meningeal layer, called the dura mater, is attached at certain points to the bones of the cranium and the sacrum. The cerebrospinal fluid forms a barrier, creating a semi-closed hydraulic system. As the system's fluid expands and contracts, pressure rises and falls, creating the craniosacral rhythm, which is palpable anywhere on the body by a trained therapist.

Craniosacral therapists assess the body head-to-toe, evaluating the entire craniosacral system. By placing hands on the body and palpating for symmetry, quality, and range and rate of motion, the practitioner can identify the source and nature of any restrictions.

Because of the structural continuity of the body through the fascia, the ability of CST to diagnose and treat extends far beyond the craniosacral system. For instance, individuals on the autism spectrum often have high tension in the meninges of the head, which puts pressure on the cerebrospinal fluid and impedes its movement. Abnormal membrane tension of the craniosacral system can restrict the visual system, causing structural, sensory, and perceptual dysfunctions in vision. Restrictions in the sphenobasilar junction, where the sphenoid bone and occiput come together, are associated with strabismus, a visual issue in many individuals with autism. CST can sometimes alleviate or even eliminate this problem.[7] See chapter 11 for more on visual issues in autism spectrum disorders.

A novel application of CST occurs at the Upledger Institute's programs in Freeport, Grand Bahama Island. There, select teams of craniosacral therapists work together in four-day Dolphin-Assisted Therapy intensive programs designed to address the specific health concerns of individuals with medical and other conditions, including ASD.

Participants spend each day in multiple-therapist sessions, both in the water where dolphins are present and free to interact with the group, and on land. Therapists find that the dolphins' innate ability to scan a person's body allows them to detect and release bodily restrictions, which the craniosacral therapist can feel. The dolphin and the therapist become a rehabilitation team. At times they defer to a dolphin's decision regarding where and when to approach a client, as the dolphin's scanning ability provides the more accurate image of the tissues than the therapist's palpation skills.

Craniosacral treatment consists of light-touch manipulation on various areas of the body, so subtle that some recipients of this therapy report feeling nothing. Manipulation encourages the meninges to release tightness, to straighten out small kinks or stuck places, to recirculate fluid between layers, and to regain their natural flexibility and symmetry of motion. Improving the environment of the nervous and endocrine systems in this way is beneficial to the entire body. Sessions can range from 15 minutes to an hour or more, depending on the child and the day.

When the cause of the symptoms is an imbalance in the craniosacral system, the response to therapy is usually excellent and can be subtle or dramatic. Some people report gradual lessening of symptoms; others report experiencing powerful images and intense somato-emotional release. Noticeable changes can occur in activity level, vision, allergies, sleep patterns, repetitive behaviors, and verbal communication. Self-destructive behavior sometimes decreases or even disappears. Symptoms caused by factors unrelated to the craniosacral system are unlikely to change.

As in any therapy, no one can predict how an individual will respond, but the gentleness and non-invasiveness of CST render it essentially risk-free. Even extremely hyperactive children do surprisingly well after a few sessions. When CST is combined with other therapies, such as dietary modification, nutritional supplementation, speech-language therapy, sensory-motor therapy, or reflex integration, synergistic benefits often emerge.

Sally Goddard Blythe, Director of the Institute for Neuro-Physiological Psychology in Chester, England, reports on a French study in which craniosacral osteopathic manipulation benefited children with abnormal reflexes. Noticeable differences were apparent after only three sessions at two-week intervals over a period of six weeks.[8] Her conjecture is that this intervention started a neurological reorganization in the body that allowed for reflex integration. She recommends that any osteopathic correction be supported by a reflex integration program, such as is described in the next chapter.[9]

A good introduction to CST, and a fascinating account of the origins of this treatment, is the book *Your Inner Physician and You*.[10] Individuals in many disciplines also take training courses from The Upledger Institute, based in Florida, which offers beginner to advanced courses all over the world. To find a practitioner or course, go to www.upledger.com.

The Anat Baniel Method

Based in the science of brain plasticity, the Anat Baniel Method focuses on the remarkable abilities of an individual's brain to change and learn until death. Developed by Anat Baniel, a student and long-time professional colleague of movement genius Moshé Feldenkrais, this breakthrough approach evolved out of Baniel's background in clinical psychology and dance, and three decades of working with adults and children who have special needs.

When Baniel was three years old, she watched Dr. Feldenkrais teach movement lessons in her parents' living room in Israel. She began doing his movement lessons with her dance teacher when she was seven. Years later, while studying to become a clinical psychologist, she looked for a method that would involve kinesthetic, body-based movement to include in her psychology work. Recalling her earlier experience with Dr. Feldenkrais's method, she looked him up.

Although an old man when she took his training program, the two quickly bonded, and Feldenkrais became her mentor. Baniel traveled the world with him, continuing her studies, teaching with him, and working jointly with clients. From the beginning she experimented daily, exploring alternate techniques and approaches while trying to help his and her clients. In 1982, shortly before his death, she began teaching Feldenkrais professional training programs in the United States and around the world.

Baniel's gentle approach focuses on waking up the brain to create new connections, rather than on a person's limitations. Instead of forcing children into achieving developmental milestones they are not ready for, which often engrains their limitations even deeper, it uses focused movement to communicate with the brain and help it heal. As a result, a child begins connecting more fully with his or her body and feelings, awakening the ability to make sense out of the world. With her method, Baniel has witnessed miraculous transformations in movement, thinking, emotions, and social skills over and over again.

Nine Essentials form the core of the Anat Baniel Method, each describing one of the brain's requirements for waking up and creating new connections.

1. *Movement with Attention*: Movement is life. It is the language of the brain—it communicates with the brain and provides it with the necessary information to form and organize itself. Without movement, the brain has no new information to work with. Through movement experiences, the brain grows, forms, and learns to organize the movements of the body, of thinking, of feeling, of emotion, and of all action.

   Movement alone is not enough. Automatic movement—movement done without attention—only grooves in the already existing patterns. When we bring attention to what we feel as we move, the brain immediately starts building billions of new neurological connections that usher in changes, learning, and transformation.

2. *The Learning Switch*: The brain is either in a learning mode or not. In other words, the switch is either on or off. Healthy young children have their learning switches on and the dials turned on high.

   Repetition, drill, and everyday stresses, as well as habitual patterns of thought, exercise, and emotions, all tend to turn the learning switch off. The same is true when a child has special challenges. For the brain to properly do its job, the learning switch needs to be on. Once on, at any age, life becomes a wonderful new adventure, filled with movement, creativity, and new possibilities.

3. *Subtlety:* The Anat Baniel Method does not subscribe to the expression "no pain, no gain." In order to overcome physical limitations, chronic pain, and to thrive, the brain needs less, not more, forceful movement and thinking. Reducing effort increases sensitivity, which enhances the brain's ability to perceive just noticeable differences. These perceptions give the brain the new information it needs to organize successful action and become more alive and vital in both body and mind.

4. *Variation:* Variety is more than just the spice of life. It is a necessity for optimum health. Variation provides the brain with rich, novel information it needs to create new possibilities for movements, feelings, thoughts, and actions. It helps increase awareness and lifts a person out of rigidity and being stuck. Variation and playfulness in virtually every activity awaken all the senses, allowing new ideas to occur and new possibilities to emerge.

5. *Slow:* Moving quickly is the body's default setting, during which the body can do only what it already knows. Moving slowly is a sign of control; that is how the brain works. To learn and master new skills and overcome limitation, the first thing to do is slow down. Moving slowly—out of the mode of automatic movements, speech, thoughts, and social interactions—actually gets the brain's attention, and stimulates the formation of rich new neural patterns. It lets us feel and experience life at a deeper, more profound level.

6. *Enthusiasm:* Enthusiasm is a self-generated skill anyone can choose to develop and become good at. It informs the brain as to what is important, amplifies and exaggerates it, and infuses it with powerful energy. Enthusiasm lights up the

brain, ushering in change, by adding meaning and generating delight, which can transform the most mundane situation or task. Enthusiasm helps make the impossible possible.

7. *Flexible Goals:* "Keeping your eyes on the prize" is a prescription for failure, according to Baniel, who recommends setting oneself free from achieving specific goals. This freedom makes one available to recognize new opportunities and new paths. Missteps and reroutes are often rich sources of valuable new information that lead the brain toward a goal. Flexible goals can reduce anxiety, increase creativity, and result in success, vitality, and joy.

8. *Imagination & Dreams:* Einstein said, "Imagination is everything. It is the preview to life's coming attractions."[11] The brain discovers new possibilities through imagination and dreams, which grow new neural connections and manifest the future. They give us the unique ability to create something new, transcending current limitations and leading to an authentic life path.

9. *Awareness:* The action of generating awareness, which Baniel calls "awaring," is to be knowledgeable about what the brain and body are doing, sensing, thinking, and experiencing. Awaring is the opposite of automaticity and compulsion. It is a unique human capacity that can catapult us to remarkable heights. When you are aware, you are fully alive and present. Your brain is working at its highest level, noticing subtle nuances of what is going on around and within you, revealing options and potentials, and greatly accelerating learning. You are enlivened and joyful, contributing to others, becoming more enlightened, and fulfilling more and more of your human destiny.

The above Nine Essentials are powerful tools that provide transformational help for children with special needs to overcome their limitations. In those with ASDs, symptoms such as compulsiveness and rigidity, difficulty relating and transitioning, and compromised coordination and poor organization of movement are seen as manifestations of the brain's inability to differentiate and form patterns like those in healthy brains.

In her book *Kids Beyond Limits* Baniel describes how to apply the Nine Essentials to individuals with a vast range of challenges, including autism, attention deficits, cerebral palsy, and complex genetic syndromes.[12] Changes in those on the autism spectrum often happen immediately. Sometimes changes build on one another and a child gradually emerges into the world. Only limited changes may occur for older children. For more information and descriptions of workshops around the world, go to www.anatbanielmethod.com.

The Brain Balance Program®

Chiropractic neurologist Robert Melillo, DC, believes that a communication breakdown between the two hemispheres of the brain is at the foundation of dysfunction in those with autism and related disorders. That is why he created the Brain Balance Program® and cofounded Brain Balance Achievement Centers, now numbering 45 in 25 states. The centers are expanding quickly, aiming to become international soon.

The Brain Balance Program® is an individualized, comprehensive, remedial program that integrates physical and cognitive exercises with effective educational and behavioral methods and easy-to-follow dietary changes. Its goal is to correct a fundamental imbalance between the two sides of the brain that may result in a range of negative symptoms and behaviors, and to promote optimum brain and body function. This program improves each individual function and then progressively integrates them.

Melillo draws from training in neurology, rehabilitation, neuropsychology, and nutrition. For more than 15 years, he has devoted himself to helping those with neuro-behavioral deficits improve their academic, social, and behavioral functions.

The Brain Balance Program® combines the best of many modalities: motor, sensory motor, language, cognitive, reflex, and other therapies. It involves an intensive thrice-a-week commitment for one-hour periods, over three months, and includes home exercises, biomedical testing, dietary changes, and nutritional supplementation. Parents have given it strong praise for moving their children with autism through developmental stages quickly and eliminating troubling symptoms.

Melillo describes his program in his books *Disconnected Kids: The Groundbreaking Brain Balance Program® for Children with Autism, ADHD, Dyslexia, and Other Neurological Disorders*,[13] *Reconnected Kids: Help Your Child Achieve Physical, Mental, and Emotional Balance*,[14] and his latest, *Autism: The Scientific Truth About Preventing, Diagnosing, and Treating Autism Spectrum Disorders – and What Parents Can Do Now*.[15]

Brain Balance Achievement Centers are an elegantly designed franchise run mostly by chiropractors. To find one near you, go to www.brainbalancecenters.com and enter your zip code.

Aquatic Therapies

For those on the autism spectrum, the pressure of water offers a safe, soothing, and supported environment in which to move without the pull of gravity, and gives therapeutic proprioceptive and tactile input that improves range of motion, body awareness, and balance.[16] Simply being in a tub or a swimming pool is a possible avenue to strengthen muscles and relieve tension.

Watsu is a specific aquatic therapy created by Harold Dull after studying some Asian bodyworks techniques. Derived by combining the words "water" and "shiatsu" (a Japanese massage technique), it is performed in a 95-degree therapy pool.

This therapy is now being used for children and adults with disabilities, including autism. The watsu therapist continuously supports a patient who floats calmly on the back, face above the water. The warm water's therapeutic benefits and freedom of movement make it an ideal medium for passive stretching. The support of the water takes weight off the spine and allows the body to be moved in ways impossible on land. Gentle, gradual twists and pulls relieve the pressure a rigid spine places on nerves, helping undo any dysfunction this pressure causes to organs serviced by those nerves. To learn more about the benefits of watsu for autism and other conditions, read Dull's book, *Watsu: Freeing the Body in Water*, now in its fourth edition.[17]

Educational Kinesiology (Edu-K) and Brain Gym®

"Kinesiology" is the study of movement, the mechanics of how muscles and bones interact to enable us to move. Educational Kinesiology (Edu-K) is a comprehensive whole-body program using specific movements, postures, and balancing procedures. By applying movement to the learning process, athletics, communication, interpersonal relations, and creativity, it integrates the brain. At school, it helps students with and without special needs be able to sit still, listen, and focus better.

Developed by Paul Dennison, PhD, from over 20 years of study and experimentation with people of all abilities, Edu-K comprises techniques from the fields of motor development, applied kinesiology, developmental optometry, Neuro-Linguistic Programming, acupuncture, yoga, martial arts, language development, psychology, academics, and brain research. One can debate whether this program belongs in this chapter or another covering one of any of the above areas. It is included here because of its broad applications.

Dennison became interested in the role of movement in learning first through his own personal struggles and later through his observations of the children at the Valley Remedial Group Learning Center in southern California, which he directed in the 1960s and '70s. There, Dennison observed direct connections between his students' subtle dysfunctional movement patterns and their learning difficulties. When physical skills are inefficient, the brain cannot attend to the demands of higher-level cognitive processing.

The relationship between dysfunctional behavior and stress is central to Educational Kinesiology. Edu-K's goal is to reduce stress and integrate the brain for enhanced learning and performance. In the early 1980s Dennison began teaching 26 specific movements designed to counter the stress response by moving attention and energy away from the survival centers of the brain. He found that more energy was then available to activate the cortex and promote integrated visual, auditory, and kinesthetic functioning.

Since Dennison and his wife Gail founded the Educational Kinesiology Foundation (now Brain Gym® International) in 1987, their belief in the interdependence of movement development, language acquisition, and academic achievement has fueled the worldwide growth of interest in their ideas and techniques. The Edu-K umbrella covers Brain Gym as well as numerous advanced techniques for enhancing learning and performance. Brain Gym® refers to the introductory level of Edu-K and the 26 activities and movements taught in the Brain Gym 101 workshop.

Modifications of Brain Gym are possible for individuals with significant special needs and severe challenges. Over a two-year period in a public school special education classroom of children with complex developmental delays, Cecilia Koester (formerly Freeman) used Brain Gym to help her students achieve both higher levels of functioning and greater inner stability and peace.

Among the eleven children, five were diagnosed with cerebral palsy, two with autism, and one each with spina bifida, Angelman's syndrome, brain damage, and mental retardation with impairment of hearing and vision. Several of them were confined to wheelchairs. Koester's work, documented in her inspirational book, *I am the Child*, demonstrates the adaptability and effectiveness of Edu-K in the hands of a talented and creative practitioner.[18]

Dennison believes that excessive involvement in two-dimensional activities popular among this generation, such as watching TV, playing video games, and even reading, are stressful to the human brain because our visual system is designed primarily for three-dimensional, not two-dimensional, vision. The trance induced by these two-dimensional activities, especially if introduced prematurely, can be so compelling that children abandon other forms of play that require depth perception.[19] The chronic stress that results pushes a child into a stressed-out pattern which, once learned, is difficult to break.

The stress that individuals on the autism spectrum experience in many everyday activities is often obvious, but sometimes sensitive exploration is necessary to tease out precisely what aspect of a task may be too challenging. To facilitate this detective work Brain Gym practitioners sometimes use a tool from applied kinesiology called muscle checking. George Goodheart, DC, the father of applied kinesiology, developed this technique in the 1960s. Muscle checking is now widely used by chiropractors, allergy specialists, optometrists, kinesiologists and many other professionals. ART, described in chapter 7, is a form of muscle checking.

All attentional, perceptual and cognitive skills have a muscular component related to the body's ability to maintain itself in an appropriate posture and to engage appropriate musculature. Brain Gym enhances this muscular component, which must be in place for efficient learning. To muscle check, Brain Gym practitioners usually use the anterior deltoid muscle. The client holds an arm out to the front at a 30-degree angle to the body, and resists against light downward pressure, causing the muscle to contract to hold its position. In the absence of stress, the muscle locks and the arm stays in place easily because the nervous system is efficiently communicating its intention to the muscle fibers. In the presence of stress, the muscle is weak and the arm wobbles or gives way under pressure.

Edu-K recognizes three primary dimensions of brain function: focus (front/back), centering (top/bottom), and laterality (left/right).

Focus Dimension

Focus involves the integration of the front and back of the body and the front (frontal lobes) and back (brainstem) of the brain. Practically, focus dimension relates to participation and comprehension—to the ability to act on the details of a situation—while at the same time understanding new information in the context of previous experience. Reading comprehension is the quintessential focus dimension task.

When children develop normally, their muscles and joints send their brains reliable information about position in and movement through space, resulting in integrated postural and spatial awareness. This basic level of neurological function is necessary for learning to take place.

Children with integrated postural and spatial awareness feel safe within their bodies. They process sensory information efficiently, easily find appropriate muscular support for their activities, and have a clear sense of physical boundaries. All of these conditions are necessary foundations for attention, concentration, and retrieval of information stored in the back of the brain.

Children on the autism spectrum often lack integration in the focus dimension and may be responding to some form of internal or external stimulation that makes them feel unsafe. Some squirm interminably — part of the fight-or-flight survival response — because their energy is all gathered in their long muscles. Some are over-attentive to peripheral visual stimulation and constantly scan their surroundings in order to detect any potential danger. Others jump up and run to the window at the sound of a car or a lawn mower because their auditory systems are constantly scanning for any sound that might signal a threat in the environment. No amount of asking these children to sit still and pay attention will work, because their bodies are maintaining them in a state of constant arousal oriented toward survival.

At the more severe end of the spectrum, bright lights, loud noises, strong odors, and certain tastes and textures can seem threatening to a poorly calibrated sensory system. A student with high-functioning autism once described his tactile hypersensitivity as living with a constant feeling that his clothing is "attacking" him.

A child who perseverates is unbalanced in the direction of over-focus rather than under-focus. In children who are either unable to be attentive or unable to keep perspective, the Dennisons would see a lack of integration in the focus dimension. Such children are sometimes labeled ADD, ADHD, or OCD (obsessive-compulsive disorder).

Centering Dimension

Centering refers to integration of the top and bottom halves of the body, and the rational top (cortex) and emotional bottom (limbic system) of the brain. This integration arises from the interrelationships among proprioception, balance, and vision, about which there is considerably more information in chapters 10 and 11. These systems work together to provide a sense of the center of one's body as a point of reference for the directions up, down, back, front, left, right, in, and out. Individuals with problems in centering often lack coordination between emotional content and abstract thought. Like some children with autism, those who are either cut off from their emotions or too easily flooded with feelings are unbalanced in this dimension.

Laterality Dimension

Laterality is concerned with the coordination of the right and left sides of the body and the right and left hemispheres of the cortex. Joined by the corpus callosum, the right hemisphere controls the left side of the body, and the left hemisphere controls the right side. Integration of the two hemispheres is essential for the development of all bilateral skills, including binocular vision and binaural hearing.

Binocularity and lateral integration become the foundations for reading, writing, and communicating. Lateral integration is also essential for fluid gross motor activity and for moving and thinking at the same time. A student with deficient bilateral skills may have difficulty crossing the midline and be labeled "learning disabled" or "dyslexic."

Some students write with their heads tipped down to one side, almost on the table, and their papers turned so that the line of script goes straight out from their noses. These students are usually processing information with only one eye and one hemisphere. Their compensatory posture helps them to suppress confusing information from the unfocused eye, but it also keeps them from activating and using the resources of the other hemisphere. In these cases, an optometric exam would probably show poor binocularity for horizontal tracking across the midline.

In the Brain Gym model, fluent oral reading with poor comprehension, hesitant error-filled oral reading with relatively good comprehension, and reversal of letters signal a lack of hemispheric balance—of poor integration in the laterality dimension. Dennison found that certain movements have the effect of bringing students with dysfunctional learning patterns into balance so they can experience that integration. Then ease in learning and performance comes naturally because the body is relaxed and good physical and mental posture support access to all parts of the brain. According to the Dennisons, Brain Gym activities promote such a state.

PACE

Four Brain Gym activities are used frequently as a warm-up. Called *PACE* for *P*ositive, *A*ctive, *C*lear, *E*nergetic, this sequence is a quick, easy, efficient way to achieve readiness for any activities from eating and dressing to athletics and academics. Anyone can complete this brain warm-up in fewer than four minutes. Brain Gym instructors recommend performing them in the order indicated below:

Energetic: Drink a sip of water. Optimal hydration enhances the brain's ability to process information efficiently. Water ionizes salts, providing the electrolyte environment needed for electrochemical conduction of nerve impulses. It increases the polarity of membranes, resulting in more effective nerve firing (a higher signal-to-noise ratio). Water also increases the affinity of hemoglobin for oxygen, improving oxygenation of the blood and brain tissues.

Clear: Massage "Brain Buttons." While holding one hand over the navel, rub thumb and finger of other hand in hollow area on either side of the sternum just below the collar bone for 30–60 seconds. Massaging the Brain Buttons, which lie above the carotid arteries, increases the flow of freshly oxygenated blood to the brain. These indentations, the kidney-27 acupressure points, connect with clusters of glial cells, which send electrical messages to the pituitary. The navel, with nerve connections to the vestibular (balance) and reticular activating (wake-up) systems, tells the brain where the body's center of equilibrium is located.

Active: "Cross Crawl." Touch hand to opposite knee, alternately moving one arm and opposite leg. Even better, touch elbow to knee. Continue for one minute. When done standing, the movement is more like marching in place than crawling. The alternating right and left hand touching the opposite knee activates the left and right sides of the brain and body simultaneously, and connects the upper and lower halves of the body. The combination of movement and touch stimulates both the motor and sensory cortex and increases hemispheric communication across the corpus callosum. Movement also promotes myelination of neurons by glial cells.

Positive: Do "Hook-Ups." Part I: Cross ankles, hold arms out with hands back to back, cross one arm over the other so that palms touch, clasp hands and bring them to the chest. Touch the roof of your mouth with your tongue. Sit this way for one-half to a full minute, listening to your breath. Part II: Uncross legs, place feet squarely on the ground, release arms, and hold finger tips together. Sit this way for another half to one minute. Hook-ups activate the sensory and motor cortex, stimulating the right and left hemispheres of the neocortex (reasoning centers). This exercise connects and balances the body's electrical circuits, allowing calm relaxation. The tongue on the roof of the mouth connects the limbic system (emotional centers) with the neocortex, allowing rational processing of emotionally charged issues and increased choice of responses and actions.

Many Edu-K practitioners and their students use PACE as a daily practice, or as needed to enhance their performance under stress. Other professionals, including educators, occupational therapists, and psychotherapists, find that they accomplish more in a lesson or therapy session when they and their students or patients start out from the internal posture of alertness and calm that the PACE exercises promote. Parents, teachers, and therapists can return to Brain Gym routines again and again when new stresses or challenges appear in the developmental process.

Although the Dennisons particularly recommend PACE, any of the 26 Brain Gym exercises can be used with those on the autism spectrum to warm up before school, meals, a doctor's appointment, a social event, or any challenging task. Some Brain Gym movements seem to be more helpful with particular skills. The Dennisons claim that once an individual learns to move correctly, integration becomes an automatic choice, and the learner does not depend upon Brain Gym movements to maintain integration.

Today Brain Gym is used in more than 80 countries and is taught in thousands of public and private schools worldwide as well as in corporate, performing arts, and athletic training programs. For more information about resources and training, go to www.braingym.org.

Take-Home Points

A number of long-recognized and emerging therapies address the structural integrity of the body and underlying functions. Chiropractic and osteopathic physicians have been working for years to realign the bodies and affect the minds of those with a variety of disorders. Applying their skills to individuals on the autism spectrum shows great promise.

Structure determines function, and function determines structure. Structure and function work hand-in-hand, especially in the bodies of those with autism spectrum disorders. Imbalances among the organs, fluids, bones, and connective tissues can disrupt the overall function of the growing organism, causing imbalances in many bodily functions. Changing the body's structure through manipulative and brain integration interventions alters its ability to function.

In addition, the work of some creative individuals such as John Upledger, Anat Baniel, Robert Melillo, and Paul and Gail Dennison is helping those with autism and related disorders function more effectively. Their work is spread through seminars to parents and therapists in many disciplines. By combining these tools with biomedical therapies to lessen an individual's Total Load, more of us can outsmart autism and help young people achieve their given potentials.

---

[1] Frymann VM. The trauma of birth. http://feelycenter.com/wp-content/uploads/2011/06/The-Trauma-of-Birth.pdf. Accessed Jan 8, 2014.

[2] Stein D, Weizman A, Ring A, Barak Y. Obstetric complications in individuals diagnosed with autism and in healthy controls. Compr Psychiatry, 2006, 47:1, 69–75.

[3] Gardener H, Spiegelman D, Buka SL. Perinatal and Neonatal Risk Factors for Autism: A Comprehensive Meta-analysis. Pediatrics, Aug 2011, 128:2, 344–55.

[4] http://www.sciencedaily.com/articles/s/sensory_neuron.htm. Accessed Jul 3, 2012.

[5] Centers S. Osteopathy: A philosophy and methodology for the effective treatment of children with autism. Autism Science Digest, Apr 2011, 1, 101–9.

[6] Block MA. No more Ritalin: Treating ADHD without drugs. New York: Kensington Books, 1996.

[7] Frey KI. Craniosacral therapy and the visual system. Journal of Behavioral Optometry, 1999, 10:2, 31–35.

[8] Cherqui S. De, L'invie a L'acquis des reflexes primitives aux reflexes posturaux. Le traitement osteopathique comme facteur d'integration des functions cerebrales. Memoire de Madame Mauriette, Sarah Chequi. Pour la soutenance du diplome d'osteopathie. DO.

[9] Goddard S. Reflexes, Learning and Behavior: A Window into the Child's Mind. Eugene, OR: Fern Ridge Press, 2005, 129.

[10] Upledger J. Your Inner Physician and You. Berkeley, CA: North Atlantic Books, 1997.

[11] www.brainyquote.com/quotes/quotes/a/alberteins384440.html. Accessed Jan 8, 2014.

[12] Baniel A. Kids without Limits. New York: Perigee Press, 2012.

[13] Melillo R. Disconnected Kids: The Groundbreaking Brain Balance Program® for Children with Autism, ADHD, Dyslexia, and Other Neurological Disorders. New York: Perigee Press, 2009.

[14] Melillo R. Reconnected Kids: Help Your Child Achieve Physical, Mental and Emotional Balance. New York: Perigee Press, 2011.

[15] Melillo R Autism: The Scientific Truth about Preventing, Diagnosing, and Treating Autism Spectrum Disorders—and What Parents Can Do Now. New York: Perigee Press, 2012.

[16] Jake L. Autism and the role of Aquatic Therapy in Recreational Therapy Treatment Services. Therapeutic Recreation Directory. Sep 1, 2003.

[17] Dull H. Watsu: Freeing the Body in Water. Middletown, CT: Watsu Publishing, 2008.

[18] Freeman C. I am the Child. Ventura, CA: Edu-Kinesthetics, Inc., 1998.

[19] Dennsion PE, Dennison GE. Brain Gym Teacher's Edition. Ventura, CA: Edu-Kinesthetics, Inc., 2010.

CHAPTER 9

Reflexes: A Blueprint
for Motor, Cognitive, and Social Development

Thank you to Eve Kodiak, MM, reflex specialist and Brain Gym®
Consultant, and Mary Rentschler, MEd, MNRI® specialist, both of whom
contributed significantly to this chapter.

Have you ever watched a baby startle, grasp an adult's finger, or turn his head toward an outstretched arm? We call these behaviors "survival" reflexes because they myelinate (build an insulating sheath) to protect the neural networks that support our ability to generate fight, flight, and freeze responses. Reflexes are not only a protective or survival response to stress or danger, but also the crucial neuro-physiological foundations for physical, emotional, and cognitive development.[1]

Eve Kodiak, a developmental specialist near Boston with a varied background in early childhood music, movement, and craniosacral therapy, calls reflexes "the Rosetta Stone" because working with them is about decoding a language.[2] After making lifestyle changes, normalizing the gut, and undergoing detoxification, embarking upon a reflex integration program could be the crucial missing step to outsmarting autism.

The good news is that almost anyone — not just specialists — can learn to recognize reflexive activity and use simple tools to alleviate it. Reflex "first aid" as therapy is yet another tool for alleviating stress and enhancing motor, cognitive, and social skills in individuals with ASD.

A Historical Overview

According to British reflex expert Sally Goddard Blythe, MSc, the earliest reference to the word "reflex" can be traced to Thomas Willis, a 17th-century medical physiologist. Willis used the terms *motus reflexus* and *refexion* to describe how "spirits" in the nerves reflected back to the muscles.[3]

The 1950s was an important time in understanding the role reflexes play in development. In Great Britain, physical therapist Berta Bobath and her husband Karel, who was both a psychiatrist and neurophysiologist, were pioneers in controlling the abnormal motor patterns of individuals with cerebral palsy. For the first time ever, they were able to inhibit reflexes and get the nervous system to transmit normal active sensorimotor experiences in young children.[4] Today their approach to neurological rehabilitation is known as "neuro-developmental treatment" (NDT) and is delivered mostly by physical therapists (PTs), occupational therapists (OTs), and speech-language pathologists (SLPs).

In Russia, social scientists including Pavlov,[5] Setchenov,[6] and L. S. Vigotsky,[7] noted that nerve impulses pass information from the sense organs to the muscles and glands, which respond reflexively to these stimuli. While researchers in the West believed that reflexes were active and then became "inhibited," Russians researchers spoke of "integration." For the reader this may appear to be a superficial semantic difference; however, it is far more, as it aids in understanding what happens in autism and related disorders, and is key in determining the direction of therapy.

The 1960s saw some interest in the relationship between the presence of hyperactive reflexes and the motor, sensory-motor, and vision problems seen in learning disabilities. Research in the field comes mostly from OTs and psychologists.

Svetlana Masgutova, PhD, a Russian psychologist currently working in Poland and the United States, has developed a system of reflex development based on the work of the experts from her native country. This well-respected model places reflexes in the framework of both higher and lower nervous system activity.

In 1989, Dr. Masgutova had just finished her PhD in psychology and began teaching in Russia when news broke about a tragic train accident nearby. She joined the large team of medical professionals to help the survivors through the event's aftermath.

The train catastrophe ultimately became a watershed event in Dr. Masgutova's life. Facing the tragedy armed with her newly acquired knowledge of learning and reflex theories, she went to work with the traumatized children, engaging simple movement and tactile activities to enhance both physical and emotional recovery. She ultimately left a promising teaching and research career to help children and adults with challenges by educating others about neurosensorimotor integration.

Today, Masgutova's techniques are practiced around the world as Masgutova Neurosensorimotor Reflex Integration (MNRI®). Much of this chapter describes her work, which is available in depth at www.masgutovamethod.com.

What Are Reflexes?

Reflexes are involuntary, stereotyped movements that a person makes in response to a stimulus. Babies are born with approximately 100 reflexes, which emerge from week nine in utero and throughout the first year of life.

Each and every reflex consists of a three-part pathway:

1. *Sensory Stimulation:* Receptors and nerve fibers recognize a stimulus and transmit it to the brain.

2. ***Brain Processing:*** The brain interprets the signals and activates an appropriate response oriented either toward protection/ survival or toward development.

3. ***Motor Response:*** Nerve fibers and organs/glands enact the appropriate reaction or motor response.

This three-step natural activation of a reflexive motor response can take place in the blink of an eye! It begins with a buildup of tension in the involved muscles and ends with the release of that tension in movement.

Infant reflexes account for a majority of the movement patterns we see during the first few months of life: turning the head, rolling over, and grasping, for instance. Neurologically, reflexes provide infants with learning experiences that lay the foundation for all motor skills and eventually motor control, which in turn are the building blocks for learning and self-control.

We acquire new skills by moving the body intentionally. If a baby misses steps in motor development or acquires unusual motor patterns, movements are neither smooth nor coordinated. Furthermore, the developing child needs intentional muscle control for essential visual skills, such as tracking the eyes from left to right, identifying what is seen, coordinating the two eyes to work together as a team, and learning how to focus and perceive. Motor control, fed by early reflex development, also leads to the ability to shape sounds with the mouth and to write letters and numbers.

Infant reflexes have a limited life span of 6 to 24 months. As each fulfills its function and integrates, more sophisticated variations of its basic motor pattern evolve under the control of the cortex. Dysfunction can exist in any part of the three steps: the sensory organs can fail to communicate with the brain; brain processing can be faulty; or the motor neurons can fail to communicate with the muscles, tendons, and ligaments. If the sensory stimulus is not recognized by the sensory apparatus and as a result is misinterpreted by the brain, or if the outgoing response is misdirected, then the reflex pattern will be inappropriate.

If we restrict the motor response by restraint, fear, or an external verbal command such as "hold still and pay attention," it may eventually lose its connection with the original sensory stimulation, or the sensory-motor connection may be weak, manifested by low muscle tone. Then, part three does not manifest as a motor response, yet the built-up muscle tension remains in the body.

A child at the mercy of such irregular motor reactions to sensory stimulation is at risk for developmental delays. Maturation and integration of the reflexes with controlled movements and skills will be slow or unreliable, especially in the presence of learning challenges and stress.

A Dual Purpose: Survival and Development

Primitive survival reflexes originate in and are controlled by the brainstem. Under threat, this ancient, early-developing, survival-oriented part of the brain mobilizes for our protection without involvement of the higher, more recently evolved cerebral cortex. Depending on the nature of the threat, the body must choose either freeze or fight-or-flight. One section of the brainstem, the Reticular Activating System, which is responsible for arousal and muscle tone, has been implicated in attention deficit disorder,[8] as has immaturity or aberrant development of the reflex system.

At first, reflexes activate the sympathetic nervous system and assist the infant in avoiding harm. As automatic, involuntary, unconscious responses to stress and danger, they serve as protective or survival mechanisms. The Grasp Reflex, for example, causes an infant to grab and hang on when it senses a loss of support.

The dexterity and artistry of a virtuoso violinist begins in the grasp of his tiny fists around his mother's fingers during his first hours of life. In the case of the musician, the Grasp Reflex is neither extinguished nor inhibited. It is integrated into mature movement patterns with all their complex and subtle variations.

Reflexes mature as their purpose is fulfilled: they integrate into the nervous system, remain available for positive protection in the presence of danger, and serve as a foundation for skillful, controlled, and intentional behavior. A fully integrated reflex eventually becomes part of an internal posture, aptitude, or skill we refer to when we use the image of a movement pattern metaphorically. Thus, integration of the various foot reflexes enable us to be grounded, to "stand on our own two feet," and to "stand tall" under stress. Maturation and elaboration of the Grasp Reflex will enable readers of this chapter to "grasp" the exciting possibilities open to professionals who embrace this concept of neurosensorimotor reflex integration and its implications for treatment of those with ASD.

Positive and Negative Protection

To describe the role of reflexes in the functioning of both typical and challenged children, Dr. Masgutova refers to "positive" and "negative" protection.

Positive protection: When a startled infant cries for help or a toddler points with his toes, reaching for the floor as his father puts him down, the reflex systems are functioning in a positive way. The involved reflexes have matured neurologically, and sensory perception functions well: the brainstem recognizes stimuli and organizes protective motor responses with no disturbance to reasoning ability and overall development.

Negative protection: When a reflex fails to mature and a dysfunctional reflex response continues beyond a time that is necessary or useful, negative protection occurs. Retained reflexes can impede normal sensory development because the brainstem interferes with cortical processing, thus interfering with volitional motor activity.

Symptoms of negative protection reactions are muscle tension, impulsivity, and involuntary movements. Outwardly, a teacher or parent might observe compensatory techniques such as an awkward pencil grasp, slumped posture, or wrapping a leg around the chair, to override the reflex. In highly dysfunctional or pathological reflex development we see more severe symptoms such as stereotypical or chaotic movements (such as in autism) or spasticity/hypertonicity in the limbs or chronic low muscle tone (such as in cerebral palsy).

The Developmental Dynamic of a Reflex

Reflex development begins during the first weeks in utero and proceeds throughout the lifespan. The importance of fully matured reflexes for optimal motor, cognitive, and social development ranges far beyond their role in infants and toddlers. Kodiak reminds us that since reflexes become active over and over again during our lives, integrating them is not necessarily a onetime event. The same reflexive gesture may need to be integrated several—or even a hundred—times because that same gesture occurred and froze at different times of life. The more integrative activity takes place, the stronger the neural networks for integration become.

Each time a reflex emerges and activates, it must go through another three-phase sequence. Maturation and integration of the reflex system is especially relevant for building the control, motivation, abstract thinking, creativity, and skillful intentional behavior necessary for smooth language, appropriate social interaction, and successful academic achievement. Every reflex must complete all three phases from emergence through growth and maturation to integration.

- *Phase one:* Basic patterns begin forming in utero, creating nerve networks that connect specific stimuli with specific functions. Early on, basic reflex patterns support the development and myelination of neurological connections in the brainstem, as well as the basis for appropriate and positive protection. Phase one continues as phases two and three begin.

- *Phase two:* This transitional phase prepares the basic pattern for further elaboration.

- *Phase three:* Variations emerge further as the cerebral cortex matures, and growth occurs in neural networks. During this phase the reflexes begin to integrate with intentional movement. Crawling on the belly as an automatic reaction, for example, becomes an intentional choice for retrieving a favorite toy. When infant reflexes remain active and have not integrated, they are considered "aberrant."

Claire Hocking, an Australian kinesiologist who has developed a Brain Gym model for integrating infant reflexes, uses the image of a sine wave to describe reflex integration.[9] Eve Kodiak explains it this way: as the wave begins, the reflex movement first emerges. Rising up the side of the wave, the reflex movements become more complex, and when the peak of the wave is reached, the reflex has developed all of the attributes it will have. Traveling down the other side of the wave, that information becomes integrated with other functions of the brain. Once these motions complete themselves and a reflex is fully integrated, the person achieves a quality of movement independence and can release his vigilance. Automatic, involuntary movement no longer drives action, and a person makes choices and moves freely.

Delay in reflex development or skipping any phase always affects the formation of future skills. Achievement reaches a plateau because the nerve networks necessary for progress are missing. A child then must develop compensations which, not being true patterns, are unreliable in situations of stress. Compensations drain energy away from the task at hand and also impede healthy motor development. Furthermore, reasoning processes in the neocortex are bypassed as the reflex system, driven by the brainstem, takes control of behavior. The brain-body system wires itself in compensatory ways around these active reflexes, causing stress.

Reflexes and Stress

We are all subject to stress. Our bodies and nervous systems are designed to tolerate the normal stressors of everyday life. In a healthy individual the autonomic nervous system engages adequate mobilization of protection to ensure near-term survival. Its sympathetic and parasympathetic subsystems function in a symbiotic fashion, regulating variations of alarm and non-alarm states, with one more or less dominant depending on the level of danger or stress presented by external conditions.

According to Kodiak, every stressful experience is accompanied by an involuntary movement. We may gasp or throw our hands up in the air (Moro Reflex), bite our nails (Babkin Palmomental), or simply feel immobilized (Fear Paralysis). We may trip (Leg Cross Flexion-Extension) or shudder (Spinal Galant) or throw back our heads in pain (Tonic Labyrinthine). Even if we keep these movements in check — for example, we feel the urge to bite our nails but don't — that reflexive response has signaled the appropriate parts of the brain to be "on alert."

Often, if we resist the stress and override the movement, the reflexive gesture gets "stuck," and the stressful incident remains fossilized in the body. An over-reaction at a later date is often because something in the present has triggered that stress reaction that was sealed in a frozen reflex movement. Eventually, the triggers become deactivated, even though the memory persists. Then, instead of a survival response, neural networks provide positive ways of dealing with stress.

When we experience an overwhelming level of stress—beyond the ability of the body and nervous system to cope—we enter the realm of trauma. Then the natural manifestations of a normal stress response may be replaced by more serious symptoms. In acute stress disorder one may experience panic reactions, confusion, dissociation, lack of trust, insomnia, and difficulty with basic self-care, work, and relationships. In trauma, painful flashbacks of the event, hyper-vigilance, and numbness occur, as well. The Total Load is simply too much for the nervous system to process.

Causes and Consequences of Reflex Abnormalities

Any pre-, peri-, or postnatal load factors can cause infant reflexes to be too weak, too strong, late, or retained. Table 9.1 shows some stressors on the system that can cause reflex abnormalities at any stage of development:

Table 9.1.

Possible Causes of Reflex Abnormalities

A traumatic birth
Forceps delivery
Prematurity
Health issues, such allergies and ear infections
A vaccine reaction
Lack of opportunities for movement
Medical interventions, such as casts to correct hip dysplasia
A serious head injury
Emotional trauma
Chronic stress of everyday life

Some of today's child-rearing practices are also probably interfering with the natural maturation of reflexes. Recommending that babies sleep only on their backs to prevent sudden infant death syndrome (SIDS), for instance, denies them of being able to use their hands to bear weight and to connect the hands with the eyes for crawling. Specialists thus must prescribe tummy time for babies whose development lags.

Lying on its tummy is essential for an infant to develop head-righting reflexes, and to learn midline awareness and bilateral integration. Children with limited time on their stomachs often experience problems with later learning tasks that require crossing the midline, such as writing.

The result of reflex abnormalities is dysfunction in future motor, cognitive, and social-emotional development. Undesirable outcomes include, but are not limited to, poor lateralization, weak muscle tone, and vestibular dysfunction, all of which are all covered in the next chapter. Vision and auditory problems can also be linked to reflex integration issues. That is why many optometrists and speech-language pathologists use reflex integration techniques in their practices.

Academic learning depends upon the automatization of basic skills at a physical level. If a child fails to develop automatic motor control, a teacher might observe symptoms such as reversals in reading and writing, mis-articulations, poor impulse control, trouble reading body language, or unsatisfactory peer relationships, all despite good intelligence. Retained infant reflexes can interfere with attention, motor, sensory, and social-emotional development. Without addressing the underlying neuro-developmental problem, smooth growth is unlikely.

Only when infant reflexes emerge strongly, integrate, and mature with all their variations, can a baby gradually gain intentional control of both the body and eyes. He or she can then achieve the right balance between automatic and intentional learning and behavior.

Reflex Integration as Therapy

A therapeutic reflex integration program can often be extremely helpful if conditions during the first year of life were not right for reflex emergence, maturation, and integration. An intervention program can be extremely beneficial for individiuals on the spectrum whose development was interrupted or compromised at any stage by immune system disorders, injury or trauma, or genetic, environmental, or social factors.

Some believe that single reflexes should be worked on sequentially, while others support a more global approach. Since the reflexes are all linked together in complex, facilitating and opposing relationships, sometimes working on one results in the spontaneous integration of another.

Parents can learn how to work with their own children, and teachers can integrate techniques into the curriculum to help all children in a class move along developmentally. YouTube has thousands of videos showing techniques. Experiment and find some that work for you! Remember, though, that anyone working with those with severe challenges should have intensive training and experience.

For those who wish to learn more about the diagnosis and remediation of reflexes, take one of the many courses offered by the Svetlana Masgutova Educational Institute (see www. mastgutovamethod.com). This website contains an enormous amount of material on the role of reflexes in learning and behavior. MNRI® is distinguished from other models of intervention by several components:

- *Safety:* If any aspect of an intervention evokes negative protection (i.e., muscle contraction, breath holding, fear, or any other sign of stress) the motor activity will be in the service of survival, not development. Therefore, the first priority is to begin in a context of trust, in which the body feels safe and ready to explore and grow.

- *Sensory stimulation, body position, and motor pattern:* The integration process begins with a precise sensory or proprioceptive stimulus to activate the reflex, followed by the exact genetically encoded motor response associated with the stimulus. For many integrating techniques the child is lying down—in the position in which he would have first experienced the motor pattern as an infant.

• *Variations:* Once the connection between the stimulus and the basic motor pattern is awakened, the opposite and all other directional variants are presented and practiced. This part of the process helps initiate the transition from basic pattern generated by the brainstem to variations under the control of the cortex.

• *Resistance:* More neurons are activated when muscles encounter resistance. At the same time, the activity should have a quality of ease and flow. Thus the resistance should elicit no more than 20% of the child's strength so that new learning can be free of stress.

• *Duration:* Individual steps of the integration process are sustained for seven seconds or more, giving the brain sufficient time to anchor the information.

Reflex integration work sometimes can result in profound and quick behavioral changes for deep, longstanding problems. Kodiak tells of a case in which immediately after the first reflex integration session, a two-year-old had stopped biting her brother. In another situation, a mother related that after the first session, her restless nine-year-old fell asleep in only ten minutes, and after one more session, the child was suddenly was able to add three digit numbers easily. Up until then, the child had struggled with both dropping off to sleep and adding two digits.[10]

Reflex integration techniques are tools in the tool chest of practitioners from many disciplines. Each has his or her own way of working with individuals on the autism spectrum. One interesting twist is Quantum Reflex Integration, developed by Bonnie Brandes, who trained in the Masgutova method. She combines reflex integration techniques with cold laser therapy on acupoints linked to the reflexes. For more information, go to www.reflexintegration.net.

Reflexes and Autism

Kodiak believes that individuals with ASD are under constant stress, and are thus reflex-driven most of the time. They are in a hyper-vigilant state, where trying to override reflex activity is like driving with the emergency brake on. They can sometimes do it, but it is stressful, inefficient, and eventually breaks down the car. Integrating reflexes is like stopping the car, taking off the emergency brake and carefully driving on, listening to make sure that everything else is functioning.

Most children on the autism spectrum still retain some infant reflexes. Lack of reflex integration could certainly account for some of these kids' odd movement and behavior patterns. Children whose bodies fail to gain full control over infant reflexes in the first six months of life grow up in a reflexive no-man's land where involuntary motor reactivity remains present, and the lifelong reflexes related to balance and stability do not fully develop. These children, who have enormous difficulty with voluntary movement patterns, are eventually labeled "dyspraxic" or "apraxic" in addition to being on the autism spectrum.

In a now-classic 1998 study of home videotapes of 17 infants later diagnosed with autism, Philip Teitelbaum, PhD, observed atypical ways of rolling over, sitting up, crawling, and walking in all subjects. Every child demonstrated at least one movement disturbance by six months of age. They had difficulty turning over and supporting themselves to crawl; they struggled to move forward, resting weight on their elbows or forearms, digging in with their toes and lifting up their rumps. Some pulled themselves along with one arm beneath the torso while attempting to crawl with the free arm. Others crawled atypically, with one leg moving and the other leg dragging behind. Most were late in walking.[11]

A follow-up study in 2002 suggested that unintegrated reflexes were at the root of the movement disturbances in Teitelbaum's subjects, especially those later diagnosed with Asperger syndrome.[12] Consistent with a Total Load approach, Teitelbaum has suggested movement analysis of infants as a means for early identification of those who might become autistic. Is it possible that a reflex remediation program could have prevented an autism diagnosis in these infants? His 2008 book, *Does Your Baby Have Autism? Detecting the Earliest Signs of Autism*, explores this possibility.[13]

Integrating Key Reflexes in ASD

Here are some of the reflexes that show up in individuals on the autism spectrum. Kodiak has found simple ways to incorporate reflex integration in rhythmic children's games and songs, as well as in some simple techniques that can be done by any caring adult. Some of these techniques are described along with each reflex.

The Fear Paralysis Reflex is triggered by a loud noise, bright light or sudden touch. It is present at birth. Fear Paralysis is a "freeze" reflex.

Techniques for integration:

• **Touch lightly on balls of the feet.** Relaxing the feet and legs send the signal to the brain that the danger is over. No need to run away or "stand your ground." Begin by holding a certain spot, which the Chinese call "Bubbling Spring," on the ball of each foot. It is below the big toe and slightly toward the second toe. Acupuncturists know it as the Kidney 1 (K-1) point, which is the beginning of the kidney meridian, and governs fear. Touch very lightly, as if you are taking a pulse (you are, even if you can't feel it!). It is usually easiest to cover these points on both feet with the thumbs. Don't worry about whether you are on exactly the right spot—the whole general area will work just fine as long as you hold a clear and peaceful intention. Eventually the muscles relax, and calm ensues.

• *Wave Hello* is a rhythmic chant that can work wonders, individually or in a group, and uses only self-touch. *Wave Hello* creates a visual stress that activates the Fear Paralysis Reflex, and the subsequent actions release that stress. Waving hello again at the end lets the system know that that trigger is no longer active—at least at that moment! *Wave Hello* has improvisatory possibilities, and you may substitute your own integrative movements for the ones in the body of the chant.[14]

Wave hello
Watch your fingers go!
Other hand!
Wave hello
Watch your fingers go!
Both hands!
Wave hello
Watch your fingers go! Now
One hand on your belly
Other one taps your chest
Tap tap tap tap, tap tap tap tap,
Tap tap tap and rest!
Switch hands!
One hand on your belly
Other one taps your chest
Tap tap tap tap, tap tap tap tap,
Tap tap tap and rest!
Now stretch —
And yawn!
One hand on your belly
Other one on your chin
Hum --------
La la la la la . . .
One hand on your back
Other one under your nose
Hum --------
La la la la la . . .
Now stretch —
And yawn!
La la la la, la la la la,
La la la la, la . . .
Wave hello,
Watch your fingers go
Wave hello,
Watch your fingers go
Mmmmm . . . .

The **Moro Reflex**, like the Fear Paralysis, it is present at birth. Another name for this reflex is the Moro *Embrace* Reflex. The Moro facilitates the first "breath of life," opening the windpipe if there is a threat of suffocation. It is composed of a series of rapid movements of the arms upward and away from the body, accompanied by rapid inhalation and a startle response.

During the first stage the hands fly up and the baby gasps for breath. The second stage is the exhalation and the hands releasing, and the third is to embrace a safe person—usually Mommy. The first stage says, "Oh no! I'm scared!" The second stage says, "I can curl up and protect myself!" The third stage says, "I can reach out for help and someone will love me!"

The Moro is triggered by a change in head or body position. It is a fight-or-flight response to threat which immediately alerts the sympathetic nervous system of danger. Blood pressure rises, stress hormones are released, the skin reddens, and an emotional outburst, such as tears or anger, results.

The Moro should integrate sometime in the first three to four months of life. Lack of integration of either the Moro or Fear Paralysis Reflex keeps an individual in a survival mode and can cause hypersensitivity to sound, light, movement, or altered position, so that the child is always "on alert."

Children on both ends of the spectrum can demonstrate Moro and Fear Paralysis Reflex problems. Children with an active Moro Reflex are constantly reacting, running, hitting, or screaming; they seem to fight calm. Adults yell, strike out, become hysterical, or run away. The energy-depleting mode of constantly fighting perceived danger leaves scanty reserves for other bodily processes, such as digestion and respiration, let alone development and learning. Moro is also implicated when children can't catch balls, because their reflexive response is to ward off the flying object rather than to grasp it.

Techniques for integration: *Something's Coming Toward Me!* by Eve Kodiak is another rhythmic chant, similar to *Wave Hello*, that enacts the Moro Reflex.[15] It ends with catching a ball.

Something's coming towards me!
(Gasp!) Hands go up!

(Exhale) It's only a leaf blowing on the wind.
Something's coming towards me!
(Gasp!) Hands go up!
(Exhale) It's only a bird flying in the sky.
Something's coming towards me!
(Gasp!) It's a ball!
(Clap!) Catch!
Yay!!!!!!

Something's Coming Toward Me! can be done as a group improvisation. The participants "go round" and say what the "fear" is, and then what it is "really." "Oh it's a monster! No, it's only a sock." "Oh, it's a T Rex! No, it's only a toy. Adults enjoy it too — "Oh, it's my taxes! No worries, my accountant will take care of it."

End Moro activities with a hug — even hugging the self is good, or a pillow or a big stuffed animal. The right people are good, too.

The **Tendon Guard Reflex (TGR)**, a maturation of the Moro and Fear Paralysis Reflexes, is a lifelong automatic whole body reaction to a message from the brainstem. Under threat, the body chooses whether to freeze, take flight, or fight.

Masgutova refers to the freeze or flight-or-fight versions of the TGR as the "Red Light" and "Green Light."[16] When the TGR sets off a Red Light (freeze) response, the body collects its resources at its core; we bend forward and stop with a narrow focus of vision. In the Green Light (fight-or-flight) response the body straightens in preparation to move; we bend backwards, the toes automatically rise as the body goes rigid, and the eyes open wide with a full field of vision.

The TGR is of extreme importance in autism. It is usually hyperactive, and implicated in toe walking, when the system chaotically sets off both Red and Green Light responses at once, resulting in the characteristic elevated heels, awkward posture, and lurching gait. When integrated and matured, its two versions provide postural templates for intense focus and analytical thinking (Red Light) and relaxed focus and gestalt processing (Green Light).

Techniques for integration: Use same techniques as for Fear Paralysis and Moro.

Tonic Labyrinthine Reflex (TLR): This reflex develops in utero, emerging around 10–11 weeks and provides an infant with a primitive way of responding to gravity. It remains active for up to four months after birth. When the head moves forward, the arms and legs flex into a "fetal position." When the head moves backwards, the arms and legs extend.

This is a "tonic" reflex, meaning that it influences muscle tone throughout the body. Continuous flexion and extension help the newborn eventually straighten out from the flexed in-utero posture and to develop head control and balance. The TLR assists the young child in head-righting.

The TLR is stimulated by activation of the vestibular system, and should integrate by about four months postnatally. A lingering TLR has wide-reaching ramifications, interfering with all activities that depend upon balance, muscle tone, and visual-motor processing. Some signs and symptoms of an unintegrated TLR include fear of heights, poor depth perception, figure/ground problems, toe walking, and motion sickness. An active TLR could be implicated in reflux if the baby throws the head backwards and stiffens. TLR is usually present when there are gut problems of any kind, so it is a big "player" for ASD.

If posture is stiff and arched, TLR is usually present. TLR is often active after dental appointments because many dental procedures require that the neck be tilted back and the mouth open for long periods of time, causing compression on the back of the skull. This often results in headaches. Interestingly enough, TLR can appear after orthodontia — even when the braces are removed! Another symptom of an active TLR is feeling unbalanced when looking up and down, say, when walking up or down stairs.

Techniques for integration:

• **Jiggle and Bounce.** Since the beginning of the human race, caregivers have recognized the benefit of bouncing and jiggling babies. These movements stimulate the flow of cerebrospinal fluid, which feeds the nerves and cushions the entire central nervous system. Magically, gas bubbles disappear, as anyone who has burped a baby knows. And it causes the vestibular system to make hundreds of micro-adjustments as the head rights itself over and over, integrating many reflexes. Children usually love being jiggled!

• **Jiggle yourself.** Lie down, pushing the feet against a wall or other hard surface and jiggle! Alternately, raise your knees and put your feet flat on the ground, and jiggle yourself up and down. You can jiggle yourself lying on your side or on your back by rolling from side to side.

• **Do yoga.** The Cat and Cow pose is great for integrating the TLR. The Cat is the TLR forward, and the Cow is the TLR backwards. Here is a rap from Eve Kodiak that narrates the movement:

Moo and Meow
Moo, I'm a cow,
And I'll show you how!
On your hands and your knees,
If you please.
Neck curves back,
Back sways down,
Look up! Whohoo!
And chew! (Chewing noises)
Mooooooooooo!

Meow, I'm a cat
I'll show you that
Back arches up
Neck drops down,
Look between your paws
And hiss!
Sssssssss . . . Meow!

Babkin Palmomental Reflex: Have you ever watched (or felt) a cat knead its paws? For mammals, who nurse their young, these kinds of "hand" (and feet!) motions are linked with movements of the mouth to improve the flow of milk. In Babkin, pressure against the fingers and palms stimulates the mouth and jaw, and vice versa.

254

A retained Babkin shows up in myriad ways. Babkin is related to security and nurturance, People with an active Babkin often didn't get the kind of early feeding experiences they needed. Just about every food-related behavior (picky or messy eaters, for example) involves some expression of this reflex. So does the compulsion to chew on things. Babkin is usually present during tantrums—the first sign that a missile is about to go flying from the hands is often a tight jaw, licked lips, or a shout! Often, when children are in the full expression of screaming and crying, the hands are working. Babkin is also present for fine motor coordination issues; again, tight hands and tight mouth go together. Difficulties articulating words are also indications of Babkin.

Some Babkin habits include nail-biting, sucking on sleeves, grinding the teeth, sticking the tongue out (especially when doing fine motor activities, like writing or drawing), wringing hands, and crying. Babkin has to do with issues of nurturance, bonding, and security.

Techniques for integration:

- **Watch for a tight jaw and licking lips.** Immediately provide some rhythmic activity that involves symmetrical pressure on the hands. Drumming on instruments or the floor, clapping hands or slapping thighs, even rubbing hands together, in rhythm, all provide positive outlets of expression for this reflex.

- **Sing song games that involve hand motions.** *Patty Cake, Miss Mary Mack,* and *Open Them, Shut Them* are a few popular ones. Look for "Step It Down: Games, Plays, Songs and Stories from the African-American Heritage" by Bessie Jones. Bess Lomax Hawes and John Feiraband (Gia Books) have published volumes of these treasures. You can also search online for hand slapping games; there are so many!

- **Combine hand and mouth motions in a variety of ways.** This creates new possibilities for hand-mouth relationships that can lay the groundwork for a more flexible response to hand-mouth stress.

- **Combine rhythmic hand motions, chewing and swallowing, and being touched or held in a nurturing way.** Sit with the child in your lap, give him a ball to squeeze or something to play with or hold, and let him eat something healthy that he likes. Hum and rock back and forth a little; it adds to the experience. You can also just have the child do something with his hands while he eats or drinks, and hold the K-1 points on the feet (see the techniques for Fear Paralysis). You can also stroke the hair or touch in any way the child finds nurturing.

- **Do the *Babkin Boogie* by Eve Kodiak:**
  Make two fists, close your mouth and Grrr!
  Make two fists, close your mouth and Grrr!
  GRRR!
  Open your hands, open your mouth and YOW!
  Open your hands, open your mouth and YOW!
  YOW!
  Knead some bread, close your mouth, say Mmmmm
  Knead some bread, close your mouth, say Mmmmm
  Mmmmmm . . .
  (These are the three basic combinations. Once you've done these, mix them up:)
  Make two fists, open your mouth and YOW! . . .
  Open your hands, close your mouth say GRRR!
  Now do anything you want . . .

Babinski Reflex: This reflex emerges during weeks 11–12 in utero and is active from birth up to two years of age, sometimes longer. It should integrate into the body's movement system by age three. The Babinski is the reflex that doctors check at birth to make sure that the neurological connections are operating normally from foot to head. Among its purposes is support for crawling and walking. Babinski has a strong cognitive component, and Masgutova considers it very important for language development.

When the Babinski Reflex is active, toes spread when the outer edge of the plantar surface of the foot is gently stroked from the heel to the toe. This touch causes a protective foot-to-body midline motion. The resultant inward rotation is accompanied by the extension of the big toe in the direction of the head and a plantar flexion of the other toes like a fan.

Lack of integration of the Babinski Reflex can interfere with the flow of cerebral spinal fluid as well as the development of stability, balance, walking, and other gross motor abilities. Babinski is one of the reflexes implicated in toe-walking; children who didn't crawl normally often have an active Babinski. Crawling is one of the ways nature ensures that this reflex will integrate.

Know anyone who constantly jiggles one knee up and down, or stands with feet turned in or out? They probably have active Babinskis. Clumsiness, frequent falling, and slow mental processing are other signs.

Techniques for integration:

• **Standing and walking, putting weight alternately on the different sides of the foot** — outside, inside, heel, and toe.

• **Press with the flats of the hands on all four sides of the foot.** Using firm but gentle pressure, slightly angle the foot "outside" and hold it there for around seven seconds. Then, do the opposite side. You can do the heel and toe this way as well. This is a lovely bedtime exercise!

• *Four-Sided Feet* by Eve Kodiak[17]
Your feet have four sides, don't you know?
Outside, inside, heel, and toe
That's outside, inside, heel, and toe
Walk outside and away we go!
(Play a drum, clap, or chant rhythmically, "Walk, Walk, Walk, and Walk . . ."
Then, repeat with "Walk inside!" "Walk on the heel!" "Walk on the toe!" and finally, "Put your whole foot down and away we go!")

Hands Supporting Reflex: Often referred to as the Parachute Reflex, this reflex emerges during the fourth month in utero and is active through the sixth month of life. To trigger the Hands Supporting Reflex, hold an infant under both arms and placed him horizontally in a face down position. At the moment the infant is lowered close to a horizontal surface, the hands should automatically reach toward the surface.

The purpose of this reflex is to break a fall and to keep danger at arm's length. When it is integrated, a person has good boundaries, a healthy sense of personal space, and a solid foundation for developing good social skills. An immature or unintegrated Hands Supporting Reflex could result in failure to recognize social "arm's length," and lack of respect for one's own and others' space, conditions often seen in autism. Another symptom of an unintegrated Hands Supporting Reflex is aggressive behavior.

If someone on the spectrum is covered with bruises and goose eggs, suspect this reflex. It is also a problem for people who unconsciously bump into objects or other people. These are individuals who seem to have difficulty gauging their distances, speed of travel, or being aware of their surroundings. An unintegrated Hands Supporting Reflex can also manifest as an inherent distrust of relationships, either by not approaching others or by not acknowledging contact.

Techniques for integration:

- **Play *Patty-Cake*.** Say the nursery rhyme while patting palms together with partner.

- **Fall towards the wall.** Standing about an elbow's length from a wall, allow yourself to fall. Break the fall with the palms of the hands, bouncing back to original position. Do this a few times, rhythmically.

- **Fall towards a partner.** Stand two elbows' lengths apart and fall towards one another, breaking the fall and meeting the resistance of the other's palms with your own. A more advanced version of this is to stand at opposite ends of a room, walk towards one another, stop at the appropriate distance and fall towards one another, breaking the fall with contact between the two pairs of hands.

Asymmetrical Tonic Neck Reflex (ATNR): The ATNR develops in utero about halfway through pregnancy and is fully present at birth. Movement of the baby's head to one side elicits extension of the arm and leg on the same side and flexion of opposite limbs. During uterine life the ATNR facilitates continuous motion, thus stimulating the vestibular system and developing muscle tone.

During labor, the ATNR teams with the Spinal Galant Reflex to help the infant "unscrew" itself and move along the birth canal. This twisting movement is the first experience of the infant in coordinating both sides of the body.

Babies born by either forceps delivery or Cesarean section did not have the opportunity to use the ATNR. Deprived of the twisting action of the birth process, they may not have experienced the early bilateral integration necessary for later development of auditory processing, and cross-lateral skills such as crawling, walking, and skipping, Results of this deprivation can include problems with balance, confusion with crossing the midline, mixed laterality, and, most significantly, poor language development. An active ATNR is also present in cases of torticollis, or any condition that includes a basis asymmetry or twist in the body, favoring one side.

Symptoms of a hyperactive ATNR can often be seen when writing, as the unintegrated reflex causes a person to tighten the dominant arm and shoulder muscles in an effort to prevent the arm from straightening out when writing on the right side of a paper. It also creates difficulties in crossing the midline and organizing work in visual or auditory midfield. When the ATNR is not integrated, the presence of new auditory information causes stress, resulting in confusion or shutting down of auditory processing.

Suspect an active ATNR in individuals who flop sideways on their chairs or even fall off. Students who turn their heads to look at the blackboard, or read with their heads to one side, also exhibit active ATNRs. Any irregular walking or crawling pattern, when a person "lists" or falls to one side is also ATNR-driven. An active ATNR is also a characteristic of insomnia, when the thoughts cannot "turn off" for sleep.

Techniques for integration:

- **Do Core Activation**, an adaptation of a Brain Gym activity that brings consciousness to the core of the body while the head is turned, reminiscent of the ATNR position. Position a child on his back, with the head turned to one side. Start by touching the four points of the rectangle of the core: shoulder, shoulder, hip, hip. Then gently but firmly press down, and then pull up on each shoulder each hip individually, as you hum a phrase of a simple tune like *Twinkle, Twinkle*. (You can also simply count to seven!) Once you have activated each shoulder and hip separately, press and pull two points at once in this order: both shoulders, both hips, right shoulder and hip, left shoulder and hip, and finish with right shoulder and left hip, left shoulder and right hip. Repeat, with the head turned to the opposite side, and finally repeat once again with the head centered.

     You can do this exercise for yourself when you are resting. Eve Kodiak swears by it as an aid to help your body calm, center, and fall asleep.

- **Do the *Baseball Boogie*** by Eve Kodiak.[18] The positions described in the rap activate and help integrate the ATNR.

Look down to the right and grab that grounder,
Look up to the right and field that fly.
Look right! Look left! Coming down the middle,
Catch that ball and throw it up high.

Spinal Galant Reflex: This reflex emerges at about ten weeks in utero, is active from three to four months after birth, and integrates between five and nine months. Its first purpose is to coordinate with the ATNR in moving the baby through birth canal. In cases of

Cesarean section, the child is deprived of this action. Results of this deprivation can include hypersensitivity along the back and spine, hyperactivity, poor posture, and sometimes bedwetting.

Sensitivity to touch is a hallmark of the Spinal Galant, so kids with an active Spinal Galant show an extreme reaction to tickling. When they involuntarily flinch, the shoulder jerks down and the hip locks to protect that soft spot in the middle of the waist.

Another sign of an unintegrated Spinal Galant is hypersensitivity to clothing; anything touching the back, including bedding, feels irritating. According to Kodiak, you can also see an active Spinal Galant in children who sit on the front of their seats, leaning diagonally backwards to rest their heads on the tops of the chair backs, not touching their backs to the chair at all!

The Spinal Galant is extremely important for posture. Children who are constantly wiggling, trying to release the irritation of real or imagined things touching them, don't tend to sit or stand up very straight because they are never calm enough to develop a sense of structure and alignment. On the emotional front, super-wiggly kids can be insecure. It's hard to feel calm and quiet if you're involuntarily twitching your back, neck, and shoulders.[19] Floppy kids, who are constantly leaning on things and people, haven't developed the core strength and posture that an integrated Spinal Galant provides.

Techniques for integration:

- **Stretch, yawn, and wiggle your shoulders.** This releases the Spinal Galant.

- **Roll the buttocks side to side.** Lying on your back and giving your buns a massage stimulates the flow of cerebrospinal fluid, which pools in the pelvis, to flow up to the brain, cushioning the spine and feeding the nerves.

- **Play *Jellyfish Jiggle*, by Eve Kodiak.** This children's game, said to a rap beat, creates a feeling of safe touch along the back side of the body.

Lie on your back
And wiggle your belly,

Jiggle jiggle jiggle
Like a bag full of jelly!
Jiggle jiggle
Jiggle jiggle jiggle!
Jiggle jiggle
Jiggle jiggle jiggle
Jiggle with your shoulders
Jiggle jiggle jiggle!
Jiggle with your hips
Jiggle jiggle jiggle!
Jiggle to one side,
Jiggle jiggle jiggle!
Jiggle to the other side,
Jiggle jiggle jiggle!
Breathe in and belly goes up
(Breathing in sounds)
Breath out and belly goes down
(Breathing out sounds)
Jellyfish are still
Floating in the water,
Breathing in,
Breathing out,
Breathing in,
Breathing out.

Symmetrical Tonic Neck Reflex (STNR): The STNR has a short lifespan, emerging around 13 weeks in utero, active from 6 to 10 months of life, and integrating between 9 and 12 months. A major purpose of the STNR is to help the infant to defy gravity and get up on hands and knees, rock, creep, and eventually crawl. When a child is on all fours, dropping the head down causes the arms to bend and legs extend; on the other hand, lifting the head up causes the arms to straighten and the legs to flex. It is this series of coordinated movements that makes crawling possible!

Many children on the autism spectrum retain the STNR. Their histories show that they rarely crawl on hands and knees; they scoot, shuffle along, or "bear walk" on their hands and feet alone. If they do crawl, they do so in an unsynchronized, unusual fashion, with rotated hands, locked elbows, and raised feet.

Creeping and crawling are essential movement patterns for sensory development. The vestibular, proprioceptive, and visual systems connect for the first time through creeping. Without going through this stage, babies end up with a poorly developed sense of balance, poor understanding of spatial relationships, and poor ability to use their eyes together, resulting in lack of depth perception.

This short-lived reflex is one of the most pesky, having the potential to interfere with many aspects of development. In *Stopping ADHD*,[20] the reading specialist authors show a relationship between a retained STNR and

- academic issues such as reading, writing, mathematics, spelling, art, and music;
- athletic problems in basketball, football, golf, hockey, soccer, skiing, swimming, tennis, volleyball, and wrestling;
- difficulties in public settings such as doctors' offices, beauty salons, restaurants, church, and sporting events; as well as
- psychological consequences such as poor peer relationships, low self-esteem, frustration, avoidance, aggression, and inflexibility.

For more information on how a retained STNR affects learning, see chapter 14.

A child with a retained STNR has difficulty sitting and may wrap his ankles around his chair legs to prevent his knees from straightening when his arms are bent. Another interesting symptom associated with an unintegrated STNR is the tendency to sit with legs splayed out behind in what therapists call the "W position," a behavior often observed in children with ASDs. Perhaps the extended legs give them better postural control. Perhaps they are trying to stabilize themselves any way they can because many of them have low muscle tone.

Australian movement consultant Brendan O'Hara believes that W-sitters process the world slowly because they cannot distinguish whether their own bodies or the world is moving. So, often, they sit and watch, unable to move forward, lowering their center of gravity to improve their balance and feel more secure.[21] Sitting in a W inhibits trunk rotation, making it impossible for a child to cross the body's midline, an important developmental milestone.

Techniques for integration:

• **Get down on the knees and elbows and rock.** Act like a baby getting ready to crawl, sliding the body back and forth. This movement affects so much! It helps the eyes to converge, as well as stimulates and balances the flow of cerebrospinal fluid.

• **Have an adult rock a child in the same position.** With one hand on the child's back, move him back and forth gently. This prepares the body to walk into the day!

Grasp and *Hands Pulling Reflexes:* The Grasp Reflex emerges at 11 weeks in utero, is active at birth, and gradually integrates by the end of the first year of life. It is elicited when touch on the top of the palm at the base of the fingers triggers grasping. Hands Pulling integrates with the Grasp Reflex at about two months of age as the baby attempts to pull himself up. To trigger it, with a person in supine position, grasp the forearms near the wrists and pull towards the feet. The response should be first flexion of the elbows, followed by head-righting and then movement of the core.

Just as children on the spectrum can have a poorly regulated sense of touch, they can be unregulated around grip. At one extreme are the kids who hold onto things limply or not at all because they may lack muscle tone in their hands. At the other end are those who grip so tightly that they can unknowingly hurt objects or other people.

The Grasp and Hands Pulling Reflexes are essential to developing good manual skills, including writing and drawing. A symptom of a nonintegrated Grasp Reflex is often an inefficient pencil grasp. A student who has skipped one of the three phases of the Grasp

Reflex might be able to write legibly, but will tire easily because of his neurologically inefficient pencil grip. He thus may experience writing as stressful and avoid it whenever possible.

Techniques for integration:

- Sing *Row, Row, Row Your Boat* with a partner sitting on the floor—feet together, holding hands, and "rowing" back and forth. Kids usually *love* this game! It also helps integrate Babinski, Babkin, and Hands Supporting Reflexes.

Reflexes and Sensory Processing

While just about any reflex can affect almost any condition, Kodiak and Masgutova associate some reflexes with certain senses. Predictable sensory processing problems may be a result of dysfunction in a specific reflex pattern. Here are a just a few examples:

- *Auditory:* Look at the ATNR, Grasp Reflex, and the Babinski.
- *Tactile:* A reflexive response to touch appears at only one week in utero, and the first impulse of the tiny embryo is to recoil from contact. After a week, under normal circumstances, the embryo no longer avoids contact with the uterine wall.
- *Visual:* Consider abnormalities with the Head Righting, STNR, and Spinal Galant if eye movements are poor, or an individual has difficulty shifting from near-point to distance.

In chapter 10, read about how the work of occupational therapist A. Jean Ayres developed from an early appreciation of the role of infant reflexes to an understanding of how the body integrates these "automatic reactions" into "a total body motor pattern" she dubbed "sensory integration." Ayres clearly agreed with the concept that "these built-in responses provide building blocks for the development of more advanced abilities."[22]

Assessment of Reflexes

Like any language, understanding reflexes occurs at different levels of complexity. Practitioners in the field may bring years of training and practice to the discipline, working at subtlety differing levels of expertise. However, because reflexes are a movement language that all people have instinctually "spoken" from infancy, simple, effective reflex recognition and integration techniques like the ones above are available to everyone.

For those interested in another step in the complexity of the reflex language, here are characteristics of the only visible, measurable link in the three-part reflex circuit: the motor response. Dr. Masgutova focuses on five characteristic parameters of each reflex:

- *Pattern:* The motor response should be exactly true to the inherent genetically encoded pattern associated with the specific sensory stimulus.

- *Direction:* Each reflex presents a precise sequence of reactions or movements that finish in a precise posture or continue in a specific direction.

- *Timing and dynamic:* The reflex circuit connects sensory input, brain processing, and motor response. To fulfill its protective function, the reflex reaction must quickly follow the onset of sensory stimulation and continue with adequate speed. Slow response time can result in injury.

- *Strength:* The energy and physical strength for movement depend on appropriate tone in the muscle/ligament system. The strength of the muscle response serving the reflex reaction must match the intensity of the stimulus. Hyperactive, hypoactive, or absent reactions are inadequate.

- *Symmetry:* The motor pattern should be balanced bilaterally. Symmetry should be evident in body structure, the organization of the body and its limbs, and the direction, timing, and strength of the motor response.[23]

Rhythmic Movement Training (RMT)

Another method of reflex integration that has its roots in Sweden is becoming popular in the US today. It is called Rhythmic Movement Training, or simply RMT. It originated with Kerstin Linde, a self-taught Swedish bodyworks therapist who developed a series of rhythmic movements inspired by those infants make spontaneously before they learn to walk.

Harald Blomberg, MD, a Swedish psychiatrist, met Kerstin Linde in 1985 and introduced her method in the psychiatric outpatient clinic where he worked. Adding this method broadened his clinic's scope with great success. During the 1990s Dr. Blomberg began treating children diagnosed with attention and learning difficulties using rhythmic movements, adding material about integrating primitive reflexes from a variety of sources, including Svetlana Masgutova. He called his method the Rhythmic Movement Training.

During his travels Blomberg met Moira Dempsey, an Australian kinesiologist, with a background in Brain Gym and other modalities. They wrote a book together, which includes a complete chapter utilizing RMT in treating autism.[24] Blomberg and Dempsey experienced a rift in their relationship, which clouds the rest of the story about what belongs to whom. RMT is easy and effective and getting more attention in the United States lately due to Sonia Story, a reflex integration specialist in Washington State.

For more information about these resources, go to http://www.blombergrmt.com, http://www.rhythmicmovement.com, and www.moveplaythrive.com.

Resources on Reflexes

Some psychologists, physiologists, developmental optometrists, occupational therapists, and educators understand the role of retained reflexes in learning difficulties, vision problems, and other developmental disorders. A growing number of professionals offer interventions that specifically target them as a key to healthy development. The following are among my favorite sources of information for identifying and evaluating reflex integration difficulties:

• Eve Kodiak's Movement Matters Blog, http://www.ecmma.org/blog.

• *Rappin' on the Reflexes: A Guide to Integrating the Senses through Music and Movement*, by Eve Kodiak. A CD and guidebook with original songs for reflex integration by this award-winning musician and therapist.

• *MNRI® Dynanmic and Postural Reflex Pattern Integration*, by Svetlana Masgutova, PhD. A course manual is available at www.masgutovamethod.com.

• *From ADD to Autism: Reaching your Child's Potential Naturally*: a DVD by optometrist Sam Berne that offers exercises to integrate the Moro, Spinal Galant, ATNR, TLR, and the STNR. Also included is a short discussion of normal motor development and the importance of diet and nutrition in ASDs.

• *Bean Bag Ditties*: a CD by Australian musician and kinesiologist, Brendan O'Hara. The songs are designed to be used for reflex integration by putting bean bags on strategic places on the body to ensure that they stay still.

• *Reflexes, Learning and Behavior*: a book by Sally Goddard Blythe, who, with her husband Peter, run the Institute for Neuro-Physiological Psychology in Chester, England. They provide workshops and intensive trainings on reflex integration, and run an annual European conference, which took place in Barcelona, Spain in 2012. See www.inpp.org.uk.

• *Physical Activities for Improving Children's Learning and Behavior*: a book by adaptive physical education teachers Billye Ann Cheatum and Alison Hammond. It includes a terrific chapter on reflexes and many group activities for reflex integration appropriate for preschool and elementary school children.

• *Primitive Reflex Training Program: Vision Therapy at Home*: a handy spiral-bound workbook and DVD combination by developmental optometrist Lori Mowbray shows you how to recognize the retained reflexes, test for them, and integrate them. Available from the Optometric Extension Program at www.oepf.org.

Take-Home Points

Survival reflexes originate in the brainstem and are automatic movements that help babies to be born and newborns to integrate the overwhelming amount of stimuli they receive once they leave their mothers' womb. Over 100 reflexes provide babies with learning experiences that build the foundations for motor, sensory, language, cognitive, and social-emotional development.

As babies develop, higher brain centers integrate basic reflex motor patterns with overall movement development and support variations that allow intentional and skillful motor activity to emerge. A child is then free from sub-cortical control over his or her muscles and able to learn, interact, and grow naturally and easily.

In many individuals with autism spectrum disorders, reflexes are absent, too weak, too strong, too slow to emerge, or linger past 6–24 months postnatally, and they are interfering with cortical processing and impeding development. Aberrant reflexes can cause babies to become "developmentally delayed," and down the road, one or more practitioners label them as having one of the disabilities on the autism spectrum.

Fortunately, at any age we can replicate missed stages of development by returning to the natural reflex movement patterns to awaken, reconnect, and strengthen neural pathways. On the foundation of matured basic patterns, the body naturally moves toward adaptive and efficient functioning.

Practitioners from a variety of disciplines have compiled reflex integration programs designed to give the brain a chance to rebuild critical neural connections that were weak or incompletely developed during the first years of life. By completing simple, quick, pleasurable motor activities on a regular basis for six months to two years, children on the autism spectrum can overcome neurological impediments to development. Their bodies and brains can then concentrate on interacting with their external—rather than internal—environments to learn, interact, and grow.

Make reflexes a priority in your therapy program. Reflex integration is the bricks and mortar in the developmental hierarchy; it comes immediately after physical health concerns, such as diet. For many on the spectrum, reflex integration may just be the missing component to outsmarting autism.

---

[1] Masgutova S. MNRI Dynamic and Postural Reflex Pattern Integration, 6th ed. Melrose, FL: SMEI, 2011, 8.

[2] Kodiak E. Reflexes 1: Emergence, Development, Integration. Movement Matters Blog. Sep 5, 2012. http://www.ecmma.org/blog/movement_matters/reflexes_i_emergence_development_integration. Accessed Jan 17, 2013.

[3] Goddard S. Reflexes, Learning and Behavior. Eugene, OR: Fern Ridge Press, 2005.

[4] Bobath B. Abnormal Postural Reflex Activity Caused by Brain Lesions. Great Britain: Heinemann Medical for the Chartered Society of Physiotherapy, 1971.

[5] Pavlov IP. Conditioned Reflexes: An Investigation of the Physiological Activity of the Cerebral Cortex. Trans and ed by Anrep GV. London: Oxford University Press, 1927.

[6] Setchenov IM. Physiology of Behavior. Ed by Jaroshevky MG. Moscow, Russia: Scientific Works, 1995.

[7] Vygotsky LS. Child Psychology: The Problems of Child Development, vol 4. Moscow, Russia, 1986.

[8] www.NewIdeas.net/adhd/neurology ADD/ADHD: Reticular Activating System. Accessed Feb 8, 2012.

[9] Hocking C. Retained Reflexes and Their Effects on Learning and Behaviours. http://www.wholebrain.com.au/uploads/1/5/9/5/15956426/manuals_form.pdf.

[10] Kodiak E. Reflexes 2: The Bricks at the Bottom of the Pyramid. Movement Matters Blog. Sep 13, 2012. http://www.ecmma.org/blog/movement_matters/reflexes_2_the_bricks_at_the_bottom_of_the_pyramid. Accessed Jan 12, 2013.

[11] Teitelbaum P, Teitelbaum O, Nye J, Fryman J, Maurer R. Movement analysis in infancy may be useful for early diagnosis of autism. Proc. Natl. Acad. Sci., Nov 1998, 95, 13982–87.

[12] Teitelbaum P, Teitelbaum O, Fryman J, Maurer R. Reflexes gone astray in autism in infancy. Journal of Developmental and Learning Disorders, 2002, 6, 15–22.

[13] Teitelbaum O, Teitelbaum P. Does Your Baby Have Autism?: Detecting the Earliest Signs of Autism. Garden City Park, NY: Square One Publishing, 2008.

[14] Kodiak E. http://www.ecmma.org/blog/movement_matters/love. Accessed Jan 11, 2014.

[15] http://www.ecmma.org/blog/movement_matters/somethings_coming_towards_me. Accessed Jan 13, 2014.

[16] Rentschler M. The Tendon Guard Reflex. New Developments Newsletter, Summer 2007, 12:4, 6.

[17] Kodiak E. Rappin' on the Reflexes: A Guide to Integrating the senses through music and Movement. Temple, NH: Sound Intelligence, 2005.

[18] Kodiak, Rappin' on the Reflexes, 81–83.

[19] Kodiak, E. Too Wiggly To Sit Still: Moving into Calm. Movement Matters Blog. Jun 24, 2012. http://www.ecmma.org/blog/movement_matters/too_wiggly_to_sit_still_moving_into_calm.

[20] O'Dell N, Cook P. Stopping ADHD: A unique and proven drug-free program for treating ADHD in children and adults. New York: Avery Publishing Co. 2004.

[21] O'Hara B. Movement and learning: Wombat and his Mates songbook. Victoria, Australia: The F# Music Company, 2003, 34.

[22] Rogers SJ, Ozonoff S. Annotation: What do we know about sensory dysfunction in autism? A critical review of the empirical evidence. Journal of Child Psychology and Psychiatry, 2005, 46, 1255–68.

[23] Rentschler M. The Masgutova Method of Neuro-Sensory-Motor and Reflex Integration: Key to Health, Development and Learning. http://masgutovamethod.com/_uploads/_media_uploads/_source/article_masgutova_method.pdf. Accessed Jan 12, 2013.

[24] Blomberg H, Dempsey M. Movements that Heal: Rhythmic Movement Training and Primitive Reflex Integration. Australia: Bookpal, 2011.

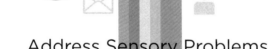

STEP 3

Address Sensory Problems

CHAPTER 10

Sensory Processing and Motor Issues

The next stage in outsmarting autism is dealing with the abundance of sensory and motor issues that plague most individuals on the spectrum. This is the last step before finally focusing directly on what adults value most: communication and socialization.

Clinicians have long recognized sensory issues in autism: psychologist Bernard Rimland, PhD, and psychiatrist Edward Ornitz, MD, are two well-known autism pioneers who observed and described these problems in the 1960s.[1] The use of contemporary measures confirms the presence of sensory processing issues in a majority of individuals with autism.[2] Refer back to chapter 2 for an introduction to the sensory connection in the Total Load, and Temple Grandin's role in raising awareness of this important area.

In earlier chapters we learned that addressing biological problems such as gut integrity, infections, and toxicity can sometimes lessen sensory issues. Likewise, as sensory and motor interventions calm the nervous system, many on the spectrum experience feeling relaxed for the first time. Circulation, breathing, and digestion improve, immunity becomes stronger, and hormones flow more freely. This process is true Total Load Theory in action: remove one impediment to functioning, and free up energy so it can work elsewhere.

This chapter is one of the densest in the book because sensory processing is *so* vital to all aspects of function. It starts with a discussion about the processing of touch, pressure, movement, taste, smell, and sound. Next, the relationships among the senses and how they integrate is introduced. The various methods for evaluating and treating sensory issues are followed by the many programs and channels for intervention: sound therapies, multisensory programs, as well as movement and fitness programs.

This chapter also includes sensory connections to sleep, picky eating, and toilet training. The conclusion of the chapter is devoted to music as a sensory tool and the interesting incidence of musical giftedness in autism. The sense of vision, an often ignored cause of dysfunction in autism, is so crucial that is has a chapter of its own, which follows.

Sensory Processing

When an individual has a sensory experience, receptors or specialized cells in the skin, tendons, muscles, joints, inner ear, and throughout the body deliver messages via the amazing nervous system to the brain. As these messages travel along neural pathways, different parts of the brain compare, combine, and interpret the sensory experiences, storing them for future reference.[3]

Each of the sensory systems has two functions: discrimination and protection. The protective function keeps people from danger. Efficient, consistent interpretation of sensations is first and foremost an essential survival mechanism. The discriminative function is important for developing sustained attention, understanding and using language, and connecting socially, as well as for all aspects of vision. Discrimination also provides detailed information about texture, temperature, shape, and size. Accurate discrimination allows a person to use objects appropriately.

How many senses are there? It depends upon who you ask! Textbooks generally teach about *five* senses: taste, smell, touch, hearing, and vision. Rudolf Steiner, a brilliant educator influential in the Waldorf School movement, taught that there are twelve senses.[4] For the purpose of this book, we will have seven. In addition to the above basic five, we include balance (also known as the vestibular system) and our "muscle sense," called proprioception.

The seven senses are described below in their approximate order of importance from birth. Understanding how typically developing individuals process sensory information is necessary to comprehend sensory dysfunction in autism.

Touch is the most basic of the senses, coming through the skin, one of the largest organs of the body. A mother's touch is the first fuel that moves us toward relationships with our family and eventually to society. Deep touch is soothing; light touch can be alerting or even frightening.

Proprioception allows the brain to interpret sensations from our muscles and joints. Have you ever picked up an empty cup that you thought was full, and your brain was surprised by how light it was? That was your proprioception at work. Our muscle sense tells us whether things are heavy, light, hard, or soft.

A baby's *vestibular system* is one of the first systems to myelinate in utero.[5] The mother's movements stimulate vestibular development in the fetus. Sometimes called the "balance system," the vestibular system is physically located in the inner ear where the labyrinths receive signals and detect the position and movement of the head relative to gravity. This sense is particularly important for muscles in the neck to regulate eye position whenever the head moves.[6] Veteran occupational therapist Josephine Moore describes this interaction as the vestibulo-oculo-cervical (VOC) triad.[7]

While all senses are important, the vestibular system is of particular interest because physiologically it is connected to the digestive tract, the language center of the brain, the limbic system, and the muscles of the eyes. A well-functioning vestibular system will thus contribute to healthy digestion, the emergence of receptive and expressive communication, emotional bonding, and visual focus, all areas of concern in individuals with autism.

Consider what happens when an adult lifts a baby off the ground playfully, holds the child overhead, and smiles and babbles at him. A child with a well-functioning vestibular system returns the smile, makes eye contact, babbles back, and in some cases, throws up! What an amazing system it is!

Auditory processing refers to how the brain interprets sounds that it hears; it is closely connected to language and communication. To be more inclusive, this chapter will use the term "sound processing." This umbrella term extends beyond the perception of sound for speech, language, and listening, and includes sound sensitivities as well.

Taste and *smell*, more primitive senses not high priority for learning and behaving for most humans, are high on the radar of those with autism. Many have highly attuned taste buds and noses upon which they depend for information because their auditory and visual systems are inefficient and unreliable. Their over-sensitivities in these areas can cause all types of behavioral issues, especially related to food, resulting in picky eating (a topic discussed at the end of this chapter).

And, of course, *vision*. Read more about how vision must become the dominant sense in chapter 11.

The seven senses rarely function alone; all behaviors are a result of the processing of one or more of the seven senses. The relationship between the vestibular and proprioceptive systems is so close that in some cases I include them together in the discussion. The brain combines incoming sensory information simultaneously, just as a conductor enables individual instruments of an orchestra make one beautiful sound. The "beautiful sounds" of efficient sensory processing are focused attention, enjoyable learning, and appropriate behavior.

Sensory Integration

Beginning in the 1960s occupational therapist A. Jean Ayres, PhD, was the pioneer in understanding how our senses work together. She coined the term "sensory integration" to describe this process. Ayres defined "sensory integration" as "the organization of sensory input for use."[8] Some of her disciples have expanded on her definition:

"Sensory integration is a neurobiological process that forms the foundation for adaptive responses to challenges imposed by the environment and learning. Sensory integration theory considers the dynamic interactions between a person's abilities/disabilities and the environment."[9]

Sensory Integration Dysfunction and Sensory Processing Disorder

If any sense is inefficient, the integration process can be disrupted and dysfunction occurs. Ayres's term for this outcome is sensory integration dysfunction, often abbreviated SID. However, because of the possibility of confusing it with the unrelated disorder Sudden Infant Death Syndrome (SIDS), in the 1980s those in the field informally began using the term DSI for dysfunction in sensory integration.

Recently, a small group of occupational therapists, led by sensory integration researcher Lucy Jane Miller, PhD, OTR, have suggested yet different terminology: sensory processing disorder, or SPD, as an umbrella term encompassing several types of sensory issues. A long-term goal of this movement is to include SPD in the Diagnostic and Statistical Manual of Mental Disorders (DSM); this effort failed, however, for the fifth edition. To learn more about SPD, go to the website of Miller's SPD Network at www.spdfoundation.net.

Former coworkers and students of Dr. Ayres are split on the use of this new terminology. In collaboration with Ayres's nephew, Brian Erwin, the successor trustee to the Jean Ayres Trust who trademarked the term *Ayres Sensory Integration®*, they established guidelines for anyone wishing to carry forth with Dr. Ayres work.

Ayres Sensory Integration includes the theory, assessment, patterns of dysfunction, and intervention concepts, principles, and techniques articulated by Dr. Ayres and applied by therapists trained in this approach worldwide. A summary of the main components of *Ayres Sensory Integration* is available on the SIGN website at www.siglobalnetwork.org.

Hypo- and hyper-reactivity. Ayres speculated that children with sensory integration dysfunction fell into one of two categories: the first includes those who are under- (hypo-) reactive to stimulation, and seek sensory experiences; the second includes those who are over- (hyper-) reactive to sensations, and show defensive behaviors. Contemporary research supports Ayres's theory and suggests that inconsistent sensory responses are due to either overly high thresholds for sensory input (hypo-) or sensory defensiveness (hyper-).[10] She further proposed that the abilities of those in both categories to register and modulate sensory stimuli varied from time to time and in different environments.[11]

Table 10.1 shows possible offenders in the environment which could trigger a defensive response from those on the autism spectrum.

Table 10.1

Frequent Environmental Offenders from Which
Hypersensitive Individuals Seek Protection

Their Own Clothing

- stiff tags
- stiff fibers (e.g., jeans)
- seams in socks
- waistbands and belts
- jewelry
- hairbands
- synthetic fibers

Clothing on Others

- synthetic fibers
- intricate patterns
- metallic look
- reflecting accessories (e.g., sequins, watches)
- noise makers (e.g., "bangle jangle" bracelets, watch alarms)

Odors

- paints, varnishes, glues
- room fresheners
- cologne, perfume, aftershave
- hair spray, gels, etc.
- clothes that have been dry-cleaned
- fabric softeners applied in the dryer
- orange peel, banana peel
- synthetics (e.g., plastic food packaging)
- fatty foods (e.g., broiled chops)
- extremely sweet odors
- extreme or unexpected body odors

Lighting

- fluorescent lights
- halogen lights
- strobe lights
- flickering sunlight (e.g., through leaves, blinds)
- severe contrast (e.g., stage productions)
- lighted mirrors
- reflective materials
- certain colors (esp. yellow-orange)
- color contrasts (e.g., red: black)
- white paper (esp. glossy magazines)
- LCD signboards
- automobile lights at night or in the rain
- automobile lights in white-tiled tunnels

Sounds	**Body-in-Space Situations**
• unexpected loud sounds	• light contact with seat, ground
• high-pitched sounds	• slightly tipped/irregular surfaces
• deeply resonating sounds	• swivel chairs
• disharmonious sounds	• open areas behind one's back
• background conversation	• close quarters
	• remaining seated while others move past

(Copyright, The HANDLE Institute; reprinted with permission)

Sometimes when multiple sensory stimuli compete for the body's attention, one sense may be hyper-responsive, while another may under-respond; there are an infinite number of sensory combinations. For instance, a child who is tactually defensive on a "bad" day and screams bloody murder at the hairdresser may tolerate a haircut if he or she is feeling more organized on another day.

Sensory Modulation and Motor Coordination

Well-functioning individuals can monitor the degree and timing of their responses to sensory information. Ayres called this automatic ability "registration," or "modulation." Many children with symptoms of sensory integration dysfunction have issues primarily in the areas of touch and movement that affect their modulation and registration. They thus have difficulty exerting consistent behavioral control over the sensory stimulus.[12]

Ayres's sensory integration theory stresses that the body's ability to process and interpret information coming in through touch, movement, balance, and body position lays the foundations for motor development. Thus, if processing of sensory input is aberrant, motor skills will be delayed.

Praxis

Praxis is one of the outcomes of motor, sensory, and sensory-motor integration all working efficiently. Simply defined as "the ability to do,"[13] Ayres wrote that praxis refers to the process underlying planning and execution of novel and complex motor patterns and sequences.[14] Praxis involves ideation, timing, sequencing, initiating, and transitioning. A dysfunction in praxis is called "dyspraxia," which can manifest itself in many ways, such as difficulty taking turns, organizing one's body and possessions, or even in trouble using speech and language. A therapist who does not recognize the role of motor planning in these end-product skills may be treating only symptoms.

Motor planning progresses from the "bottom-up" and the "inside-out." Good organizational skills and appropriate social interaction are two valued results of praxis. When motor development progresses smoothly, a child gains control over his or her body in the following order: lower body, upper body, shoulders and neck, upper arm, lower arm, hands, fingers.

Picture a one-year-old child beginning to walk with a wide-based gait, arms raised for balance and stability. As lower limbs strengthen and the trunk becomes more stable, arms drop to the sides. At first a child is unable to both walk and hold something in her hand. Eventually, as the trunk stabilizes, walking becomes more automatic, and the hands and arms can perform actions without fear of falling. As the upper body strengthens, the arms and hands become more coordinated.

Watch a three-year-old paint at an easel. The legs are positioned in a wide stance, the brush is held in a fisted grasp, and the movement is with the whole arm. Usually the eyes are not focused on the easel; if they are, they are looking at the finished product, not the active painting. Eventually, as the upper arm stabilizes, the grasp improves, and the standing posture narrows and is more flexible.

As motor development continues to take place, a child can sit comfortably at a table to write or draw, with trunk held upright and not collapsed. Both sides of the body begin to work together as two eyes and two hands coordinate, one to execute, and one to support the task at hand. The shoulders are still, an elbow may rest on the table, and the joints of the fingers work independently to engage the writing implement.

That predictable sequence of motor development allows a child to gradually be able to control big muscles and use smaller and smaller muscles with good coordination. This ability develops with everyday sensory and motor experiences. Compare this to those on the spectrum, many of whom are still "whole body," even as adults.

Sensory Processing in Autism

"If the senses are musical instruments, in autism, they lack a conductor. They are not able to play together."[15] An estimated 80–90% of individuals with autism experience atypical and problematic sensory processing.[16] Both hypo- and hyper-reactions to touch, movement, pressure, sound, smell, taste, and vision are the hallmarks of autistic behavior. Some are nauseated by the odors of a garbage truck; others insist upon wearing the same soft, loose sweat pants every day. Some crave deep touch and pressure; others cannot stand hugs.

Table 10.2 shows typical behaviors of those on the autism spectrum classified by sense and whether they represent hypo- or hyper-reactivity.

Table 10.2.

Autistic Behaviors Resulting from Hyper- and Hypo-Reactivity to Each Sense

SENSE	HYPER-REACTIVITY	HYPO-REACTIVITY
HEARING	Covers ears Dislikes haircuts Crying or tantrums	Attracted to sounds Likes vibrations Turns up volume
TOUCH	Avoids messy foods Ticklish Picky about clothing Won't walk on grass or sand	Ignores food on face Self-injurious behavior Touches everything High pain tolerance
TASTE & SMELL	Gags at new foods Reacts to odors Picky eater	Prefers spicy foods Smells clothing, self Mouths objects
VISION	Blinks excessively Covers eyes Picks up specks of dust Poor eye contact	Poor focus Lacks awareness Fascinated by reflectic Flicks fingers by eyes
VESTIBULAR/ PROPRIOCEPTIVE	Fearful of movement Gets car-sick Fear of being upside-down	Seeks deep pressure Spins or rocks Wiggles and squirms

Inappropriate reactions—such as flinching when touched, tuning out, hiding under the furniture, and covering eyes and ears—to the thousands of daily sensations from foods, clothing, and all aspects of the environment can all be the result of sensory overload. All of these responses interfere with further development and can cause additional problems with eating, dressing, bonding, learning, and just "being."

Many with autism function at a low sensory level, often preferring to rely upon the primitive senses of smell and touch; they use their mouths, instead of ears and eyes, to gain information about their worlds. They might sniff inedible objects (or people), put objects in their mouths, and touch things to learn where they and the objects are in space.

They also have vestibular dysfunction. Signs of vestibular problems are poor balance, hyperactivity due to gravitational insecurity, coordination difficulties, low muscle tone, and slumped posture. An underdeveloped vestibular system can be a contributing factor to faulty digestion, delayed language, poor social interaction, and lack of eye contact. Confining a mother with a high-risk pregnancy to bed rest (a practice that is now being questioned[17]) could result in a baby being born with an underdeveloped vestibular system.

Dysfunction in any part of the vestibulo-oculo-cervical (VOC) triad disrupts function in the others, resulting in compromised adaptive responses to environmental demands. Why is this important in autism? Because many children with ASDs experience *gravitational insecurity*, which creates significant feelings of anxiety and fear in response to vestibular-proprioceptive stimulation such as being tilted back in a chair or simply walking on uneven surfaces. If the secondary emotional responses are treated without addressing the probable underlying sensory causes, further incidents are inevitable.

Sound processing difficulties in autism manifest themselves as the impaired ability to perceive, process, or respond to sound appropriately. Children might experience

- **speech and language issues**, such as difficulties with articulation; memory; auditory discrimination, sequencing, rhythm, and timing; learning a foreign language; stuttering; or dysfluency;

- **social/emotional problems**, such as excessive crying, inability to make and keep friends, or using inappropriate words; or

- **academic issues**, such problems with decoding, reading comprehension, spelling, writing, or math.

As children grow up, further issues become apparent, such as difficulties tuning out background noise and following conversations, lack of self-confidence, and poor organization, public-speaking, and singing skills.

Many individuals with autism also demonstrate problems with sound sensitivities. Both under- and over-responsivity to sound are common. Those who are hypo-responsive may "tune out" and appear deaf at times. Others may be under-responsive and experience certain environmental sounds, such as the humming of a fluorescent bulb, as intolerable or even painful. Birthday parties, shopping malls, restaurants, sporting events and other gatherings can be particularly troublesome for them because of the unpredictability of sound.

Distorted processing of auditory signals impairs the brain's ability to focus on and give meaning to that which is heard. Inconsistencies in hearing the various frequencies of sound, or lack of synchronicity of the two ears, can result in behavior that is distractible, avoidant, hyperactive, inattentive, or bizarre.

School can be a sensory nightmare for those with autism. Sitting at circle time, standing in line, and negotiating moving bodies in the hallways and on the playground can involve human contact that is intermittent and unpredictable. For the child who experiences tactile over-sensitivity and who has difficulty reading cues that tell him what to expect next, these situations are likely to create anxiety and discomfort.[18]

The late psychiatrist Stanley Greenspan, MD, and psychologist Serena Wieder, PhD, found that 95% of 200 children with autism exhibited sensory modulation difficulties.[19] Australian psychologist Jan Piek and her colleagues showed that deficits in sensory integration contribute to problems in motor coordination and visual perception in students with autism spectrum disorders.[20] Another study compared eight boys with autism to eight controls and found that those with ASD had sensory issues that contributed to balance issues.[21]

On a cognitive level, those with autism have significant difficulty with higher-level sensory processing tasks, such as organization, because these activities require efficient sensory integration to give meaning to their world. With extreme sensory overload, one or more of the sensory systems eventually "shuts down."[22]

Research shows that gross, fine, and visual-motor deficits are common in children with ASDs.[23] They are considered clumsy and uncoordinated, often being the last chosen for any team sport or game. They have trouble isolating a foot to kick, an arm to throw, or a finger to write. They are "whole body."

One report found motor problems, including low muscle tone, motor planning problems, and other issues in over 80% of cases of autism.[24] Movement analysis by Philip Teitelbaum and his colleagues cited in the previous chapter also shows that children later diagnosed with autism showed persistent asymmetries in lying, righting, crawling, and sitting before the age of six months.[25]

The etiology of these sensory issues is unclear and varies person to person. If, as with many babies later diagnosed as autistic, high levels of toxins are present, they could very well be related to environmental factors. Another option is the repeated inner ear infections that many experienced as babies, as well as the treatments used to ameliorate them. Since senses are all immature at birth, they compete for the body's energy during those crucial first two years of life. Little energy is left for the demanding tasks of processing sight, sound, touch, and movement, let alone for language, feelings, social-emotional cues, and academics.

Sensory Diet

Many individuals with autism whose sensory processing is compromised find it hard to achieve and maintain an appropriate arousal level. They move from sensory-seeking to sensory-avoidance behaviors, which can be problematic for authority figures even though they serve a purpose for the individual. But what if kids with autism were given opportunities to rock, touch, move, and jump? Maybe they would be satiated and not act out inappropriately.

This is the stance taken by many occupational therapists who show parents how to use a "sensory diet." Just as a nutritionist recommends certain foods and supplements, the OT recommends readily available opportunities to be physical, and supplements them with a prescription of the "just right" combination of sensory activities for a particular child. Essential ingredients of a rich sensory diet are heavy work, physical activity, muscle exertion, movement, and firm, comforting touch.

A good sensory diet is food for the nervous system and includes activities such as swinging, climbing, digging, and molding play dough. Including vestibular stimulation activities as part of the daily diet for a child on the autism spectrum can be extremely powerful. Working against gravity on suspended equipment could result in secondary gains in the crucial areas of digestion, visual function (including eye contact), communication, and socialization.

Here are some ways to give kids of all ages and abilities more sensory experiences throughout the day:

- *Modify routine activities:* Add weight, move things out of reach, go the longer way over uneven terrain, put pressure on shoulders to activate neck receptors for proprioception while walking, give tighter hugs.

- *Modify objects to increase sensory demands*: Provide obstacles to climb over, crawl under, or walk around; make door catches tighter so one has to pull or push harder; use objects of differing sizes and weights to require frequent readjustment of exertion; offer larger versions of tasks, such as writing on a chalkboard instead of paper.

- *Create new opportunities:* Take breaks for moving, pushing, or pulling; wrap ace bandages around limbs for extra touch pressure; do isometric exercises and chair push-ups; do Brain Gym® before challenging activities (see chapter 8); sit quietly to settle down after excitement, while hugging knees and taking deep breaths.

- *Add sensation to a non-sensory activity:* Review academics while swinging or while balancing on a T-Stool, answer questions while pushing or pulling, sit on a vibrating pad or slightly inflated ball while reading or taking a test.

A rich sensory diet can make a big difference in how everyone experiences and relates to the world. A balanced "meal" of sensation could leave students with autism feeling replenished, settled, organized, and empowered.

How sensory diet and nutrition interact. While a good sensory diet is critical to correcting sensory imbalances, its effectiveness is limited by the quality of an individual's neural connections. Typical children have well-nourished nervous systems, which are strong and flexible. The nervous systems of many with autism, however, are composed of "malnourished" wires. For them, sensory therapies can be insufficient to produce efficient sensory integration.

Thus, a rich sensory diet must be supplemented with those minerals, essential fats, B-vitamins, and antioxidants discussed in earlier chapters. For instance, the nervous system needs magnesium to transmit electrical information. If a child has a magnesium deficiency, nerve signal transmission can be inefficient, resulting in poor sensory processing.

Kids with sensory issues have higher needs for both sensory input and nutritional intake than their typical peers. A limited sensory diet plus a self-limited food diet leaves them empty. Parents and therapists must thus broaden both areas to modify behavior. Kelly Dorfman suggests starting by removing the worst, empty-calorie foods from the pantry, and closing the nutrient gap with basic supplements.

Changing the structure and function of the nervous system takes time, and direct results may be hard to measure or tie directly to nutrition.

The good news is that "nutritious" sensory stimulation can actually improve the body's ability to use vitamins and minerals! Deep pressure, using weighted blankets and vests, and rhythmic activities such as dance, release oxytocin and may explain some of the repetitive rocking that many with autism seem to enjoy.[26]

Think "diet" in broad terms. By providing both a nutritious food diet and a healthy sensory diet, parents can ensure a strong, well-regulated nervous system, which in turn supports efficient cognition and behavior.

Dyspraxia in Autism

Dysfunction in praxis, or dyspraxia, is becoming more widely recognized as one of the critical functional deficits in autism spectrum disorders. While motor planning issues certainly present problems in isolation, their dramatic effect on functional skills cannot be underestimated. Dyspraxia could account for a number of the symptoms of autism; inappropriate social-emotional behavior (especially involving interpersonal relatedness), language development, and symbolic play are reported to be the areas most affected.[27] Turn-taking, the pragmatics of language, and reading social cues most certainly involve ideation, timing, and sequencing.

At any point in the above developmental sequence, if the demands for production exceed motor and visual maturity or if a reflex has not integrated, the child's body must physically compensate, and aberrant postures will emerge. This is often what happens in autism. A teacher may then observe a child slumping at the desk, wrapping her foot around the table leg, laying her head on an arm to write, or demonstrating other symptoms indicative of the lack of motor and visual readiness.

Uneven or spotty development, such as low tone and poor motor control, can result in missing important developmental steps over time, such as poor eating or omitted crawling. Parents, teachers, and therapists must be patient and focus on improving these lower-level skills rather than moving prematurely to higher skill levels. Pushing academics prematurely can result in diagnosed learning disabilities, attentional issues, or autistic-like behavior later on.

Sensory Evaluations

Sensory evaluations can be administered by qualified occupational therapists, physical therapists, optometrists, and others working with motor and visual skills. They usually include both formal and informal assessments of tactile, proprioceptive, and vestibular processing; motor planning, kinesthesia, muscle strength and tone, and motor control; attention to task; and visual perception and visual-motor integration.[28] Those on the autism spectrum experience difficulties in many or all of these areas. Therapists also depend upon their informal clinical observations, especially for those who cannot comply with the demands of formal testing.

Evaluating sensory processing is an ongoing process, as behaviors change day-to-day and in different settings with varying demands and people. To ensure a complete history and observation of sensory responses, information should be gathered at home and school, from teachers and parents, and from any other setting where the child can be observed. For those on the severe end of the spectrum, whose behaviors are the most challenging, informal assessments, questionnaires, and checklists yield more information than formal testing.

Some OTs have developed forms for taking sensory histories, as well as checklists and questionnaires to evaluate the sensory functioning of those on the autism spectrum. A popular informal instrument is *"Questions to Guide Classroom Observations"* by Kientz and Miller.[29] Teachers respond to a series of 38 questions about the child, specific tasks, the physical environment, and the social and cultural context. This questionnaire is most commonly used to informally guide teachers and therapists on how to improve a child's performance at school. It is especially helpful in identifying environmental issues, such as noises from heating and air conditioning, difficulties with lighting, or excessive visual stimulation. Altering any of these factors can improve a student's potential for success.

Another popular instrument for use with this population is the *Sensory Profile* by Winnie Dunn.[30] This instrument is available in two forms: Infant/Toddler and Adolescent/Adult. Using a Likert scale, caregivers rate an individual's responsivity to 125 items. Information is categorized into six domains of sensory processing (auditory, visual, vestibular, tactile, multisensory, and oral), five domains of modulation (tone, body position, activity level, and visual input affecting emotional responses and activity level), and three domains of behavioral outcomes (typical, probably atypical, or definitely atypical).

Studies are ongoing using the *Sensory Profile* for both making a differential diagnosis and for remediation recommendations. One study found that this instrument was able to discriminate with 90% accuracy among those with pervasive developmental disorders, attention deficits, and those who were not disabled.[31] The *Sensory Profile* is also excellent for monitoring progress and adapting intervention techniques.

The newest informal assessment tool is the *Sensory Processing Measure (SPM)*, published by Western Psychological Services (WPS).[32] Available in three forms—for home, classroom, and the school environment—this comprehensive instrument makes it possible to obtain a complete picture of sensory functioning for children ages two through twelve.

A child's parent or home-based care provider completes the 75-item "Home Form," and the primary classroom teacher fills in the "Main Classroom Form" (62 items). Adjunct school personnel complete the "School Environments Form" (10–15 items per environment) to assess sensory processing in six environments: during art, music, physical education, and recess, in the cafeteria, and on the school bus. Because it solicits input from school staff members who are not typically involved in assessment—the art teacher and school bus driver, for example—the "School Environments Form" serves a team-building function. It educates school personnel about sensory processing disorders and uses their input. Results yield scores in

- social participation
- vision
- hearing

- touch
- body awareness (proprioception)
- balance and motion (vestibular function)
- planning and ideas (praxis)
- total sensory systems

Scores for each scale fall into one of three interpretive ranges: "Typical," "Some Problems," or "Definite Dysfunction." Within each sense, the SPM offers descriptive clinical information on processing vulnerabilities, including under- and over-responsiveness, sensory-seeking behavior, and perceptual problems. Comparison of the child's sensory functioning at home and at school is available.

If a child is able to comply with the demands of standardized testing, most OTs administer a formal measure. Formal tests, coupled with the examiner's clinical observations, can elicit a great deal of information about a child's response to sensory stimulation, posture, balance, coordination, and movement activities. These reactions are compared to norms established for the child's age. After carefully analyzing data and putting them in the context of the child's home and school environments, the therapist can make recommendations.

The standardized instrument of choice for children age four through eight is the *Sensory Integration and Praxis Test (SIPT)*.[33] Specially trained and certified occupational or physical therapists can conduct a formal evaluation using this test, which can serve to establish a baseline of functioning in each of the sensory systems. The SIPT is an extremely comprehensive measure based on factor analysis, and is computer scored. It consists of 17 subtests measuring space visualization, figure-ground perception, standing/walking balance, design copying, postural praxis, bilateral motor coordination, praxis on verbal command, constructional praxis, post-rotary nystagmus, motor accuracy, sequencing praxis, oral praxis, manual form perception, kinesthesia, finger indentification, graphesthesia, and localization of tactile stimuli.

In a study all of the subtests of the SIPT discriminated significantly between children who were developing typically and those with high-functioning autism. Those with autism demonstrated significant difficulties in praxis, bilateral integration, sequencing, and some aspects of vestibular function.[34]

For children who are outside the age norms of the SIPT, or who cannot comply with standardization procedures, OTs observe spontaneous play with toys and equipment, coordination, tone, laterality, goal orientation, and initiation of actions. These clinical observations are sometimes equally or more valuable than the test results.

Screening for Sensory Integration Dysfunction

A faster way of checking for sensory issues is to do a sensory screening. Lynn A. Balzer-Martin, PhD, OTR, a veteran with over 30 years' experience, has designed a screening tool for preschool children based on sensory integration principles. She administers it annually to all the three-, four-, and five-year-olds at several nursery schools in the Washington, DC, area. It includes not only the direct screening of children, two-by-two, but also parent and teacher questionnaires. All of the data is combined to provide recommendations for the adults in the child's life. Entitled the *Balzer-Martin Preschool Screening (BAPS)*, it is published by St. Columba's Nursery School, 4201 Albemarle St NW, Washington, DC 20016.

Two other formal measures for screening young children are *The DeGangi-Berk Test of Sensory Integration (TSI)*[35] and the *Miller PreSchool Screening Test*.[36] Both are designed for use with three- to five-year-old children, and are available from Western Psychological Services (WPS).

Interventions for Sensory Processing Issues

In the 1970s Carl Delacato, an educational psychologist, was the first to propose that the sensory abnormalities of those with autism were treatable.[37] Today, OTs are the most likely profession to treat sensory problems in autism, although practitioners from a variety of disciplines, including physical therapy, audiology, and optometry, have designed numerous sensory-based approaches, which are included in this chapter. Vision therapy is covered in chapter 11.

One OT who spent her professional life applying sensory integration theory to patients with autism and other developmental disabilities is the late Lorna Jean King, OTR/L, FAOTA, founder and director of the Children's Center for Neurodevelopmental Studies in Glendale, Arizona. Beginning with just one student in 1978, this model center has served thousands of children ages 3 through 22, who are treated by various therapists utilizing sensory integration techniques. **To learn more about King's legacy go to** www.thechildrenscenteraz. org.

Sensory integration based occupational therapy consists of guided activities that challenge and enhance the body's ability to respond appropriately to one or more senses. Certification is required for those performing evaluations, but not for doing sensory integration therapy. Therapists use controlled tactile, proprioceptive, and/ or vestibular input to elicit the simplest adaptive responses. Some activities are aimed at improving the processing of an individual sense, while others facilitate components of praxis, such as initiation, sequencing, bilateral coordination, timing, and imitation.

At first the child participates in simple, safe, and purposeful sensory activities, such as swinging, receiving deep pressure under pillows, and being touched with a soft cloth. Eventually, with gentle guidance, the child might tolerate increasingly stimulating activities such as merry-go-rounds, hair brushing, and new foods. Soon a child may independently recognize that swinging on the playground fulfills the same sensory need as running in circles, and then choose a socially appropriate, rather than an inappropriate, activity. As efficient, organized responses occur more frequently and become more consistent, they ultimately heighten a child's ability to pay attention, relate, sit still, organize language, and focus.[38].

Therapy does not focus on the training of specific skills, because then the underlying problems are not resolved, and the body does not learn how to adapt to future similar activities, but rather just how to do that single task. A variety of tools, including suspended equipment, is necessary. Table 10.3 shows some of the tools occupational therapists use to normalize each system.

Table 10.3.

Tools for Normalizing Sensory Processing

AUDITORY Whistles, musical instruments, CDs, environmental
sounds

TACTILE Stretch fabrics including lycra & spandex, finger paints,
play dough, ball pits

TASTE & SMELL Salty, sweet, sour, crunchy foods; aromatherapy
oils; NOXO Autism Alleviation™ balm from Olfactory
Biosciences Corp. (http://noxoinfo.com/sensory)

VISUAL Slant boards

VESTIBULAR Hammocks, swings, slings, scooters, teeter-totters,
gliders, skates, bikes, rockers

PROPRIOCEPTIVE Weighted vests or blankets, ankle and wrist
weights, seat cushions, beanbag chairs

In the book *Asperger Syndrome and Sensory* Issues,[39] the authors
include over 25 pages of behaviors, such as "has rituals," "won't
eat certain foods," and "poor eye contact," with possible sensory
interpretations and suggested interventions. This section of the
book is a great reference for parents to help them understand the
role of touch, movement, vision, and the other senses in the aberrant
behavior they see in their kids.

Sound Therapies

Utilizing sound to facilitate bodily change is not new. For centuries,
almost every culture on earth has developed methods using sound
and song to heal. Unfortunately, many of these tools are associated
with superstition and mysticism. Today's sophisticated computerized
technology allows us to document what is happening in the body
and brain, thus removing the mystery.

Modern sound-based therapies include interventions that address
auditory, listening, and vestibular issues. Some call sound-based
therapies "listening therapies" or "auditory retraining therapies."
However, they are much more than "listening" to music or
"retraining" the ear. The term "sound-based therapies" embraces all

components of the other terms as well as includes other therapies that utilize sound and vibration on the body through special equipment, modified music, and/or specific tones or beats.

In the past 20 years, an increasing number of professionals from a variety of disciplines, including audiology, occupational therapy, psychology, and speech-language pathology, are recommending and incorporating sound-based therapies to improve the auditory, listening, and vestibular skills of children with ASDs. While some programs are designed to take place in a therapist's office, others can be used at home under a therapist's supervision.

A renowned expert in every aspect of sound therapy is audiologist Dorinne Davis, MA, CCC-A, F-AAA, who for more than 30 years has been using sound to rehabilitate individuals with autism and other disabilities. She is credentialed in 20 different sound-based therapies, including Tomatis®, Berard, Solisten™, Fast ForWord®, Digital Auditory Aerobics®, EnListen®, JoEE®-h, JoEE®-v, HiFi Brain Fitness®, Samonas® I, Therapeutic Listening, EaSE™, Dynamic Listening System®, REI®, Lindamood-Bell Learning Processes Program, and Medical Resonance Therapy Music®.

Davis always begins with her *Diagnostic Evaluation for Therapy Protocol (DETP®)* from which she determines which sound-based therapies may be appropriate. While all sound therapies have efficacy, Davis believes that long-standing changes are possible only when therapies are administered in the correct order.

Based in New Jersey, the Davis Center is one of the world's premier sound therapy centers and attracts patients from all over the world. Readers interested in learning more about this powerful intervention should read one of Davis's five books and go to her website at www.thedaviscenter.com.

Two of the most common methods of sound therapy used with autism are the Tomatis Method, named after French otolaryngologist and the father of sound-based therapies, Alfred Tomatis, MD, and Auditory Integration Training (AIT), which was founded in 1992 by Guy Berard, MD, (age 98 at this writing!) a French physician who studied with Tomatis. Tomatis therapy supports a connection between the voice, the ear, and the brain first identified by Tomatis in the 1950s. AIT retrains the acoustic reflex muscle in the middle ear, allowing better transmission of "clearer" sound to the cochlea and subsequently to the brain for comprehension.

Tomatis® is appropriate for anyone interested in improving balance, coordination, motor skills, sensory integration, academics, communication, attention, memory, or organization, or for anyone desiring to enhance overall development and personal growth. A typical core program consists of two intensive sessions of 30 hours each: two hours per day for 15 days, with a month break in between. Tomatis can also be delivered as a personalized sound stimulation program called The Listening Program™, a series of eight to ten CDs engineered with classical music selections and nature sounds that naturally enhance function of the ear and brain.

When Tomatis died in 2001, his protégé, Canadian psychologist Dr. Paul Madaule, became the disciple for his work. For Madaule, the ear is the conductor of the sensory orchestra. When he speaks of the ear, he means the organ as well as all of its connections to the nervous system and the whole body.

Madaule has written about his experiences and his life's work practicing and adapting the Tomatis method in his book, *When Listening Comes Alive: A Guide to Effective Learning and Communication.*[40] It is also available in Spanish as *Terapia de Escucha.*[41] Madaule's adaptation of the Tomatis Method is called Listening Fitness Training or LiFT®. Madaule owns and operates the Listening Centre in Toronto, Ontario, Canada, which he founded in 1978. At the Listening Centre, he evaluates and helps many individuals with autism spectrum diagnoses. Go to www.listeningcentre.com for more info.

Another important Tomatis disciple is Pierre Sollier, who studied with Tomatis and has translated his works. His book, Listening for Wellness: An Introduction to the Tomatis Method, is a great way to learn about this intervention.[42] You can find a certified Tomatis provider on his website at www.tomatis.com.

Finally, read Sharon Ruben's heartfelt story about her daughter who recovered from autism using the Tomatis Method: *Awakening Ashley: Mozart Knocks Autism on its Ear.*[43]

Berard Auditory Integration Training (AIT) is appropriate for those with hypersensitivity to sound, lack of awareness of sound, and the inability to discriminate sound differences. Originally called "Auditory Training," the word "integration" was added later, making it AIT. This intervention randomly introduces low- and high-pitched sounds to the auditory system; these sounds increase blood flow to the brain, adding to the overall positive effect. Therapy consists of twenty half-hour sessions, twice daily for ten days.

Berard postulated that the quality of the perception of sound that one hears is equal to the behavior of the individual. He formulated his own theory that "human behavior is greatly conditioned by the way one hears." Berard's theory evolved further as he observed how the audiograms of children with disabilities change along with their behavior.

Berard developed his own "hearing retraining device" to treat patients with auditory problems that were more subtle than hearing loss. He originally described his method as one of "hearing re-education" in *Hearing Equals Behavior*,[44] which was recently updated and expanded in collaboration with Sally Brockett, MS.[45] Brockett trained under Berard in 1991, and is currently director of the IDEA Training Center in Connecticut. Annabel Stehli introduced AIT for those with autism in the early 1990s after her daughter Georgiana's remarkable improvement.[46]

In 2004, Stephen M. Edelson, PhD, and the late Bernard Rimland, PhD of the Autism Research Institute (ARI) reviewed 28 published studies investigating the effectiveness of AIT in autism spectrum disorders. Most research shows that AIT clearly confers improvement for a significant proportion of those with ASDs. Positive changes include reduced hyperactivity, social withdrawal, restlessness, anxiety, and sound sensitivity; increased attention span and language output; and improved speech perception. One study also showed biochemical changes, specifically, an increase in norepinephrine and decrease in serotonin levels.[47] Abstracts of all studies are available online.[48] To find a Berard practitioner worldwide, go to www. berardaitwebsite.com.

Interactive Metronome® (IM) is not a true sound therapy, but it is included here because it combines sound with a computer-based monitor, and requires a motor response. It is a true measure of sensory integration! Created by James Cassily, a sound engineer, IM is based on the premise that improving one's ability to plan and sequence motor actions enhances cognitive, learning, and social skills. Professionals in a number of disciplines have added it to their tool chests for those with autism.

A subject wears a special headset that emits signals. The IM computerized program challenges the participant to precisely match the computer's rhythm by tapping hand or foot sensors. A different set of tones gives the person feedback as to whether his or her response is too early, too late, or just right. The computer immediately analyzes the difference in milliseconds between the actual beat and the person's motor response, and then averages his or her ability to maintain focus over an extended period of time. During a full training, a person could respond over 35,000 times.

IM takes fifteen days, listening one hour per day over three to five weeks. Some people need up to as many as ten additional sessions. Interactive Metronome is now in use in more than 5,000 clinics in North America. To find a practitioner and to learn more, go to www.interactivemetronome.com.

Multisensory Programs from Occupational Therapists

A number of occupational therapists have developed packaged programs that address the sensory needs of their patients. While not specifically for those on the autism spectrum, these are very adaptable for those with high-functioning autism. Two particularly good programs are the *Alert Program for Self-Regulation*, also known as "How Does Your Engine Run?"[49] and the *Tool Chest for Teachers, Parents and Students*.[50]

The Alert Program, developed by occupational therapists Mary Sue Williams and Sherry Shellenberger, empowers students to learn how to regulate their own arousal systems. Comparing their bodies to cars, kids rev up their engines for active times of day, such as recess, and rev down for re-entering the classroom for reading. The techniques can also be used to prepare for anxiety-producing situations, such as going to the doctor, and over-stimulating environments, like restaurants and shopping malls.

In their book, *Take Five! Staying Alert at Home and School,* these innovative therapists provide a myriad of activities for the hypo- and hyper-sensitive child in five areas: touch, movement, vision, audition, and oral-motor.[51] Some of these activities are appropriate for in-office use to maximize an exam or enhance therapy. The manual also includes an extremely valuable checklist for adults with sensory issues.

Tool Chest, developed by Diana Henry, OT, includes comprehensive handbooks and DVDs offering many activities for home and school. Her focus is on mitigating undesirable behaviors by addressing their sensory roots. She travels around the world giving workshops for school systems. Her techniques are worth seeing if she is ever in your area. Go to her website at www.ateachabout.com to see her schedule.

Sensory-Based Programs from Other Professions

Sensory Learning is a unique program developed in 1997 by Mary Bolles, a mother who was seeking help for her son. Not speaking at age three, Jason was exhibiting behaviors consistent with children on the autism spectrum. Mary discovered that combining three individual modalities (visual, auditory, and vestibular) into one multisensory experience provided the positive results she had been seeking for Jason.

This intervention targets students at both ends of the autism spectrum. Based on an evaluation of an individual's auditory, visual, and vestibular function, computer-assisted technology prescribes an individualized remediation program. The visual component uses syntonics—colored lights that pulse on and off about six times per minute (read more about syntonics in the next chapter). The vestibular stimulation is delivered on a motion table that rotates in various planes. The auditory part uses headphones that contain modulated music.

Over 30 Sensory Learning Program centers around the world provide clients with two 30-minute sessions each day for 12 consecutive days, including weekends and holidays. Each session is an individual sensory experience that simultaneously engages visual, auditory, and vestibular systems to work in an integrated way. The repetitive sensory activation of each session builds on the session before. After 12 days of sessions, the individual returns home with a portable light instrument to continue the program with a 20-minute session each morning and evening for the next 18 days. For more information on Sensory Learning and locations of centers, go to www.sensorylearning.com.

HANDLE is another international program not designed by an OT, that focuses on the sensory issues in autism along with the accompanying nutritional and digestive problems. An acronym for the Holistic Approach to NeuroDevelopment and Learning Efficiency, the concept for this approach grew out of the need for its late founder, Judith Bluestone, to understand and heal her own challenges. Since 1994 the HANDLE Institute in Seattle, Washington, has certified hundreds of trainers and treated thousands of individuals with learning disabilities, attention deficits, autism, PDD, dyspraxia, language disorders, Tourette syndrome, and a plethora of perceptual and behavioral disorders.

Strengthening the vestibular system, enhancing muscle tone, and increasing differentiation are the goals of HANDLE. These are all accomplished through deceptively simplistic activities that are sensitive to the client's physical and social-emotional needs. Small, measured doses of specific activities are incorporated into daily activities in the home, daycare, or school setting. Therapy time typically requires approximately a half hour, preferably interspersed throughout the day. Some of the more frequently suggested activities involve

- drinking from a crazy straw
- playing follow-the-leader with a flashlight
- rhythmic ball bouncing
- copying designs by only feeling them
- catching a suspended ball
- stepping through a hula hoop maze

For more information on HANDLE, read *The Fabric of Autism: Weaving the Threads into a Cogent Theory*[52] and visit www.handle.org.

The Squeeze Machine was invented by Temple Grandin, PhD, probably the most well-known and successful adult with autism in the world. As a child she regularly visited a relative's farm, where she was attracted to the machine used to restrain cows while they were branded. She loved the deep pressure the machine provided her body, and found that it calmed her and decreased her severe tactile defensiveness. This life-changing experience led to her career as the world's authority on livestock handling equipment.

The squeeze machine appears to lessen tension and anxiety in young children with modulation issues by delivering deep touch pressure to the trunk. For improvement, six to twelve sessions are necessary.[53]

Today, families of children with autism can purchase a prototype she designed, available for use in homes and schools from the Therafin Corporation at www.therafin.com. The Squeeze Machine allows the individual to control the amount of and need for pressure. According to the website, "This ingenious system is used for deep touch stimulation and produces a calming effect on hyperactive and autistic individuals."

Movement and Fitness Programs for Autism

If you are clumsy, can't catch your breath, and don't know where your body is in space, how do you learn? In the "olden days" when I went to school, we had gym class *every day*. No longer! Daily gym has been replaced by weekly physical education (PE), and general fitness has been replaced by sports. But what if you cannot play competitive sports?

For those on the autism spectrum, fitness is an important life skill that is missing in many IEPs and special education curricula. Some schools have adaptive physical education for students with special needs, but again they meet once or twice a week. Everyone, no matter their age, needs to move *every* single day! Use it or lose it. We *must* move to keep our muscles and joints oiled, our hearts pumping, and our digestion flowing. Moving against gravity easily, effortlessly, and without pain is being fit.

Here are some model programs that combine professional evaluations, individual goal setting, and a customized programming of coordination, sensory, and motor activities to improve fitness, motivation, self-esteem, self-advocacy, socialization, and overall physical wellness. Ultimately those on the spectrum gain joy in movement and healthy motor activity for a lifetime.

Autism Movement Therapy (AMT), including the Aut-erobics® DVD, is a movement and music integration program developed by Joanne Lara, MA, a California special educator and dancer. AMT combines motor patterning, movement auditory processing, rhythm, and sequencing in a unique and fun way with the goal of improving behavioral, emotional, academic, social, speech, and language skills. Available in three levels designed for those with "emerging," "developing," and "proficient" skills, each group goes through warm-ups, stationary movements, locomotion, improvisation, and cool down. Learn more about training, certification and using this exciting program at www.AutismMovementTherapy.com.

A couple of great programs in the Washington, DC area provide movement and sensory opportunities for those with autism and motor challenges. Joye Newman, MA, the founder of Kids Moving Company (www.kidsmovingco.com) in Bethesda, MD, and Dov Judd, the owner of MOCO Movement Center (www.MOCOmc.com) understand that kids with autism spectrum diagnoses can benefit greatly from climbing, jumping, moving and balancing. Their programs are multi-faceted, and include intensive camps, classes, and individual sessions. Activities are non-competitive and reach success through a progressive skill acquisition process using of state-of-the-art equipment.

Newman has partnered with Carol Kranowitz, MA, author of the best seller *The Out-of-Sync Child*,[54] to produce *Growing an In-Sync Child: Simple, Fun Activities to Help Every Child Develop, Learn, and Grow*,[55] and accompanying In-Sync activity cards.[56]

MOCO Movement Center in Kensington, MD takes pediatric therapy out into the "field" where the child can practice skills in the real world. They learn at a climbing center, ice skating rink, playground, hiking/biking trails, and even in music and art studios. One of their therapists is a very smart and friendly trained therapy dog named Ziza.

Marc Sickel, ATC, founded *Fitness for Health* in Rockville, MD, to promote fitness for those with autism and other special needs. Sickel had personal experience in special education. Today he is committed to helping this generation of children (and seniors!) maximize their physical potential, improve self-esteem, and achieve goals previously thought unattainable.

Special equipment includes a laser maze that teaches athletes where their bodies are in space and builds motor planning, coordination, and balance as they crouch under and step over laser beams. They receive instant auditory feedback if they err in their movements. Participants can play virtual reality sports games with actual body movements, scale an 80-foot transverse climbing wall at different levels, harness up and climb a 10-foot-tall, glow-in-the-dark climbing wall, bounce down a 30-foot trampoline while playing mini-basketball, negotiate a ropes course, bat in a batting cage with an indoor pitching machine, play glow-in-the-dark soccer, test skills against a high-tech reaction and coordination game, and be introduced to a variety of games and equipment involving visual perception and motor planning. To learn more, go to www.fitnessforhealth.org.

Two unique programs in metropolitan New York City are Autism Fitness on Long Island and WeeZee World in Westchester County. **Autism Fitness** was founded 10 years ago by Eric Chessen, MS, YCS. To Chessen, fitness is the ability to navigate successfully through everyday motor challenges. It is at the foundation of all human performance, and includes life skills such as getting dressed independently, taking out the garbage, maneuvering the monkey bars on a playground, and, yes, playing sports.

Chessen began working with kids on the spectrum as a camp counselor, and after a graduate education in psychology, he combined his background in fitness with his training in Applied Behavior Analysis to develop a successful fitness program for children with autism. Today he is a national motivational speaker who teaches about fitness for individuals with autism of all ages.

How does Chessen get kids on the autism spectrum off the couch—away from their beloved video games—and help them overcome their movement deficits? By establishing a relationship and setting up reasonable expectations. Recognizing that their perceptions and experiences are different, his number one goal is to alleviate frustration and anxiety. Some favorite questions are: What do you want to do? Which piece of equipment should we use first? What kinds of jumps should we do? He wants them to own their individual physical abilities and be able to use them in a wide variety of situations.

Chessen has developed a set of activities, which he offers as a DVD, that incorporate five essential movement patterns: pushing, pulling, rotating, squatting, and locomotion. These might use sandbells, stability balls, hurdles, or other equipment. He also has a distance mentoring program for fitness professionals who wish to work with individuals with autism and related disorders. His newest product is his Autism Fitness e-book, designed to provide parents, educators, fitness professionals, and therapists with a blueprint for creating a successful fitness program for individuals or groups. All of these are available on his websites, www.AutismFitness.com and www.ericchessen.com.

Louise Weadock, a licensed nurse with one of the world's largest staffing companies, saw the need for a family-friendly gym to serve individuals of all ages and abilities. She transformed 18,000 square feet of unused office space in Chappaqua, NY, into a sensory paradise called **WeeZee World: The World of "YES I Can"** (www. WeeZeeWorld.com). Her mission is to create sensory adventures that improve academic performance, develop athletic coordination, and enhance social relationships.

Even though WeeZee does not target those on the autism spectrum, it is autism-friendly. WeeZee incorporates techniques, equipment, and research from the field of sensory integration and translates them into a fun and exciting exploratory environment. Kids move and explore under the guidance of sensory coaches who have skills ranging from musical talent to athletic accomplishment and backgrounds in teaching, coaching, or working with children.

WeeZee blends elements of a children's museum, an indoor playground, and a multi-station learning center. Members move from sense to sense and room to room exploring drums, guitar, and piano through karaoke; climbing rock walls; and jumping into ball pits and on trampolines. Each time they walk down the hall, they receive therapeutic brushing from plastic bristles on the chair rail.

Some prefer water play in the Rain Room; others chill on massage chairs in the Zen Den. A separate room for the youngest and those who prefer less stimulation is available. The Groove Grove, Vibration Station, Art Room, GalaxZee, and Brain Games all lend themselves to group interaction, through which kids can gradually develop confidence in social situations.

Animals as Sensory Integration Therapy Tools

"People and animals are supposed to be together," states Temple Grandin in *Animals in Translation*.[57] Thus, partnering with animals in sensory therapies is natural! While almost any animal will do, the most commonly used animals are dolphins, dogs, and horses.

Dolphins are true sensory processing machines! Laboratory studies confirm that they use sound, taste, touch, and vision to communicate and navigate their environment.[58] Using dogs for people with disabilities is not new; Seeing Eye dogs have helped those with limited sight for decades. A dog can provide considerable sensory stimulation, most of which is comforting. Just the smell of a familiar dog can be calming for some children on the spectrum. Recently, well-trained service dogs have become trusted companions for those with autism. Read more about both of these animals in chapter 12, where they are included because of their strong impact on improved communication and social interactions in individuals with autism.

Therapeutic horseback riding, or "hippotherapy," is practiced by specially trained occupational, physical, and speech therapists. Therapists' goals do not focus on specific riding skills, but rather on establishing the neurological foundations for improved function and sensory processing. Participants groom, dress, ride, care for, and love their horses, but do not control their horses' movements.

The horse's walk provides proprioceptive, vestibular, tactile, visual, auditory, and olfactory stimuli that are beneficial to the rider through movement which is variable, rhythmic, and repetitive.[59] Through adapting to the horse's movements, the rider develops better balance and coordination, as well as flexibility, posture, muscle strength, mobility, and overall physical function.[60] These skills often generalize to other areas, including increased independence, which fosters improved performance in a wide range of daily activities. To find a stable near you, go to www.pathintl.org, the website of the Professional Association of Therapeutic Horsemanship International.

Music

According to neurologist and best-selling author, Oliver Sacks, MD, pathways for music occupy more areas of the brain than for language.[61] Sally Goddard Blythe calls music "one of life's earliest teachers." Prenatally, the fetus reacts to music with movement; infants respond to music and can imitate simple rhythms, like Paddy Cake, before they develop speech. Music supplies the architecture for many aspects of learning.[62]

Music can be very organizing and can assist in the remediation of any skills by providing calming or alerting background sounds. It can enhance cognitive function, language comprehension and usage, and perceptual-, gross-, and fine motor skills. For those on the autism spectrum it can make the difference between being able to participate in an activity and avoiding it.

Music Therapy

Music therapy, quite different from sound therapy, "provides a variety of multi-sensory experiences in an intentional and developmentally appropriate manner" for those on the autism spectrum.[63] Certified music therapists use a variety of instruments, including their voices, to deliver concrete, auditory, visual, tactile, proprioceptive, and vestibular stimulation to both hemispheres of the brain.

Several types of music therapy are showing success with individuals on the autism spectrum.[64] To learn about them and to find music therapists in your area, go to www.musictherapy.org.

Developmental Music Therapy

Joe Romano invented the profession "developmental music therapist" to describe how he helps children and adults on the autism spectrum and others most professionals have given up on, to function at higher levels and lead more enjoyable lives. For Joe, music is the engine that makes people run. Working closely with behavioral optometrists to maximize his results (see next chapter), Joe combines music with movement, visual processing, and other techniques that he invented, to understand children's minds and to move their development forward.

As a young child, Joe had a severe eye turn; one eye often pointed at his nose instead of aiming with the other eye. Doctors recommended surgery to straighten the turned eye, but Joe's mother, not convinced, declined. Alone in his room, in secret, by the light of the streetlight outside his bedroom window, Joe worked night after night training his brain to process his eyes together. As a young musician, he learned songs with specific rhythm patterns that affected a listener's heart rate and breathing patterns.

Rather than use his newfound knowledge selfishly, for the past 20 years Joe has selflessly been applying these subtle but powerful sound and rhythm techniques to working with children on the autism spectrum. Rhythm is an integral part of life, and many children with autism are unaware of rhythm. The ability to consciously tap into rhythm can enhance a person's capacity to think and move more successfully; rhythm can slow down the mind.

A couple of years ago, Joe had a vision: to create an engaging story CD called "The Kingdom of Should" filled with songs and music that positively affect attention and behavior for those on the autism spectrum. The story's three heroes are children on the spectrum. The adults are an optometrist and developmental music therapist.

Romano has also created the music CD, "Dreaming in The Land of Can," an exceptional and innovative therapeutic tool for kids who have trouble falling and staying asleep. Because these pieces are designed to loop over and over throughout the night, they promote deep, restful, and relaxing sleep. To order his products, go to www.kingdomofshould.com.

Occupational Therapy to Music

OTs discovered that music can be both calming and alerting; several have composed songs to enhance sensory integration. Here are two of my favorites:

- *Genevieve Jereb, OTR,* was born "down under" in Australia, so her songs have a bit of a different flair. Kids of all developmental levels love "Songs for Sensory Regulation," "Say G'Day," "No Worries," "Cool Bananas," and "Jumpin' Jellybeans." These CDs are packed with fun and engaging, ready-to-use rhythmic songs and activities to support learning, transitions, sleep, attention, focus, and self-regulation. Listen to them and choose your favorites at www.sensorytools.net.

- *Aubrey Carton Lande, OTR,* and **Lois Hickman, MS, OTR, FAOTA,** teamed with musician Bob Wiz to make "SongGames for Sensory Processing." This delightful CD has 25 songs that engage young children in active play, calms them down, and can decrease tactile, auditory, visual, and sensory defensiveness. Order from www.fhautism.com.

Musical Giftedness

Many individuals with autism are intrinsically attracted to music. Some are musically gifted, like David Helfgott, featured in the movie *Shine*. Matt Savage, called the "Mozart of jazz" by the late Dave Brubeck, and Stephen Shore, PhD, a very accomplished adult on the spectrum, have musical gifts as well.

Savage was diagnosed with PDD at the age of three and in his teens became a professional jazz pianist with his own trio. He plays all over the world alongside the best adult musicians of our time.

Shore, who teaches music to those with autism, writes eloquently about the role music played in his childhood. In his autobiography, *Beyond the Wall*, he explains how, when he could not learn the Hebrew necessary for his Bar Mitzvah, he perfectly mimicked an audiotape of a cantor singing the prayers, which he accompanied with the necessary ceremonial, rhythmic, rocking called *davening*.[65]

Sensory Connections to Other Problems in Autism

Sleep disturbances, picky eating, and toilet training, three of the most problematic issues in autism spectrum disorders, all have sensory connections. Parents frequently call upon therapists to intervene in these troublesome areas.

Sleep

Children at both ends of the spectrum have difficulties falling asleep, staying asleep, and waking up. Professionals in the field attribute these difficulties to sensory regulatory issues. Physical therapist Debra Dickson and occupational therapist Anne Buckley-Reen conceived a sleep hygiene program called SANE. The SANE approach facilitates change through restorative **S**leep, **A**ctivities to reduce stress, balanced **N**utrition, and nurturing **E**nvironments.

Buckley-Reen and Dickson contend that following their routine at the same time every night, results in significant changes in one to two weeks.[66] Refer back to chapter 3 to see their guidelines.

Picky Eating

The nutritional issues in autism are covered in earlier chapters. Nutritional deficiencies often begin as early as in the preemie nursery where tubes taped to the faces of tiny babies produce sensitivities on the lips, tongue, cheeks, and face. A combination of sensory and oral motor issues, such as limited lip and tongue mobility, difficulties swallowing, chewing, and teeth grinding are common.

Babies can emerge from the neonatal intensive care unit (NICU) with tactile defensiveness, low tone, or hyposensitivity in the very areas responsible for their survival. Nursing from a breast or a bottle may be difficult. As feeding becomes a challenge, infants and mothers become anxious. The train has just left the station for a possible lifetime of eating disorders.

When nutritional issues combine with sensory problems, picky eating results, and toddlers reject foods because of their flavors, odors, or textures. Kelly Dorfman, a nutritionist in suburban Washington, DC, and author of *Cure Your Child with Food*,[67] is an expert on picky eating. She focuses on both nutritional and oral motor deficits, as well as on the psycho-emotional and behavioral issues in picky eating, and recommends a team approach.

Dorfman believes that children with autism, especially those with significant sensory issues, refuse food because this is one way they can control their surroundings in order to lessen their anxiety. She cites sensory misreading in the mouth as one factor that can contribute to picky eating.

Some hospitals have "feeding clinics" featuring multidisciplinary teams composed of oral motor specialists like occupational therapists, speech-language pathologists, and nutritionists. Without early expert oral motor therapy, many infants are destined to become picky eaters.

Toilet Training

Moving from diapers to the bathroom is one of the most elusive milestones for many families working with children on the autism spectrum. Sensing that the bladder or intestine is full and acting upon it requires a high level of sensory integration. When children with autism are calm, they may be able to feel the sensations that they need to urinate or defecate, but if they experience sensory overload they may not be able to feel that urge. Thus, sometimes these kids can use the toilet correctly; at other times they will not.

Dr. Temple Grandin believes that severe sensory processing problems play a large role in toileting issues. Some children like to flush the toilet repeatedly as pleasurable sensory stimulation. For others with severe hearing sensitivities, the sound of the toilet flushing may hurt their ears or simply terrify them.

Grandin states two major causes of toilet training problems in children with autism: they are either afraid of the toilet or they do not know what they are supposed to do. Sometimes the highly sensitive child can learn to use a potty chair located a short distance from the frightening toilet. Most need to see someone else use the toilet in order to learn.[68]

Several excellent references enumerate management strategies for toilet training the child with autism. A chapter is devoted to this subject in *Autism: A Sensorimotor Approach to Management.*[69] *Toilet Training for Individuals with Autism and Related Disorders* is a complete book on the subject.[70] Both focus first on habit training and determining readiness, then on sensory strategies and generalizing to unfamiliar environments.

Flower Essences and Essential Oils

A final intervention that can affect all aspects of functioning, from breathing and digestion to emotional and immunological healing, are flower essences and essential oils. The beginning of this chapter introduced smell as a primitive sense upon which humans rarely depend for information. Because those on the autism spectrum often have strongly attuned noses, and often *do* respond quickly to products that tap into olfaction, flower essences and essential oils can profoundly change their behavior.

For thousands of years people have looked to plants for healing. Outside of the United States, where we depend more upon pharmaceuticals than on natural products, these plant products are considered serious options in medicine. Ironically, most drugs are the result of a discovery of healing from a plant.

Extracting or steam-distilling the plant essences results in highly concentrated substances that can be ingested, inhaled, diffused, or absorbed by the skin. Studies show that, when taken in through the olfactory system, the strong effects of these products travels quickly through the body, and can cross the blood-brain barrier, thus affecting us physically, emotionally, and even spiritually.

Single oils that may be useful for individuals on the spectrum are:
- *Bergamot essential oil* to improve motor coordination
- *Crocus flower essence* for diarrhea, excess gas, and bloating associated with yeast overgrowth
- *Calendula flower essence* for normalizing responses to touch (by things or people)
- *Geranium essential oil* for anxiety and increasing eye contact

- *Lavender essential oil* to calm agitation, rage, or temper tantrums
- *Neroli essential oil* for urinary bed wetting

One company, Young Living, offers combinations of oils with names such as "Brain Power", "Common Sense," and "Valor" under "Oils for Autism."

Oils are *highly* concentrated. *One* drop is usually adequate to rub on your hands and let a child smell. Depending upon the child and circumstances, offer a massage with an essential oil like lavender mixed with coconut oil at bedtime, a sniff of the oil during a temper tantrum, or diffuse the oil to keep germs away. Rubbing a drop onto the wrist or on the bottoms of the feet during the day can also have a calming effect.

All oils are not equal, just as supplements vary in quality. To learn more go to www.learningabouteos.com or refer to a guidebook on the subject. Flower essences and essential oils are available in health food stores and online at www.youngliving.com and www.mydoterra.com. Speak to a knowledgeable aromatherapist before proceeding.

Take-Home Points

Like nutritional issues in autism, sensory problems are often responsible for behaviors that are socially unacceptable. Instead of trying to extinguish them, therapists taking a sensory approach evaluate behaviors, always looking for possible underlying causes.

Once specialists determine which senses are hyper-reactive, which may be hypo-responsive, and how the integration of sensory processing is being affected, they can design an appropriate intervention program. When sensory issues are resolved, coordination, sleep, picky eating, and even toilet training can be less difficult. Targeting problem senses such as touch, sound, balance, and pressure can result in more organized, integrated sensory processing and more appropriate behavior.

Resources

In order to fully understand what goes wrong sensorily in autism spectrum disorders, the reader is referred to several publications that cover this topic in-depth. All of these books published 10 or more years ago are still sound in their extensive explanations of theory and techniques, and the intention of this chapter is not to repeat the information they contain.

During the beginning of the autism epidemic, the American Occupational Therapy Association (AOTA) published its first compendium on treating sensory issues in autism for OTs. This book, *Autism: A Comprehensive Occupational Therapy Approach*, now in its third edition, provides information about both autism and the role of the occupational therapist throughout the lifespan.[71] Other excellent resources include the following:

- *Understanding the Nature of Sensory Integration with Diverse Populations*[72]
- *Exploring the Spectrum of Autism and Pervasive Developmental Disorders: Intervention Strategies*[73]
- *Autism: A Sensorimotor Approach to Management*[74]

Two books that explain to the public the unusual sensory perceptions present in autism are:

- *Sensory Perceptual Issues in Autism and Asperger Syndrome*[75]
- *Asperger Syndrome and Sensory Issues*[76]

---

[1] Rimland B. Infantile Autism: The syndrome and its Implications for a Neural Therapy of Behavior. New York: Appleton Century Crofts, 1964; Ornitz EM. Disorders of perception common to early infantile autism and schizophrenia. Comprehensive Psychiatr, 1969, 10, 259–74.

[2] Tomchek SD, Dunn W. Sensory Processing in Children With and Without Autism: A Comparative Study Using the Short Sensory Profile. American Journal of Occupational Therapy, Mar/Apr 2007, 61, 190–200.

[3] Murray-Slutsky C, Paris BA. Exploring the Spectrum of Autism and Pervasive Developmental Disorders: Intervention Strategies. San Antonio, TX: Therapy Skill Builders, 2000.

[4] Steiner R. Man's Twelve Senses in Their Relation to Imagination, Inspiration, and Intuition. http://www.waldorflibrary.org/. Accessed Mar 19, 2014.

[5] Ayres AJ. Sensory Integration and Learning Disorders. Los Angeles: Western Psychological Services, 1972, 113–29.

[6] Kawar M. Oculomotor Control: An Integral Part of Sensory Integration. In Bundy AC, Lane SJ, Murray E, eds. Sensory Integration: Theory and Practice, 2nd ed. Philadelphia, PA: FA Davis Company, 2002.

[7] Moore JC. The Functional Components of the Nervous System: Part I. Sensory Integration Qrly, 1994, 22, 1–7.

[8] Ayres AJ. Sensory Integration and the Child. Los Angeles: Western Psychological Services, 1979, 184.

[9] Spitzer S, Smith Roley S. Sensory integration revisited: a philosophy of practice. In Smith Roley S, Blanche EI, Schaaf RC, eds. Understanding the Nature of Sensory Integration in Diverse Populations. Tucson, AZ: Therapy Skill Builders, 2001, 5.

[10] Baranek GT, Foster LG, Berkson G. Tactile defensiveness and stereotyped behaviors. Am J Occup Ther, 1997, 51, 91–5.

[11] Ayres AJ. Hyper-responsivity to touch and vestibular stimuli as a predictor of positive response to sensory integration procedures in autistic children. Am J Occup Ther, 1980, 34, 375–86.

[12] Ayres AJ., Sensory Integration and the Child, 124.

[13] Trecker A. Play and Praxis in Children with an Autism Spectrum Disorder. In Miller-Kuhaneck H, ed. Autism, A Comprehensive Occupational Therapy Approach, 2nd ed. Bethesda, MD: AOTA Press, 2004.

[14] Ayres AJ. Developmental Dyspraxia and Adult Onset Apraxia. Torrance, CA: Sensory Integration International, 1985.

[15] Marohn, S. The Natural Medicine Guide to Autism. Charlottesville, VA: Hampton Roads Publishing Co., 2002, 194.

[16] Rogers SJ, Ozonoff S. Annotation: What do we know about sensory dysfunction in autism? A critical review of the empirical evidence. Journal of Child Psychology and Psychiatry, 2005, 46, 1255–68.

[17] Biggio JR. Bed Rest in Pregnancy: Time to Put the Issue to Rest. Obstetrics and Gynecology, Jun 2013, 121:6, 1158–60.

[18] Mailloux Z. Sensory integrative principles in intervention with children with autistic disorder. In Smith Roley S, Blanche EI, Schaaf RC, eds. Understanding the Nature of Sensory Integration in Diverse Populations. Tucson, AZ: Therapy Skill Builders, 2001, 365–84.

[19] Greenspan SI, Wieder S. Developmental patterns and outcomes in infants and children with disorders in relating and communicating: A chart review of 200 cases of children with autistic spectrum diagnoses. J Dev Learn Dis, 1997, 1:1, 87–142.

[20] Piek JP, Dyck M.J. Sensory-motor deficits in children with developmental coordination disorder, attention deficit hyperactivity disorder and autistic disorder. Hum Movement Sci, 2004, 23, 475–88.

[21] Molloy CA, Kietrich KN, Bhattacharya A. Postural stability in children with autism spectrum disorder. J Aut Dev Dis, 2003, 33:6, 643–52.

[22] Bogdashina O. Sensory Perceptual Issues in Autism and Asperger Syndrome. Different Sensory Experiences, Different Perceptual Worlds. London: Jessica Kingsley Publishers, 2003.

[23] Jones V, Prior, M. Motor imitation abilities and neurological signs in autistic children. J Aut Dev Dis, 1985, 15, 37–46.

[24] Case-Smith J, Miller H. Occupational therapy with children with pervasive developmental disorders. Am J Occup Ther, 1999, 53, 506–13.

[25] Teitelbaum P, Teitelbaum O, Nye N, Fryman J, Maurer R. Movement analysis in infancy may be useful for early diagnosis of autism. Proc. Natl. Acad. Sci USA, 1998, 95, 13982–87.

[26] Peretti C. Oxytocin and Autism. Interview with Dr.Luis Martinez, International Autism Summit, Cairo, Egypt, 2009.

[27] Rogers SJ, Bennetto L, McEvoy R, et. al. Imitation and pantomine in high functioning adolescents with autism spectrum disorders, Child. Dev, 1996, 67, 2060–73.

[28] Hessellund K, Nutto J. Understanding Occupational Therapy's Role in Sensory Integration. In Barber A, ed. Vision and Sensory Integration. Santa Ana, CA: Optometric Extension Program, 1999.

[29] Kientz MA, Miller H. Classroom evaluation of the child with autism. School System Special Interest Section Qtly, 1999, 6:1, 1–4.

[30] Dunn W. The Sensory Profile. San Antonio, TX: The Psychological Corporation, 1999.

[31] Ermer J, Dunn W. The Sensory Profile: A discriminant analysis of children with and without disabilities. Am J Occup Ther, 1998, 52, 283–90.

[32] Miller-Kuhaneck H, Henry D, Glennon TJ, Parham D, Ecker CL. The Sensory Processing Measure. Los Angeles: Western Psychological Services, 2007.

[33] Ayres AJ. Sensory Integration and Praxis Test. Los Angeles, CA: Western Psychological Services, 1989.

[34] Parham D, Mailloux Z, Smith Roley S. Sensory processing and praxis in high functioning children with autism. Paper presented at Research 2000, Feb 4–5, 2000, Redondo Beach, CA.

[35] Degangi GA, Berk RA. The DeGangi-Berk Test of Sensory Integration (TSI). Los Angeles: Western Psychological Services, 1999.

[36] Miller LJ. Miller PreSchool Screening Test. Los Angeles: Western Psychological Services, 1999.

[37] Delacato C. The Ultimate Stranger: The Autistic Child. Novato, CA: Acad Therapy Pub, 1974.

[38] Mailloux Z., Sensory integrative principles, 365–84.

[39] Myles BS, Cook KT, Miller N, et al. Asperger Syndrome and Sensory Issues. Shawnee Mission, KS: Autism Asperger Publishing Co., 2000.

[40] Madaule P. When listening comes alive. Norval, Ontario, Canada: Moulin Publishing, 1994.

[41] Madaule P. Terapia de escucha. Mexico: Editorialis Trillas, 2005.

[42] Sollier P. Listening for Wellness: An Introduction to the Tomatis Method. Walnut Creek, CA: The Mozart Center Press, 2005.

[43] Ruben S. Awakening Ashley: Mozart Knocks Autism on its Ear. Lincoln, NE: iUniverse, 2004.

[44] Berard G. Hearing Equals Behavior. Georgiana Foundation. Pre-publication issue, 1992, 1.

[45] Berard G and Brockett S. Hearing Equals Behavior, Updated and Expanded. Manchester Center, VT: Shires Press, 2011.

[46] Stehli A. The sound of a miracle: A child's triumph over autism. New York: Doubleday, 1991.

[47] Panksepp J, Rossi J, Narayanan TK. Biochemical Changes As a result of AIT-type modulated and unmodulated music. Lost & Found: Perspectives on Brain, Emotion, and Culture, 1996/7, 2:1&4.

[48] http://www.berardaitwebsite.com/sait/aitsummary.html. Accessed Jan 23, 2013.

[49] Williams MS, Shellenberger S. How Does Your Engine Run? A Leaders' Guide to the Alert Program for Sensory Regulation. Albuquerque, NM: Therapy Works, 1996.

[50] Henry D. Tool Chest for Teachers, Parents and Students. Youngtown, AZ: Henry OT Services, 1999.

[51] Williams MS, Shellenberger S. Take Five! Staying Alert at Home and School. Albuquerque, NM: Therapy Works, 2001.

[52] Bluestone J. The Fabric of Autism: Weaving the Threads into a Cogent Theory. Seattle, WA: The HANDLE Institute, 2004.

[53] Edelson SM, Edelson MG, Kerr DC, Grandin T. Behavioral and physiological effects of deep pressure on individuals with autism: A pilot study investigating the efficacy of Grandin's "hug machine." Amer Jrl of OT, 1999, 53, 145–52.

[54] Kranowitz C. The Out-of-Sync Child: Recognizing and Coping with Sensory Processing Disorder, Rev Ed. New York: Perigee Press, 2006.

[55] Kranowitz C, Newman J. Growing an In-Sync Child: Simple, Fun Activities to Help Every Child Develop, Learn, and Grow. New York: Perigee Books, 2010.

[56] Newman J, Kranowitz C. In-Sync Activity Cards. Arlington, TX: Sensory World, 2012.

[57] Grandin, T. Animals in Translation. New York: Scribner, 2005, 6–8.

[58] Pack AA, Herman LM. Sensory integration in the bottlenosed dolphin: Immediate recognition of complex shapes across the senses of echolocation and vision. Journal of the Acoustical Society of America, 1995, 98, 722–33.

[59] Shkedi A. Sensory input through riding. Proceedings for the 7th International Therapeutic Riding Congress, Aarhus, Denmark, 1991, 129–32.

[60] Biery MJ, Kauffman N. The effects of therapeutic horseback riding on balance. Adapted physical activity quarterly, 1989, 6, 221–29.

[61] Sacks O. Musicophilia: Tales of music and the brain. New York: Vintage, 2008.

[62] Goddard S. Reflexes, learning and behavior. Eugene, OR: Fern Ridge Press, 2005, 108–9.

[63] AMTA. "Music Therapy as a Treatment Modality for Autism Spectrum Disorders." 2012. http://www.musictherapy.org/assets/1/7/MT_Autism_2012.pdf. Accessed Jan 24, 2013.

[64] Whipple J. Music in intervention for children and adolescents with autism: A meta-analysis. J Music Ther, Summer 2004, 41:2, 90–106.

65 Shore S. Beyond the Wall. Shawnee Mission, KS: Autism Asperger Publishing Co., 2003, 68–83.

[66] Broadfoot A. The S.A.N.E. approach helps alleviate sleep problems in kids with developmental delays. Family & Parenting, May 4, 2010. http://www.examiner.com. Accessed Jan 22, 2013.

[67] Dorfman K. Cure your child with food. New York: Workman Press, 2013.

[68] http://legacy.autism.com/autism/grandinfaq.htm. Accessed Jan 22, 2013.

[69] Leone EF, Rogers SL. Sensory applications for sleep and toilet training. In Huebner RA, ed. Autism: A Sensorimotor Approach to Management. Gaithersburg, MD: Aspen Publishers, 2001, 355–63.

[70] Wheeler M. Toilet Training for Individuals with Autism and Related Disorders: A Comprehensive Guide for Parents and Teachers. Arlington, TX: Future Horizons, 2001.

[71] Miller-Kuhaneck H, ed. Autism, A Comprehensive Occupational Therapy Approach, 3rd ed. Bethesda, MD: AOTA Press, 2010.

[72] Smith Roley S, Blanche EI, Schaaf RC, eds. Understanding the Nature of Sensory Integration in Diverse Populations. Tucson, AZ: Therapy Skill Builders, 2001.

[73] Murray-Slutsky C, Paris BA. Exploring the Spectrum of Autism and Pervasive Developmental Disorders: Intervention Strategies. San Antonio, TX: Therapy Skill Builders, 2000.

[74] Huebner RA, ed. Autism: A Sensorimotor Approach to Management. Gaithersburg, MD: Aspen Publishers, 2001.

[75] Bogdashina O. Sensory Perceptual Issues in Autism and Asperger Syndrome. Different Sensory Experiences, Different Perceptual Worlds. London: Jessica Kingsley Publishers, 2003.

[76] Myles BS, Cook KT, Miller N, et al. Asperger Syndrome and Sensory Issues. Shawnee Mission, KS: Autism Asperger Publishing Co., 2000.

CHAPTER 11

Focusing on Vision: The Dominant Sense

Do you know someone who has "vision?" What do we mean when we say, "I see?" If we say someone is "myopic," are we referring to his glasses prescription, his thinking, or both? Vision words are a part of our everyday vocabulary!

For almost 30 years vision and its relationship to learning and behavior have fascinated me. Why do so many individuals with special needs, especially autism, have poor eye contact, flick their fingers in front of their eyes, or demonstrate poor coordination? No, it is not because they are autistic! They are autistic, in part, because their vision malfunctions, resulting in "odd" behaviors.

My training as a mental health professional did not satisfy my thirst for information about vision, so I turned to other disciplines for answers. In the 1980s I was fortunate to meet several brilliant optometrists who opened my eyes (literally and figuratively!) to how the brain, body, and eyes work together. They became my mentors, my friends, and my family; without them, my career would have been much less exciting.

Vision deserves its own chapter in this book because, in addition to being a strong interest of mine, it plays a huge, generally ignored role in development. Furthermore, visual processing problems add a very large stress factor to the Total Loads of many individuals on the autism spectrum.

This chapter defines and explains vision in all of its aspects and shows what happens in typical development. Next, it demonstrates how vision processing problems can interfere with many areas of development in individuals with ASDs, and how these problems are at the root of many undesirable behaviors.

Finally, the chapter explains how vision therapy using lenses, prisms, and motor activities can often ameliorate underlying visual problems, removing them as a Load Factor. Remediating visual issues frees up energy for immune system function, communication, and social interaction. In many cases behavior becomes more desirable, language emerges, even allergies disappear, and the long-awaited social-emotional skills mature. If you are going to outsmart autism, you must have vision!

What Is Vision?

Vision is the learned developmental process of focusing on and giving meaning to what is seen. The operative words in this definition are "learned" and "developmental." Vision involves the eyes, body, and brain; it is much more than 20/20 eyesight, which describes only the clarity of what we see at a distance. Vision allows us to attend to, focus on, organize, understand, and interact with the world around us; it is both perceptual and conceptual.

Vision is Learned

We learn to use our vision in the same way that we learn to walk, talk, and write: through sensory experiences that teach us how to select which targets to touch, pick up, identify, think about, and talk about.[1] According to pioneer optometrist G. N. Getman, a child learns how to use the body by fully participating in and exploring his world for the first two or three years of his life. During this time his entire body, hands, eyes, mouth, and ears are his tools for learning. "The movement of self through space, the manual and visual exploration and inspection of his world and its contents, vocalization of names, labels, needs and desires are the full-time occupation of the small child." He spends every waking moment visually inspecting his three-dimensional surroundings.[2]

For Getman and his colleague, developmental psychologist and physician Arnold Gesell, MD, PhD, the visual experiences a child has in his early years lay the foundation for his ability to be successful in society. Gesell is the founder of the world renowned child development center at Yale University. Autism historians would be interested to note that the Director of the Gesell Institute of Child Development from 1978 to 1985 was Sidney MacDonald Baker, MD, one of the founders of the Defeat Autism Now! movement. Baker, a brilliant physician with a heart of gold, is one of the most respected leaders in the field of autism treatment today.

Getman and Gesell could never have imagined that two-dimensional tablets, computers, and smartphones with their touchscreens and cursors would replace three-dimensional wooden blocks, pots and pans, and balls as the playthings of childhood. They would probably be horrified by, but not surprised about, the less-than-positive outcomes these modern-day technological wonders have on the visual skills of today's young children. For these developmentalists, visual experiences in three dimensions drive imagination and creativity, and even many types of intelligence.

Vision Develops

Vision develops every time the brain integrates sensory input from the tactile, proprioceptive, olfactory, gustatory, and balance receptors, as well as from the ears, eyes, body, and brain, eventually emerging hierarchically as the dominant sense in well-functioning people. Gesell, along with his colleagues at Yale, pediatrician Frances Ilg, MD, and psychologist Louise Bate Ames, PhD, understood how babies learn. Their impeccable work on the predictable sequential development of children from infancy is immortalized in *Infant and Child in the Culture of Today*, first published in 1943 and revised in 1971.[3]

Getman, the eye care professional on the Gesell team, wrote about the importance of sensory experiences a generation ago in his classic, *How to Develop Your Child's Intelligence*.[4] This tiny book comes with an amazing chart documenting developmental patterns in many areas. At each age level, 6 through 54 months, the chart shows expected motor, visual-motor, visual-tactual, visual-language, cognitive, and guidance patterns, giving developmental guidelines to parents and educators. Getman maps rhythm, emotional, ethical, hygiene, eating, play, and guidance patterns for older children. The book is well worth owning for this amazing chart alone that allows you to track all aspects of children's development from 6 months through almost 14 years of age.

All of these pioneers undoubtedly recognized that during a typical child's development, the motor system stabilizes from the inside-out: from the body's core and the midline outwards, and from large muscles to small ones—head, neck, shoulders, arms, elbows, wrists, hands, fingers, joints. Vision develops from the bottom-up: from whole body to lower, then upper body, trunk, neck, head, and eyes. Each body part, including the eyes, eventually functions independently of the core, head, and upper body. Enter Swiss developmental psychologist, Jean Piaget.

Piaget's Developmental Hierarchy

Piaget, who practiced for over 20 years after Gesell's death, devoted his career to investigating stages of child development. He argued that motor and visual development take place in tandem, in a predictable hierarchy. He conceptualized a series of progressive stages from sensorimotor (age birth to two), to preoperational (age two to seven), to concrete (age seven to eleven), to abstract (age twelve and up), leading to higher and higher levels of cognition.[5]

The *motor stage* comes first, during which individuals move primarily without purpose as the receptors for touch, proprioception, balance, vision, and hearing are maturing. At this stage, the baby is simply a motor being: the motor system drives vision. As tone heightens, sensory integration takes place and movement becomes more directed by the body and brain.

The *motor-visual stage* follows. For months, the typical infant's and toddler's movements take the eyes along for a ride as the brain learns to control the upper and lower body. The eyes process what they see wherever they are directed.

Next comes the *visual-motor stage*. Progressing to this level is a major hurdle in development. Vision now directs movement. Instead of moving purposelessly through space, children at a visual-motor stage take inventory of the space around them, focus on a target, and move toward it. Movement and drawing become purposeful. Preschoolers see the block corner, recall the tower they had built the day before, and race there to re-experience the pleasure it had given them. They take the crayon and draw a person, one body part at a time. The motor and emotional experience have become one.

During this very critical time frame, vision begins to dominate the movement system, to coordinate the proprioceptive, vestibular, and tactile systems. If there is faulty information processing in any of the primitive sensory systems—perhaps further complicated by retained primitive reflexes—visual dysfunction is inevitable. Because their visual systems are inefficient, these patients still need to touch and move to be secure in their environment.

The last step is the *visual stage*. At this level, people no longer need the actual bodily movements for experience; rather, they can "move" in their mind's eye. A child at this stage tells his mother, prior to going to school, that when he arrives, he will go right to block corner to make a tower. His sensory, motor, visual, and emotional brains have memory of the experience and want to have it again. This step is the beginning of the ability to plan, organize, conceptualize, and ideate: all results of the senses and motor abilities are integrating efficiently.[6]

For a child to be academically "ready," the above steps take place in sequence, resulting in the development of a dominant eye and hand (not always on the same side) and the ability to use the two sides of the body together. Success at end-product skills, such as holding down the paper with one hand and writing with the other, or using paper and scissors together, are examples of bilateral tasks that developmentally emerge as the motor and visual systems work together.

The Two Parts of the Visual System

As the body and eyes work together sending messages to the brain, magic happens. Neurological connections form, allowing the visual system to develop two parts:

Focal or "central" vision, which allows an individual to determine "what is it?" Optometrists sometimes call this "parvo" vision. Focal vision is primarily a conscious function, allowing one to see clearly, to recognize objects, and eventually to read.

Ambient or peripheral vision which answers "where am I?" or "where is it?" Optometrists sometimes call this "magno" vision. It is a subconscious function, and its role is to orient an individual and object in space.

When vision is functioning normally, magno and parvo vision integrate. Dysfunction results when a person uses one part more frequently than the other or has trouble engaging and disengaging between the two systems, as do many people with ASD.

Fundamental Visual Skills

During normal development, many important visual skills necessary for all aspects of functioning emerge. Table 11.1 lists all essential visual skills.

Table 11.1.
Essential Visual Skills

Accommodation: Ability to activate focus for near-visual space to attain clarity, and to shift focus between near point and far point to maintain clarity

Acuity: Sharpness or clarity at both distance and reading distance

Binocularity: Ability to move the two eyes together as a team—up, down, in, and out—to coordinate their messages and send one distinct image to the brain

Convergence: Ability to move both eyes together inward simultaneously toward the nose (cross the eyes)

Divergence: Ability to move eyes together outward away from the nose

Focusing: Ability to maintain clarity while changing distances

Eye Tracking and Fixation: Ability to look at and accurately follow an object

Binocular Vision or Fusion: Ability to use both eyes together efficiently

Eye Teaming: Ability to aim, move, and work the eyes as a coordinated team

Visual-Motor Integration: Ability to combine visual input with input from the other senses and respond motorically

Visual-Spatial Understanding: Ability to know where one is in relationship to objects and people.

When the two eyes are working together properly, the brain tells the eyes what to look for, the eyes take in information, and the brain stores and uses it efficiently. Language emerges as we conceptualize what we see.[7]

Skeffington Circles

The father of modern developmental optometry, A. M. Skeffington, OD, meshed knowledge about vision and the other senses in the 1960s and '70s. According to innovative developmental optometrist Leonard Press, OD, FAOO, FCOVD, what Skeffington conceived was the interplay between the ambient and focal processes, as well as between the eyes, brain, and body to generate the basic the "what," "where" and "how" of vision.[8] Figure 11.1 shows this interaction.

Figure 11.1.

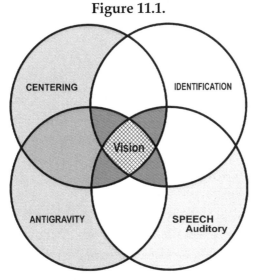

Skeffington Circles

Skeffington's brilliant model demonstrates that what we call "vision" results from the overlap of the four circles, which represent the integration of the senses. In this diagram, "Centering" is ambient vision, "Identification" represents focal vision, "Antigravity" describes balance and spatial orientation (vestibular function), and "Speech/Auditory" is self-explanatory. An understanding of this model demonstrates how vision eventually emerges as the dominant sense.

A. M. Skeffington was to developmental vision what A. Jean Ayres was to a sensory integration approach to occupational therapy. No one knows if they ever met, but if they did, they certainly would have had some very interesting conversations!

Vision and Autism

Visual Symptoms in Autism

If genetic or environmental factors interfere with a child's growth, a cascade of events takes place, starting with health issues, which interrupt the emergence of reflexes, motor development, and sensory processing, including vision. At some point, a parent, grandparent, day care provider, or teacher notices one or more of the following vision symptoms that occur frequently in those with autism:
- Has difficulty making eye contact
- Tilts head when observing closely
- Squints or closes an eye
- Is fascinated by lights, spinning objects, shadows, or patterns
- Looks through hands
- Flaps hands, flicks objects in front of eyes
- Looks at objects sideways, very closely, or with quick glances
- Shows sensitivity to light (photophobia)
- Becomes confused at changes in flooring or on stairways
- Pushes or rubs eyes
- Widens eyes or squints when asked to look
- Bumps into objects or touches walls while moving through space

What Causes Visual Symptoms in Autism?

Vision affects and is affected by genetics, the environment, and lifestyle choices. While it is difficult to separate nature from nurture, nearsightedness (myopia) and a turned eye (strabismus) are believed to run in families.[9] Some contemporary societal practices that restrict babies' and young children's movements for safety reasons may also be responsible in part.

Safety measures such as back sleeping (even when remediated by "tummy time"), car seats, backpacks, strollers, infant seats, and baby exercisers can impede the emergence of important reflexes necessary for motor development. An increased early use of electronics, such as computers, TV, and video games, that force visual focus at inappropriate distances and for extended periods of time, may also contribute in subtle ways.

The eyes are profoundly affected by vitamin deficiencies. In fact, the eyes are one of the most nutritionally demanding organs of the body and are often the first place disease, such as diabetes, appears.[10] In the late 1990s, Mary Megson, MD, discovered that a deficiency of vitamins A and D played a role in regressive autism. Megson saw great progress when supplementing the diets of her patients with cod liver oil, an excellent source of the deficient vitamins.[11]

Heavy metals, many medications, and the foods we eat and drink—especially aspartame, alcohol, and excitotoxins such as MSG—quickly affect vision. Visual side effects include blurring, double vision, or even blindness. Did you know that dilated pupils are a sign of possible mercury poisoning?[12]

Oxygen deprivation from many sources can affect vision. Whether it is from anoxia at birth or shallow breathing at any time of the day or night, visual function will suffer. According to Melvin Kaplan, OD, a high percentage of patients on the autism spectrum exhibit dysfunctional breathing patterns.[13] Their inability to integrate movement and breathing stresses their muscles and nervous systems, and reduces attention. The muscle tension and stressed nervous system impair vision, leading to mismatches in how the brain interprets where things are relative to where they appear to be.

Some symptoms of breathing issues in those with autism spectrum disorders are:

327

- **Poor blowing skills,** such as with candles on a cake, bubbles, or a musical instrument;
- **Yawning and/or sighing** in an attempt to get more oxygen;
- **Rocking,** which compensates for lack of synergistic neural control of the eyes, head, and body;
- **Holding of the breath** when giving effort to motor and visual activities, including reading and writing; and
- **Hyperventilation** related to fear and anxiety.[14]

Because constraints on breathing affect every aspect of performance, Kaplan believes that an effective vision remediation program must incorporate teaching appropriate breathing patterns. Breathing properly is an inherent part of Educational Kinesiology and reflex integration, as well. Read about the importance of the breath in these therapies in chapters 8 and 9, respectively.

Difficulty integrating central and peripheral vision. One of the most significant issues for individuals with autism is coordinating central and peripheral vision. Just as all individuals with autism differ in their nutritional deficits and needs, each is unique visually. Trying to determine where one is in space uses time and energy.

People with autism tend to use one part of their vision, but not both simultaneously and efficiently. Some who are more "focal" may play with specks of dust, obsess over details, or demonstrate savant abilities. Others are "ambient" — fascinated by contrast, lights, shadows, and shiny objects. Some with autism constrict their peripheral vision to cope. Without integration, the body is under stress.

If the eyes are not working together as a team or are processing information inefficiently, the brain must decide what to do with the partial information. Kaplan thinks that hyperactivity might just be a survival mechanism for those with autism who attempt to establish the limits of "self" by locking onto objects in space with such intensity that they lose awareness of self when standing.[15]

Likewise, poor integration of ambient and focal vision could cause other behavioral symptoms such as extreme inflexibility. These visual problems, along with poor binocularity, inefficient and slow focusing, poor integration of vision with other senses, and poor visualization come crashing together to manifest themselves as poor attention, memory, spatial awareness, visual-motor integration, perception, or visualization: all symptoms of autism!

Convergence insufficiency. Many individuals with autism spectrum disorders have convergence insufficiency (CI), the inability to coordinate the eyes for any length of time at a near distance, such as in reading.[16] In those with CI, eyes tend to drift outward; crossing the eyes is difficult, if not impossible, to hold for more than a few seconds. Symptoms of CI include headaches, blurred vision, sleepiness while reading, and difficulty concentrating.

The ability to converge is an essential skill that keeps the eyes binocular and allows the brain to receive and interpret one integrated image. CI interferes with focusing, so it can easily be missed and is commonly misdiagnosed as attention deficit disorder.[17]

Convergence insufficiency is not uncommon; it occurs in about 5% of the population.[18] Unfortunately, it is rarely picked up in routine vision screenings, so those affected rarely know they have it, and it does not get treated.

Strabismus. Kaplan's experience is that about half of individuals with an ASD diagnosis evidence an eye turn, called a "strabismus."[19] The numbers are astounding when compared to only 4% of the population in general with this problem.[20] An eye may turn in (esotropia) or out (exotropia). A strabismus is sometimes seen after a traumatic birth, an infection, a high fever, surgery, heavy metal toxicity, sensory deprivation, or any assault on the growing nervous system. Strabismus always requires attention.

A common recommendation for treating a strabismus is patching, and, if this intervention is unsuccessful, surgery to "straighten" the eye(s). While this approach may create a cosmetically straight eye, it rarely achieves binocularity.[21] This is not surprising, given that Nobel Prize-winning neurophysiologists David Hubel, MD, and Torsten Wiesel, MD, concluded that patching eventually leads to the elimination of the visual cells that respond to both eyes simultaneously, eventually leading an individual to attend to the input of only one eye at a time.[22]

A strabismus affects learning and behavior. In strabismus, one eye accurately aims at the object of regard, while the other eye misses it by aiming above, below, or to the left or right of it. Double vision (diplopia) results, and the brain must learn how to cope and adapt. The misalignment may be constant or intermittent, and thus not always noticeable. Disorganization and confusion follow as the brain struggles to integrate competing messages.

In order to minimize the disorganization and confusion, sometimes the unconscious mind adapts to strabismus by suppressing signals from the faulty-aiming eye. Eventually, visual suppression leads to amblyopia or "lazy eye," in which the nerves that transport and interpret visual information lose some of their ability. The result is poor vision in one eye due to an interference in the neurological interpretive mechanism.

In many instances the reduced eyesight cannot be corrected with glasses or surgery. With the eyes functioning at less than 100% efficiency, any sustained visual activity such as reading may require extra effort and strain. In about half of cases, amblyopia occurs with strabismus, but in the remaining half doctors can find no sign that one eye sees more poorly than the other. However, some people with amblyopia may turn their heads to see certain things or close one eye when reading.[23]

Optometrist Melvin Kaplan, whose book is the source of much of this information, believes that the body and brain's adaptations to a strabismus are wide-ranging, especially for individuals with autism. They experience three basic losses, which overlap:
- loss of control of the environment and of the self in relationship to the environment,
- loss of mobility, and
- limitation of the range and variety of visual concepts.

All of these losses result from the eyes not working together as a team. When perception does not occur as an end product of a dynamic process involving the use and integration of **all** sensory receptors, including the eyes, the best outcome that a strabismic individual can attain is the construct of space, not the true perception of space.[24]

Since a good number of the eye's neural fibers bring information to the body's balance system, it follows that a person's sense of where he or she is in space is compromised if these fibers deliver inaccurate information. A child who is disoriented in space experiences himself and his environment as unstable and unpredictable. He may grow increasingly inward, become belligerent, or demonstrate sensory defensiveness. Because space perception also affects movement, language development, social skills, reading, writing, mathematics, and many untold other areas, these end-product skills all suffer as well. Strabismic behavior, like mercury poisoning, has very, very similar symptoms as autism.

For more information on strabismus, go to www.strabismus.org.

Applying Piaget's Developmental Hierarchy to Autism

Refer back to Piaget's hierarchy of motor-visual development described earlier in the chapter. From a Piagetian developmental point of view, many children with autism, regardless of chronological age, are stuck at the *motor-visual stage*. They "look" with their whole bodies. Ask them to follow a moving object, and observe that they move not only their eyes, but heads and trunks, as well. They read with head and body movements across the page.

Those at the motor-visual stage often wander aimlessly around their classrooms, finding themselves somehow in the block corner, where they may line up instead of build with blocks. When an adult offers crayons or markers to children at this stage, they scribble, sometimes not even looking at their hands or what they are drawing. They may start out with an idea of drawing a person but end up with a tree as their motor skills override their visualization abilities.

Some of their "aberrant" behaviors, such as flapping and other self-stimulatory hand and arm gestures seen in kids at a motor-visual stage, may actually serve the purpose of allowing them to interact with their world, albeit in a strange way that tells the brain where the body is in space.

To move to the next step, the *visual-motor stage*, the body must know where it is in space and move automatically. If a child does not know where he or she is in space, it will be extremely difficult — even impossible — for him to know where objects, such as his backpack, homework, or letters on a page are in space. Kids with autism who have organizational difficulties are usually "lost in space" as a result of underlying visual dysfunction.

The *visual stage* is a long-term goal for those with autism. A very few, like Temple Grandin, have figured out how to "think in pictures."[25] Others have photographic memories and can draw whole cities or recall where a word is on a page. Usually, though, these talents are "splinter skills" that do not generalize to real life or allow them to organize themselves, conceptualize ideas, and think abstractly.

Research on Vision and Autism

Not surprisingly, there is a dearth of research on the visual status of children with autism. Most studies, including the more recent ones, have small sample sizes even though individuals with autism abound. More research is available on those with less severe diagnoses, such as learning disabilities and attention deficits. Those interested in research studies documenting the role of vision in learning disabilities and dyslexia can read a review of over 300 references that affirm a positive relationship between learning problems and the following: poor eye movement skills, convergence insufficiency, faulty binocular vision, farsightedness, lazy eye, poor visual processing, weak visual motor skills, and suppression of one eye.[26]

Pioneer behavioral optometrist John Streff was one of the first to write about optometric care for a child with autism in 1975; he described a case of an almost-five-year-old boy who he had evaluated at the aforementioned Gesell Institute.[27] Because of little interest in autism for the next 20 years, no known articles on vision and autism appeared again until the early 1990s.

In 1992, a Chicago team of Janice Scharre, OD, and psychologist Margaret Creedon, PhD, did a study of 34 children with autism, aged 2 to 11 years. They found strabismus in 21% and acuity problems at near in 44%.[28] Other studies show that eye movement problems are also common.[29]

In the early 1990s, Melvin Kaplan and psychologist Stephen M. Edelson, PhD, now of the Autism Research Institute, found that using special lenses (see below) on 18 children with autism ages 7 to 18 improved behavior, attention, posture, coordination, and spatial orientation.[30]

A recent study was done on a sample of 36 children, mostly ages 4 to 16, with autism diagnoses in Nepal. Consistent with earlier studies, both refractive errors and strabismus were more common in those with autism diagnoses than in the general population.[31]

The ultimate go-to reference on vision issues in autism is *Seeing through New Eyes: Changing the Lives of Children with Autism, Asperger Syndrome and Other Developmental Disabilities through Vision Therapy*, by Melvin Kaplan, who offers a more detailed explanation of the problems, as well as many, many innovative therapy approaches.[32]

Vision Exams

Choosing an Eye Doctor

Anyone with an autism spectrum diagnosis should have a complete vision evaluation as soon after the diagnosis as possible. Different professions "view" vision differently, due to their widely diverse training.

Ophthalmologists, who are MDs, define vision largely in terms of structural pathology. They are the best option if surgery is being considered.

Optometrists, or ODs, take a functional approach to vision. Their training emphasizes that vision operates in relationship to the rest of the body. These professionals look at the visual skills necessary for learning, including visual perception. Optometrists are the best choice for a vision exam for individuals with autism, because for them, function — not structure or eye health — is the concern.

A small subset of optometrists have advanced training and have passed rigorous tests qualifying them as Fellows of the College of Optometrists in Vision Development (FCOVD). In their evaluations, in addition to checking for eye health and structural pathology, these doctors also run a full set of tests measuring visual skills. Most also provide remediation to guide the patient so he can learn how to use vision more efficiently (see below). To find a qualified doctor near you, go to www.covd.org.

Optometrists interested in learning more about working with patients on the autism spectrum can read "Autism Spectrum Disorders: A Primer for the Optometrist" and "Serving the Needs of the Patient with Autism."[33] To become proficient, optometrists may take postgraduate courses from the Optometric Extension Program (OEP), the continuing education arm of optometry.

Vision Exams for Individuals with Autism

Depending upon the developmental age and cooperation of the patient, an exam consists of both informal observations and formal testing. Identifying and treating underlying visual issues requires a complete developmental vision evaluation that includes acuity and eye health, as well as all aspects of visual function. The skill and training of the examining doctor are key to obtaining important information about a particular individual's visual skills.

For those at the low end of the spectrum, the optometrist might simply watch the patient move and play, first with large motor skills and then with fine motor activities. They may present the individual with objects such as puzzles, balls, or attention-getting objects such as puppets, balloons, and bubbles.

Many behavioral optometrists are administering reflex evaluations with increasing frequency. They may ask the patient to lie on the floor, and then see how strong his or her core is and whether he or she can follow verbal commands to move the whole body or to isolate component parts, such as the right leg only.

If the individual is able to comply with demands, the eye doctor may use some special equipment to look at the essential visual skills, such as binocularity and convergence. He or she may also try different lenses and prisms, noting carefully a patient's change in focus, posture, breathing patterns, and even language. Even if the patient cannot tolerate testing glasses on the face, a doctor can measure a response by holding flippers in front of the eyes.

If visual function is low, testing may resemble an occupational therapy evaluation more than a vision test. In patients with higher-level skills, vision testing will be more obvious. The ultimate goal is to see how well an individual uses vision to direct behavior, to identify which Piagetian level he or she is functioning on, and to determine if dysfunctional vision is an issue in development. If so, specific visual interventions can be invaluable in treating underlying visual lags that impact a child's development and behavior.

Change Behavior by Changing Vision

Following the examination, the eye doctor will determine if vision therapy is the top priority, since treatment usually takes place in the sequence presented in this book. Some patients with major health issues need to return Step One of this book and deal with biomedical issues. Those for whom reflexes remain problematic must work on them. Occasionally, an optometrist will prescribe lenses and a home program for the patient while the family pursues other therapies, and schedule a progress evaluation in three to six months.

If the optometrist believes that vision therapy is warranted, he or she will pinpoint problem areas and develop a vision therapy program that includes activities to help the patient learn to use vision more efficiently. This program may include reflex integration.

Vision Therapy (VT) for Individuals with Autism

Vision therapy (VT), also known as "vision training," can be an astounding missing piece in outsmarting autism. Specially trained optometrists and their assistants offer in-office and at-home VT all over the world. Their ultimate goal is to teach the eyes, body, and brain to work together. Since children do not outgrow delays in visual development without intervention, VT can never start too young.

For anyone with a strabismus, vision therapy can be life-changing. Optometrists view strabismus not as a structural deficit of the eye but rather as a functional motor-sensory misalignment caused by a person's unconscious adaptive response to neural dysfunction. VT recodes how the brain interprets the new information in the new visual-spatial framework. As the patient's mind recognizes the difference between the "old" way of processing and the "new" way, neural pathways develop that result in higher-level visual performance.

By laying down new neural pathways, VT is far superior to patching or surgery, which often do not improve — and may in fact impair — visual processing. That was the experience of Sue Barry, PhD, a neuroscience professor at Mount Holyoke College, whose life changed forever when she used her eyes together and saw in three dimensions for the first time at 50 years of age! Barry, nicknamed "Stereo Sue" by neurologist Oliver Sacks, MD, was born with severe strabismus and underwent several unsuccessful surgeries as a child to straighten her crossed eyes and give her depth perception. She believed, as do most of her neuroscientist colleagues, that for her eyes to work as a team with the brain to see 3-D was impossible at her age.[34]

Enter behavioral optometrist Theresa Ruggiero, OD, FCOVD, who told her that it is never too late, and that with determined effort for a long time, Sue might be able to become binocular through vision therapy. Sue liked challenges (she is married to an astronaut!), so she decided, "Why not try?"

Her amazing book, *Fixing My Gaze: A Scientist's Journey into Seeing in Three Dimensions*[35] is the story of how she learned to see the shapes of flowers in a vase, individual snowflakes falling instead of a white sheet, and the steering wheel of her car jump out from the dashboard.

Vision Therapy Activities

VT generally includes motor, motor-visual, visual-motor, and visual activities, with or without the use of lenses and prisms (see below). It typically takes place once or twice a week in a doctor's office, supplemented with 15–30 minutes per day of home therapy to reinforce skills. While improvement is often seen in a month or so, therapy frequently continues for an average of three to nine months, and sometimes for as long as a couple of years, to stabilize and solidify learned skills, depending on the child and the severity of the visual dysfunction.

For the lowest-functioning patients with autism, a skilled optometrist might begin VT with simple, gentle visual arousal activities, such as blowing bubbles, playing flashlight tag, beanbag games, or Lite Brite, with or without lenses. For nonverbal individuals and those with significant cognitive, language, and social-emotional challenges, these simple VT activities can sometimes turn on attention.

Early treatment for the most significantly impaired might also include whole-body movement procedures like walking and marching, eventually integrating movement with listening and seeing by adding rhythm and balance challenges, such as walking on a rail to the beat of a metronome. Enhancing these visual skills often results in improved consistency and frequency of eye contact and social interaction outside of the VT room.

As a person learns to use the two eyes more efficiently, therapy moves to more visually-directed motor tasks such as throwing a beanbag at a target or putting pegs in holes on a rotating board. These activities are often done both with and without lenses and prisms to break up old habits and establish new ones.

For higher-functioning students, VT can enhance organizational skills, visual thinking (see below), and language. Incremental gains in these areas could be sufficient to allow a student with autism to move outside of a self-contained special education class and work independently in a mainstream setting.

At the heart of vision therapy are activities individually designed to teach a person's eyes to move, align, fixate, and focus as a team. The ultimate purpose of VT in autism is to increase visual and spatial awareness and to develop and stimulate using both eyes together. The brain learns to coordinate new messages from the eyes for improved perception and cognition.

During vision therapy, learning to use the eyes together first requires a conscious effort. The ability to perform complex visual-motor activities—like skiing or writing—develops gradually. The ultimate goal is for patients to learn to use the two eyes together effectively, and to integrate vision with movement and the other senses effortlessly and automatically.

As in any treatment, VT providers need to be cognizant of a patient's sensory issues and possible overload. Often, the optometrist involves a parent, caregiver, or therapist who knows the patient well in the therapy sessions.

Optometrists usually schedule periodic progress evaluations about every twelve sessions, or at least every six months, to evaluate visual skills, to review improvements in related areas, and to determine if further therapy is needed. Some patients improve quickly, others only gradually.

Lenses and Prisms

Counter to what many believe, lens prescribing is an art, not a science. While a machine might indicate one Rx, that prescription might make a patient dizzy or nauseous. Lenses are for particular purposes: to do a specific job, such as reading in the sun, or driving a truck in the rain at night. Unfortunately, for most people, one lens cannot solve both problems. Different prescriptions are thus necessary, depending upon the task.

Ophthalmologists use compensatory lenses to improve eyesight for specific purposes, such as those just described. Many people reading this chapter are wearing compensatory lenses. Optometrists, however, often use lenses not to correct eyesight, but rather therapeutically to correct vision.

Some prescribe "learning lenses" or "training lenses" to give an individual with autism a new point of view. These lenses may be used temporarily to give the brain a preview of what to expect, and eventually it can perceive differently without the lens. However, motor experiences are necessary for consolidation and permanent changes in perception.

All lenses displace light. Single lenses address focal vision and help us see "What is it?" Ambient prism lenses operate on the "Where is it?" function. They deflect the light rays differently through a thin edge at the top and a thick edge at the base, influencing how the brain interprets where the body is in space. Prisms are available in various magnitudes from "weak" to "strong," measured in diopters. The optometrist can change a patient's perception by altering both the magnitude and the direction of the prism.

The use of prism lenses for behavioral and learning problems goes back only to the 1970s when optometric pioneers began using these tools at the Gesell Institute. Prisms can be powerful temporary tools for individuals with autism and other delays because they alter neural processing of the brain, creating an unconscious change in posture or attention.

Yoked prisms. When the prisms' bases face in the same direction in both eyes, they are called "yoked." Designed to alter neural organization, yoked prisms are powerful tools that can have a dramatic impact on the lives of those with autism. Yoked prisms address a patient's ability to organize space and create a coherent body schema — the "Where is it?" and "Where am I?" functions. These lenses are used therapeutically to change the neuromotor processing of the brain; after rehabilitation occurs, they are no longer needed.[36].

Yoked prisms can cause the environment to appear to be shifted up, down, left, or right. Objects may thus appear closer, farther away, or sloped. These prisms also stimulate spatial awareness, redirect visual focus, increase visual attention, and facilitate visual change, all by working on the ambient or peripheral visual system. Most importantly, yoked prisms can make those who have tuned out their visual surroundings begin to notice their environment, thus leading to generally increased attention and awareness.

As the eyes reorient, the motor system adjusts, sending information to the brain, which comprehends that the individual must adapt his or her body to this new position in space. This readjustment causes a reorganization of the motor and sensory data in the cortex. In time, and with vision therapy, this reorganization becomes permanent.

According to Kaplan, success in making the shift in motor orientation occurs not simply because the eye muscles change in alignment, but also because the brain matches the visual information, while at the same time connecting vision, the motor components of vision, the vestibular process, the kinesthetic process, and proprioception. The prisms thus serve to establish balance among all the senses.[37]

Kaplan has used prism lenses with great success on many populations, including those with anxiety and other psychiatric disorders. One of his most dramatic cases, and one that permanently altered the course of his work more than 30 years ago, was Rickie, the daughter of a prominent psychiatrist. At age 13 she developed symptoms of schizophrenia, requiring hospitalization. After 10 years of failed attempts at medications, electroshock treatments, and psychotherapy, she found her way to Kaplan's office.

Upon examination, Rickie, a beautiful and intelligent young girl, acted like a frightened animal. Kaplan found severely impaired visual processing skills, including tunnel vision, lack of binocularity, and lack of depth perception. Her history showed visual dysfunction at age three, which continued with significant learning disabilities. Eventually, Rickie's highly stressed-out visual system collapsed and relapsed into a psychiatrically diagnosed state.

Rickie completed a year of intensive vision therapy combined with nutritional support and counseling. The results were amazing: Rickie blossomed. She gradually gained independence, returned to school, trained as a practical nurse, married, and had several children.[38]

Rickie's father, Frederic Flach, MD, and Kaplan later collaborated on several projects. Their research revealed that two-thirds of psychiatric patients suffer from some form of visual dysfunction. Nearly 85% of patients with severe, chronic "mental" illness exhibited marked impairments in spatial organization. Those with the most severe visual problems exhibited the highest levels of social withdrawal, academic failure, and employment difficulties.[39]

Kaplan believes that patients with autism develop strategies such as eye turns, postural warps, and self-stimulating behaviors to compensate for their underlying visual deficits. By the time they reach an optometrist who can help, these behaviors are habitual and ingrained. His experience is that yoked prisms alter perception and bring about behavioral changes that are instantaneous and dramatic. Prism lenses instantly create a new visual world in which their adaptive mechanisms are no longer necessary or relevant. As a result, these patients rapidly begin to use previously suppressed visual processing abilities in order to make sense out of their altered environment.[40]

Kaplan and Stephen Edelson of the Autism Research Institute completed a double-blind crossover study in which they divided a group of 20 students with autism and used yoked prisms on one half and a placebo on the others. Those wearing prism lenses showed a decrease in behavior problems after two months, compared to those wearing placebo lenses.[41]

Colored lenses. The medical use of colored light to treat conditions such as jaundiced newborns and Seasonal Affective Disorder (SAD) is well-known. Optometrists use color to treat visual dysfunctions of all types, including strabismus, amblyopia, focusing and convergence problems, learning disorders, and effects of stress and trauma. The name of this method is Syntonics, also known as optometric phototherapy. It is showing promise in the treatment of brain injuries, emotional disorders, and yes, autism.

Syntonics uses many frequencies of light to enhance visual information processing and overall visual performance. Each frequency is a different color. The colors can be delivered to a patient's eyes by having him stare at a colored filter placed over a light bulb or in a special light box. Some patients prefer to wear temporary cardboard glasses frames with the colored filter in them for 5–10 minutes a day.

Reported results are increased binocularity and focusing, and improved use of peripheral vision. For more on this interesting method, and to find a practitioner, go to www.collegeofsyntonicoptometry. com.

Eye doctors and other professionals sometimes tint or color lenses to help patients deal with glare or visual sensitivities. Almost 30 years ago, Helen L. Irlen, a California psychologist interested in visual sensitivities, named the underlying problem "Scotopic Sensitivity Syndrome"; today, the condition is simply called Irlen Syndrome. Irlen found that a subgroup of individuals who were sensitive to light, especially light from fluorescent bulbs, showed a marked improvement in their reading ability when they covered what they were reading with colored acetate sheets.

Irlen has trained hundreds of screeners and diagnosticians around the world to use her method, which filters out the wave lengths of light that create visual stress, allowing the brain to make the normal adjustments for various lighting conditions, glare, and brightness.

One study in the UK showed that in a sample of 36 boys ages 9 to 15, 74% of children with autism increased reading speed by 5% when using an overlay chosen for clarity, and 38% read more than 25% faster. In comparison, only 23% of the controls improved performance, and the improvement was less pronounced than in the ASD group, with only 6% showing more than a 25% increase.[42]

While covered overlays may indeed make it easier for some to read, these overlays may just be Ritalin for the eyes, in that they are treating symptoms but not getting to the underlying problem. Research by optometrists at the Pennsylvania College of Optometry found that 90% of 39 subjects ages 10 to 49 had significant underlying vision problems.[43] A review of 13 research papers on this subject by eminent optometrists at the Learning Disabilities Unit of the State University of New York College of Optometry corroborated that those with Irlen syndrome had various refractive, binocular, and accommodative disorders.[44]

Bifocal lenses. Optometrists frequently prescribe bifocal lenses, which can have an enormous immediate impact on functioning. Bifocals allow the eyes and the brain to readjust and respond differently as they move together into a new visual field (about every eight inches). Some children with autism wear bifocals for the convenience of having two different prescriptions in one frame, one for near work and one for distance. These two prescriptions could be either for correcting an eyesight problem or to take the stress off of the eyes and brain working together.

The Vision-Vestibular Connection

The previous chapter described the relationship between vestibular function and vision. Many with impaired vestibular systems depend upon vision for balance. With eyes closed, the balance system works even less efficiently.[45] Not surprisingly, research shows that children who received therapy for both vestibular and visual function made the best progress. While vestibular intervention alone improved balance, sensory integration, and socialization, adding visual therapy and including the use of lenses and prisms also improved binocular function.[46]

Melvin Kaplan has been particularly interested in the effects of yoked prisms on the visual-vestibular feedback loop. He compares this loop to the telephone, in that incoming and outgoing "calls" move from one sensory system to another. Visual input affects vestibular function, and vestibular input affects visual function. Using prisms to stabilize eye movements also resulted in decreased motion sickness and anxiety.[47]

Many developmental optometrists collaborate with occupational therapists (OTs) today to improve the vestibular and motor coordination of their patients. Optometry stresses the role of vision as primary and movement skills as foundational. Occupational therapy focuses on movement and balance, viewing vision as one of the most important sensory systems.

In 1990 and again in 1999, Lynn Hellerstein, OD, FCOVD, and Beth Fishman, OTR, wrote about the synergistic relationship that can develop between behavioral ODs and OTs.[48] Workshops on OT/OD collaboration have spawned numerous OT/OD pairs whose collaborative work may be familiar to the reader. Few areas of application are more suited to these alliances than autism spectrum disorders.

Vision's Role in Language Development and Social Skills

Pragmatic language and social skill development, two areas that are of great concern to parents of children with autism, are the most complex outcomes of tactile-motor-visual integration. Many years ago, I wrote an article entitled "Say Hi to Patty." In it I elaborate upon how efficient vision allows a child to focus on someone who greets him or her; give the obligatory handshake, hug, or kiss; listen to what the person is saying, even if seeing double; give those words meaning; and respond — all in a matter of seconds!

Speech-language pathologists and mental health professionals sometimes collaborate with optometrists. At the optometrists' suggestions, many even add breathing exercises to their therapy programs because they recognize that natural and spontaneous breathing brings increased amounts of oxygen to the cells and the brain, leading to improved movement, language, vision, cognition, learning, and behavior.

Most professionals working with ODs find that lenses, prisms, and vision therapy complement and enhance their own interventions by treating underlying dysfunctions of the visual system that are load factors in an individual's Total Load. They thus see positive changes in muscle tone, posture, movement, and cognitive function, as well as visual-motor, visual-spatial, visual-perceptual, language, and social-emotional skills that cannot be attributed to their therapy alone.

Vision in the Schools

An educational model defines vision as acuity, and offers "vision" services for students with "low vision" or eyesight problems. School-based occupational therapists (OTs), special educators, and school psychologists can all evaluate visual perception and write IEP goals to enhance visual perception as it relates to academic achievement. However, if the eyes are not working together or if there are other functional vision issues, school-based professionals cannot evaluate or remediate these problems, but rather only look at and work on skills that they impede.

School Vision Screenings

In 1999, the National PTA passed a resolution stating that the screening tests that most schools offer are merely measures of eyesight at distance and are insufficient to identify students with underlying vision problems. This leads to mistaken conclusions that academic deficiencies are a result of behavior or poor motivation rather than caused by serious vision issues, such as convergence insufficiency.[49]

How then can schools know if they are doing a good job of picking up students with underlying vision problems? By testing students' acuity at both distance *and* near point, and by looking at essential visual skills such as focus, accommodation, and convergence in addition to acuity at 20 feet.

School nurses or teachers can use a screening machine that costs about $1,000, called a Keystone Telebinocular, to do thorough vision screenings. This instrument is portable and can move from school to school. It is well worth the price to ensure that all students are working with efficient visual skills. For more information, go to www.keystoneview.com.

Kindergarten readiness tests can also include items that screen vision. A favorite copying test is "cat's whiskers," a horizontal line intersected by an X. Developmentally, the ability to reproduce this design occurs at about age five and one-half, the age at which most children enter kindergarten. A child should copy the design in three strokes, preferably from left to right and top to bottom. Most important is that the rays of the design are not fragmented and that the three lines intersect at a single point. Any variation, such as six rays, the letter "V", or right-to-left drawing shows lack of visual readiness for reading and writing, and the need for intervention. Being able to copy this correctly is a sign that a student is probably using both eyes together and crossing the midline of his or her body.

Environmental Changes that Enhance Vision

Many modifications of the classroom environment will enhance vision not only for students with autism and other disabilities, but for all students. Consider the following:

- *Ensure quality lighting* — Natural light is best; full spectrum bulbs help. Fluorescent lighting is the least desirable.[50]

- *Decrease visual "busyness" of room and written work* — For students with autism, avoid mobiles, venetian blinds, wallpaper, and clutter; they are all distractors. Make sure photocopied materials are fully legible.

- *Provide seating options* — Some kids do better on special cushions and beanbag chairs than on hard, ill-fitting, unforgiving wooden chairs. Make sure that the table or desk is not too high or low, so both feet fully touch the floor and the child's lap is at a right angle.

- *Allow breaks*—When children can move around, they also have the opportunity to rest their eyes.

Classroom Visual Activities

Some of the motor, motor-visual, visual-motor, and visualization activities done in vision therapy with special lenses and prisms can easily be incorporated into the curricula of special education programs, especially at the preschool and elementary levels. Game-like activities with beanbags, balls, balloons, and other items help vision develop, solidify emerging visual skills and consolidate vision for everyone. A number of books directed at teachers and occupational therapists offer suggestions:

- *Begin Where They Are*,[51] is an activity workbook designed to assist parents and professionals who work with individuals with autism of all ages. Written by two vision therapists familiar with in-office vision therapy, it offers very simple exercises for the lowest-functioning kids and explains how to make each game more difficult by adding balance, rhythm, and cognitive distractors like counting to 100 while walking on a balance beam.

- *Classroom Visual Activities: A Manual to Enhance the Development of Visual Skills*,[52] was written under the guidance of a developmental optometrist, and emphasizes chalkboard activities that are done standing. Hopefully, you can find an old-fashioned blackboard; if not, a white board or white paper taped at eye level to the wall will do, using markers instead of chalk.

- *Developing Your Child for Success*,[53] is a cookbook of hundreds of activities from a seasoned optometrist, that move from motor to motor-visual to visual-motor. Many exercises have instructions on how to adapt them for different developmental levels. Excellent drawings make the instructions very clear.

Visual Thinking: Our Goal

Visual thinking, the ability to generate and use imagery, is the culmination of efficient vision development. The skill of running movies in the mind's eye is important for reading comprehension, written language, and understanding mathematics concepts. Temple Grandin is masterful at "seeing in pictures." However, many children with autism do not have her gifts and are attracted to video games, television, and computers to fill the empty space in their minds' eye where imagination should be. Far better than electronic images are those that come out of their own sensory experiences of moving through space.

Harry Wachs, OD, an optometrist who has devoted his long life to combining knowledge of vision with Piagetian theory, is one of the pioneers of visual thinking. Almost 40 years ago, he collaborated with Swiss developmental psychologist Hans Furth to produce *Thinking Goes to School*,[54] a classic still in print. It is a truly remarkable book of over 200 activities that pair vision with every other sense for those of all ages. Chapter headings include "Movement Thinking," "Hand Thinking," "Logical Thinking," and "Tongue and Lip Thinking." Anyone doing intervention with those on the spectrum will find this a valuable addition to their therapy libraries.

At 90 years old, Wachs has recently produced another extraordinary manual of visual/spatial/cognitive exercises with psychologist Serena Wieder, PhD, cofounder with the late Stanley Greenspan, MD, of the DIR method, described in the next chapter. With the cumbersome but all-inclusive title of *Visual/Spatial Portals to Thinking/Feeling and Movement: Advancing Competencies and Emotional Development in Children with Learning and Autism Spectrum Disorders*, it is another gem. Categorically similar to *Thinking Goes to School*, it includes comprehensive photos and drawings explaining Wachs's model.

Wachs uses classic vision therapy tools such as a Marsden ball (a small ball hanging on a string, with letters and numbers on it) as well as more familiar items such as parquetry blocks. He starts with simple patterns and eventually presents constructions from different points of view because taking another's perspective is an abstract concept that starts visually and concretely, and then develops into abstract thought. Read more about this book in the next chapter, which discusses Dr. Wieder's contribution.

Another professional with many years' experience enhancing and improving visual thinking is Colorado optometrist Lynn Hellerstein, OD, FCOVD. Hellerstein has packaged her ideas under the brand "See It, Say It, Do It." She offers a book, workbook, and other materials for use at home and school. Her website is www.lynnhellerstein.com.

For the relationship between visual thinking and academics, go to chapter 14. Note the importance of this foundational skill, especially for reading comprehension and putting one's thoughts on paper. Reading and writing are the culmination of strong visualization skills.

Take-Home Points

Focusing on vision is the next step in remediating foundational sensory issues in individuals with autism spectrum disorders. Addressing and correcting visual dysfunction that underlies so many learning and behavioral problems is the missing link in the healing of many children, especially those on the higher end of the spectrum.

Whether used for part- or full-time wear, and/or during vision therapy activities, lenses and prisms can be very powerful tools for increasing visual awareness and redirecting and extending the range of vision in a person at either end of the spectrum. Using them therapeutically can be life-changing for patients with autism, as it was for neuroscientist Sue Barry.

Vision therapy must be part of an overall treatment plan that includes biomedical intervention and other sensory and motor therapies. Each child is unique, and the therapies for an individual must be appropriate for his or her developmental age and history. As Charles Hart of the Autism Society has written, "To understand autism, or any other human condition you must observe the individual, not just the stereotypes. Our most talented teachers agree when they say, 'to reach a child with autism, you must first learn to see the world through the student's eye.'"[55]

Parents, educators, therapists, physicians, counselors, or others not familiar with vision therapy, may wish to consult additional references for the basics of vision. Some good resources are www. oep.org, www.children-special-needs.org, http://www.covd.org, and www.visiontherapy.org.

Oh, yes, to answer those questions at the beginning of the chapter are: Steve Jobs had vision. "I see" is in your mind's eyes, and people who are myopic in their glasses prescriptions are often also myopic in their thinking.

---

[1] Noe A. Out of Our Heads: Why You Are Not Your Brain, and Other Lessons from the Biology of Consciousness. New York: Hill and Wang, 2009.

[2] Getman GN, Gesell A. Vision, its development in infant and child. New York: Harper & Brothers, 1949.

[3] Ilg F, Ames LB, Gesell A. Infant and Child in the Culture of Today. New York: Harper & Brothers, 1943.

[4] Getman GN. How to Develop Your Child's Intelligence. Santa Ana, CA: Optometric Extension Program, 1993.

[5] Flavell J. The developmental psychology of Jean Piaget. New York: D. Van Nostrand Company, 1967.

[6] Suchoff IB. Cognitive Development: Piaget's Theory. Santa Ana, CA: Optometric Extension Program; 1978.

[7] McDonald LW. Some Considerations When Developing Visual Abilities. Santa Ana, CA: Optometric Extension Program Foundation, 1964, 2, 189–94.

[8] Press LJ. Sensorimotor dynamics and two visual systems: Shades of Skeffington and Brock. Part 1. Visionhelp, May 22, 2011. http://visionhelp.wordpress. com/2011/05/22/sensorimotor-dynamics-and-two-visual-systems-shades-of-skeffington-brock-part-1/.

[9] Hornbeak DM, Young TL. Myopia genetics: A review of current research and emerging trends. Curr Opin Ophthalmol. Sep 2009, 20:5, 356–62; Engle EC. Genetic Basis of Congenital Strabismus. JAMA Ophthalmology, Feb 2007, 125, 2.

[10] Diabetes Discovery—Via the Eyes. https://www.vsp.com/diabetes.html. Accessed Jan 31, 2013.

[11] Megson M. The biological basis for perceptual deficits in autism. http://megson. com/readings/BiologicalBasis.pdf Accessed Jan 31, 2013.

[12] Carman KB, Tutkun E, Yilmaz H, Dilber C. Acute mercury poisoning among children in two provinces of Turkey. Eur J Pediatr. Jun 2013, 172:6, 821–27.

[13] Kaplan, M. Seeing Through New Eyes: Changing the lives of children with autism, Asperger syndrome and other developmental disabilities through vision therapy. Philadelphia: Jessica Kingsley Publishers, 2006, 126.

[14] Kaplan. Seeing Through New Eyes. 10-16.

[15] Kaplan. Seeing Through New Eyes.

[16] Milne E, Griffiths H, Buckley D, Scope A. Vision in children and adolescents with autistic spectrum disorder: Evidence for reduced convergence. J Autism Dev Disord. Jul 2009: 39:7, 965–75.

[17] Novak L. Not autistic or hyperactive. Just seeing double at times. http://www.nytimes.com/2007/09/11/health/11visi.html, Accessed Feb 3, 2013; Granet D, Gomi C, Ventura R, Miller-Scholte A. The relationship between convergence insufficiency and ADHD. Strabismus, Dec 2005, 13:4, 163–68.

[18] Cooper J, Duckman R. Convergence insufficiency: Incidence, diagnosis, and treatment. J Am Optom Assoc, 1978, 49, 673–80.

[19] Kaplan M, Rimland B, Edelson S. Strabismus in Autism Spectrum Disorder. Focus on Autism and Other Developmental Disabilities, Summer 1999, 14:2, 101–5.

[20] Friedman DS, Repka MX, Katz J, Giordano L, et al. Prevalence of amblyopia and strabismus in white and African American children aged 6 through 71 months the Baltimore Pediatric Eye Disease Study. Ophthalmology, Nov 2009, 116:11, 2128–34.

[21] Press LJ. Topical review: Strabismus. J Optom Vis Dev, 1999, 22, 5–20.

[22] P Venkhatesh. Do we Learn to see? Resonance, Jan 2011, 16:1, 88–99.

[23] Kavner, RM. Strabismus and Amblyopia. New Developments, Winter 2002–03, 8:2, 5.

[24] Kaplan. Seeing Through New Eyes.

[25] Grandin T. Thinking in pictures and other reports of my life with autism. New York: Vintage, 1996.

[26] Bowan MB. Learning disabilities, dyslexia and vision: A subject review. J Am Opt Assoc, Sep 2002, 73:9, 553–70.

[27] Streff JW. Optometric care for a child manifesting qualities of autism. J Am Optom Assoc, 1979, 46:6, 592–97.

[28] Scharre JE, Creedon MP. Assessment of visual function in autistic children. Optom Vis Sci, Jun 1992, 69:6, 433–39.

[29] Rosenhall U, Johansson E, Gillberg C. Oculomotor findings in autistic children. J Laryngol Otol, May 1988 102:5, 435–39; Kemner C, Verbaten MN, Cuperus JM, et al. Abnormal saccadic eye movements in autistic children. J Autism Dev Disord, Feb 1998, 28:1, 61–7.

[30] Kaplan M, Edelson DP, Gaydos AM. Postural orientation modifications in autism in response to ambient lenses. Child Psychiatr Hum Dev, 1996, 27:2, 81–91.

[31] Neupane S, Bhandari G, Shrestha GS. Ocular morbidity in children with autism. Optometric & Visual Performance Jrl, 2012, 1:1, 32–42.

[32] Kaplan, Seeing Through New Eyes.

[33] Taub M, Russell, R. Autism Spectrum Disorders: A Primer for the Optometrist. Review of Optometry, May 2007; Coulter RA. Serving the needs of the patient with autism. Optom Vis Dev, 2009; 40:3, 136–40.

[34] Sacks O. Stereo Sue. New Yorker Magazine, June 19, 2006, 64–73.

[35] Barry S. Fixing My Gaze: A Scientist's Journey into Seeing in Three Dimensions. New York: Basic Books, 2010.

[36] Kaplan. Seeing Through New Eyes, 81.

[37] Kaplan. Seeing Through New Eyes, 47.

[38] Kaplan. Seeing Through New Eyes, 37–41.

[39] Flach FF, Kaplan M. Visual Perceptual Dysfunction in Psychiatric Patients. Comprehensive Psychiatry, 1983, 24:4, 304–311.

[40] Taub and Russell. Autism Spectrum Disorders.

[41] Kaplan M, Edelson SM, Seip JA. Behavioral changes in autistic individuals as a result of wearing ambient transitional prism lenses. Child Psychiatry Hum Dev, 1998. 29:1, 65–76.

[42] Ludlow AK, Wilkins AJ, Heaton P. Colored overlays enhance visual perceptual performance in children with autism spectrum disorders. Research in Autism Spectrum Disorders 2, 2008, 498–515.

[43] Scheiman M, Blaskey P, Ciner EB, Gallaway M, et al. Vision characteristics of individuals identified as Irlen Filter candidates. J Am Optom Assoc, Aug 1990, 61:8, 600–5.

[44] Solan H, Richmond J. Irlen Lenses: A critical appraisal. J Am Optom Assoc, Oct 1990, 61:10, 789–96.

[45] Molloy CA, Kietrich KN, Bhattacharya A. Postural stability in children with autism spectrum disorder. J Aut Dev Dis, 2003, 33:6, 643–52.

[46] Solan HA, Shelley-Tremblay J, Larson S. Vestibular function, sensory integration and balance anomalies: A brief literature review. Optom Vis Dev, 2007, 38, 1–5.

[47] Taub and Russell. Autism Spectrum Disorders

[48] Hellerstein LF, Fishman B. Vision therapy and occupational therapy: An integrated approach. J Behav Optom, 1990, 1:5, 122–26; Hellerstein LF, Fishman B. Collaboration between occupational therapists and optometrists. J Behav Optom, 1999, 10:6, 147–52.

[49] National PTA. Learning Related Vision Problems Education and Evaluation. 1999.

[50] Mumford R. Improving visual efficiency with selected lighting. JOVD, 2002, 33:3.

[51] Nurek K, Wendelburg D. Begin where they are. Santa Ana, CA: Optometric Extension Program Foundation, 1993.

[52] Richards R, Remick K. CVA: Classroom Visual Activities: A Manual to Enhance the Development of Visual Skills. Novato, CA: Academic Therapy Press, 1988.

[53] Lane K. Developing your child for success. Lewisville, TX: Learning Potentials Pub, 1991.

[54] Furth H, Wachs H. Thinking Goes to School. New York: Oxford Univ Press, 1975.

[55] Hart, C. A parent's guide to autism. New York: Simon and Schuster, 1993, 1.

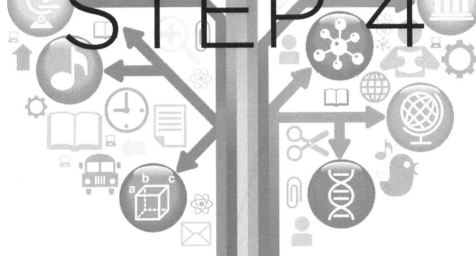

STEP 4

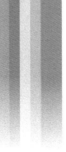

Focus on Communicating,
Interacting, and Learning

CHAPTER 12

Communication:
Improving Social Skills through Play

Finally! Three-quarters of the way through this book, we get to what parents value most: communication and social skills. Poor, unusual, and absent communication skills and poor, unusual, and absent interpersonal relationships are the hallmarks of autism spectrum disorders. To review information presented in chapter 1, symptoms of autism include:

Impairment in social interaction
- Inappropriate eye contact or facial expression
- Failure to develop peer relationships
- Lack of spontaneous sharing of enjoyment or interests

Impairment in communication
- Delayed or non-existent language development
- Poor conversational abilities if language is present
- Lack of make-believe or social imitative play

Repetitive and stereotyped behavior, interests, and activities
- Abnormally intense preoccupation with one or more interests
- Mannerisms such as hand or finger flapping or twisting or whole body movements
- Preoccupations with object parts

Foundations for Language and Social Skills

By now, you should have gotten the point: the emergence of language and social skills depends upon *everything* discussed in the previous chapters. Biomedical treatments remove stressors from the body by normalizing digestion, detoxification, and other bodily functions, thus releasing energies for sensory processing. Visual, auditory, and occupational therapies can then be most effective and produce secondary benefits in communication and social-emotional interaction. Before proceeding further reconsider whether:

• *The child's Total Load is sucking up significant energy, leaving little available for talking and interacting.* Remember: the body's top priority is staying well. If the physical body is battling chemicals, heavy metals, gut bugs, viruses, bacteria, mold, or any other unwelcome toxins, it is difficult to focus outward. Consider running laboratory testing to evaluate these areas, as described in Step One. In the long run, testing will save considerable time and money.

• *The child is eating, drinking, or breathing something to which his body is reacting.* This possibility is an extension of the first. Allergies to food or environmental pests, such as bee stings and pollen, show a weakened immune system. If a child's behavior changes markedly with the seasons of the year, consider this possibility, and strengthen immune functioning with dietary modification and supplementation.

• *Oxytocin and vasopressin levels are abnormal.* Oxytocin and vasopressin are hormones that play key roles in emotional and social behaviors and bonding. Oxytocin can improve social behavior in individuals with autism. Refer back to chapter 6 for more on this subject and on how to implement therapy.

• *The family has experienced significant stressors for several generations.* Deep psychological wounds that go back generations are common in families of children with ASDs.

Read about family constellations, the remarkable work of German psychiatrist Bert Hellinger to heal these energetic traumas, in chapter 7.

• *Structural or reflex abnormalities are interfering with language processing.* If a child was born by C-section, or the birth was otherwise traumatic, these areas should be considered. (See chapters 8 and 9.)

• *Sensory and motor development are not strong and reliable.* Low tone throughout the body may also be causing oral motor issues, making it difficult to form words. Vestibular and auditory processing problems often interfere with language and social skills. Review these areas in chapter 10.

• *Vision difficulties such as lack of binocularity have not been resolved.* A developmental vision exam is an essential prerequisite to addressing language and social skills. If a child's eyes are not working together properly, communication and behavior will be severely affected. Refer back to chapter 11 for more on this subject.

Prior to embarking upon the long-awaited relationship-based therapies that act directly upon delayed language and social-emotional skills, let's review how children develop all the skills necessary to talk, engage, relate, and converse through play. According to Rebecca Klaw, MS, MEd, an autism specialist in Pittsburgh, Pennsylvania, play begins "small and simple" for typically developing children. With input from parents, teachers, siblings, and friends, simple play gradually expands over time, becoming rich and very complex.

The elaboration of play is fueled by positive social interactions, and serves as the basis for early learning. The child at play is not idle or aimless, boring or bored, or wasting time. The child is, in fact, engaged in complex activities that develop skills and build, bit by bit, concepts as complicated as physics and as essential as empathy.[1]

Sensory Integration and Mirror Neurons

Play occurs as the senses integrate through endless experiences. Three senses are primarily responsible for good social-emotional development: touch, balance, and vision. Eventually, as these sensory processing systems mature and integrate, language and social interactions deepen.

Touch is grounding, and the ability to tolerate it is essential for feeling secure and confident. "The child with tactile defensiveness sends out signals that he is unfriendly and prefers to be left alone."[2]

An efficient balance system allows a child to feel grounded and know where his or her body is in space. When one is gravitationally insecure, feeling emotionally secure is difficult, if not impossible.

Children with efficient vision not only see another person, but also are able to give appropriate meaning to subtle facial expressions and gestures. They focus *on* the person's face, not *in front of* her or over her shoulder, and can judge appropriate social distance for conversation. Dysfunctions such as double vision, lack of visual flexibility, and difficulty focusing can interfere significantly with social interaction. Eventually, vision emerges as the dominant sense.

Efficient sensory integration is imperative for receptive and expressive language development; it is also vitally important for appropriate social interactions. Dr. Daniel J. Siegel states, "Our brains use sensory information to create representations of others' minds. Based on these sensory inputs, we can mirror not only the behavioral intentions of others, but also their emotional states."[3]

In the mid-1990s Italian neuroscientists discovered the mechanism that allows the brain to perform this remarkable feat: "mirror neurons," cells in the premotor cortex that fire both when a person performs an action itself and when he observes another living creature perform that same action. These "monkey-see, monkey-do" parts of the brain appear to be vitally important in understanding social skills and empathy. While a 2005 study showed deficits in the mirror neuron system in those with autism,[4] researchers are still debating this theory.

Figure 12.1

Ways to Engage Children with Autism in Play

- Heighten interest
- Be persistent
- Include repetition
- Establish routines
- Add sensory stimulation
- Minimize language
- Have fun

Autism and Relationship Building

Children with ASDs tend to play alone in unusual and repetitive ways. They often have difficulty learning how to expand their play from others. They might be good at creating sounds, sights, and motions for their own pleasure and at manipulating objects and figuring out how they work. What they are not good at, however, is playing with someone else, because they miss the social components of play. Children with autism spectrum disorders tend to get stuck in their play, and they need to learn, through patient and skilled adults, how to play.

How do you play with a child who wants to be left alone? Insist that they play with you, using persistence, intelligence, flexibility, and humor. Children with ASDs need to be guided in memorable ways to explore all aspects of their world, not just how to manipulate objects, but how to share, build, pretend, elaborate, invent, describe, and create. Klaw offers strategies that utilize the guidelines from some of the methods elaborated upon in this chapter in figure 12.1.

Social Skills Training for Autism

Speech-language pathologists, mental health professionals, educators, and others have used a variety of social skills training programs for years. Despite the popularity of social skills training in schools, a review of the literature shows that it is only minimally effective for children with ASD![5] That finding may come as a surprise to those who work so hard to teach appropriate social behaviors to their clients on the autism spectrum. The latest study referenced above is consistent with other previous studies on the subject.

Why do social skills training programs fail? Probably because one or more of the load factors listed above is interfering with the emergence of play and interactive language. If we train social skills from the outside-in, rather than let children develop them from the inside-out, we teach them to distrust their own sensory processing.

But *some* programs must work, or there would not be a chapter on the subject in this book. What *are* the components of those that make a difference? A group of researchers at the University of Utah evaluated several programs and came up with some guidelines. Effective programs

- break down complex social behaviors into concrete steps and rules that kids can practice in a variety of settings;
- concretize abstract concepts through a variety of visual, tangible, "hands-on" activities that make socialization fun; and
- provide a variety of learning opportunities that allow skills to integrate and generalize.

All of the programs described in this chapter meet these criteria.

Relationship-Based Approaches to Autism

Relationship-based approaches are appropriate for children at any age and any developmental level. It is never too early or too late to use them because they all respect a child's interests and hold the belief that all behavior is meaningful. In addition, all programs in this chapter recognize the role of efficient sensory processing in language and social-emotional development. Therapists focus on building trusting relationships by following a child's lead, rather than have a strict agenda, thus developing intrinsic motivation. The programs for relationship building and communication covered in depth here are:

- DIR/Floortime
- Profectum and FCD™
- The Affect-Based Language Curriculum
- RDI®
- The Son-Rise Program®
- Social Stories™
- The Miller Method®

This chapter also includes some less well-known programs, including SCERTS® and the Polyvagal Theory. Finally, utilizing animals as channels for communication and relationship building is explored.

Therapies in this chapter can be added to or combined with other therapies in this book, especially those focusing on biological foundations for behavior. However, the best approach is often to use dietary modification and nutritional supplementation first, and then wait; often relationships and communication improve spontaneously, rendering additional therapy unnecessary.

Greenspan's DIR® and Floortime™

The **D**evelopmental, **I**ndividual Difference, **R**elationship-based Approach (DIR®), is a comprehensive, intensive interdisciplinary approach developed by the late child psychiatrist Stanley Greenspan, MD, and psychologist, Serena Wieder, PhD. Greenspan and Wieder are the coauthors of *The Child with Special Needs*[6] and *Engaging Autism*,[7] from which I have drawn much of the information in this section.

DIR builds healthy foundations for social, emotional, and intellectual capacities rather than focusing on skills and isolated behaviors. It incorporates and is fully compatible with many of the therapeutic programs described in previous chapters, including biomedical intervention, occupational therapy, sound-based therapies, and vision therapy.

According to Greenspan and Wieder, all individuals categorize experiences by their sensory and affective qualities simultaneously. Affective categories essentially function as sense organs. As experiences accumulate, sensory impressions become increasingly tied to feelings. Making sense of an experience is an immediate emotional reaction, which probably precedes any cognition. Intelligence is the connection between a feeling (or a desire) and an action (or a symbol).

Whereas a majority of mental health professionals consider emotional reactions secondary to cognitive perceptions, Greenspan believed that in many instances they are primary. Dual coding of experiences is the key to understanding how emotions organize intellectual capacity and create a sense of self, because the learning process allows children to "cross-reference" each memory or experience in a mental catalogue of phenomena and feelings, and to reconstruct it when needed. This process theoretically also provides the basis for generalization, abstraction, logic, and reasoning.

DIR Theory and Autism

The DIR/Floortime model is useful in working with children at all levels of severity on the autism spectrum. Greenspan and Wieder found that the degree of autism does not necessarily determine prognosis with DIR.

In the Greenspan model of autism, aberrant sensory perceptions are processed by a brain that has not mastered the ability to attach emotions to relevant experiences. When sensory processing is disrupted, the emotional organization of experiences can be compromised.

The first goal in the DIR approach is to help the child work around sensory processing difficulties to establish a meaningful relationship with parents. For a child who is in his own world and not relating to others, the emphasis is on enticing him into the world by giving him a greater degree of pleasure in relating.

DIR takes into account the child's feelings, relationships with caregivers, developmental level, and individual differences in his ability to process and respond to sensory information. It focuses on the child's skills in all developmental areas, including social-emotional functioning, communication, thinking and learning, motor skills, body awareness, and attention. It is less focused on specific skills such as reading and writing, recognizing that those skills will develop more readily when the child has a solid foundation from which to learn. Because the development of symbol formation, language, and intelligence is based on a series of critical emotional interactions early in life, when a child does not master these emotional interactions, essential learning abilities and behavior suffer.

Components of DIR®

Developmental. The Developmental part of the model describes the building blocks. Understanding where the child is developmentally is critical to planning a treatment program.

DIR takes into account six sequential stages of development that denote how well a child engages with others, initiates interaction, and uses gestures to communicate. First, a child masters the early nonverbal developmental stages of communication and learns to maintain a continuous flow of interaction and engagement. Early on, DIR focuses on getting the child to play symbolically. At the second stage, a child moves to understanding the full range of feelings and develops interpersonal problem solving. The latter stages focus on helping children develop abstract thinking through making comparisons and judgments based on their own emotional experiences. The six stages are:

1. *Shared attention:* Utilize all the senses and motor abilities, stretching the child's capabilities for interaction.
2. *Engagement:* Follow the child's lead, building upon pleasurable interactions. Match the child's rhythm, deepen the warmth, add physical closeness.
3. *Two-way purposeful interaction with gestures:* Exaggerate emotion, become animated, support initiative, facilitate goal achievement.
4. *Two-way purposeful problem-solving interaction:* Add extra steps to play, such as acting dumb, playing obstructively, and creating barriers, forcing the child to solve problems.
5. *Emotional ideas:* Encourage imaginary play, combining words with ideas and affect with action.
6. *Emotional thinking:* Build bridges between ideas and development of abstract reasoning. Challenge with "wh" questions. This high level of development is the ultimate goal for all children.

Individual differences. The *I* in DIR stands for individual differences and describes the unique ways each child takes in, regulates, responds to, and comprehends sensations and the planning and sequencing of actions and ideas. While the DIR model tailors intervention to the individual needs of each child, it also focuses on the entire family, thus often resolving family issues that may be interfering with a child's growth and development.

Relationship-based. The Relationship component refers to the interactions with caregivers, educators, therapists, peers, and others who tailor their behavior to the child's individual differences and developmental capacities to enable progress. A child's unique individual differences and developmental challenges combine to affect how he or she relates to others. Understanding each child's unique set is crucial in planning emotionally-based interactions, which are at the heart of intervention. The DIR approach assists caregivers in developing adult/child relationships, which then allow a child to develop meaningful relationships with peers and siblings.

Floortime™

At the heart of the DIR approach is Floortime™, a specific technique to both follow the child's lead and at the same time challenge the child towards greater and greater mastery of social, emotional, and intellectual capacities. The guidelines for Floortime allow the child to develop spontaneous interactive behaviors that are purposeful and intentional. The basic principles of Floortime are to:

1. *Follow a child's lead.* The child is the leader; do what the child does. The role of the adult is to facilitate communication and problem solving and to keep the play interactive, not to direct the child's play. Use every opportunity to encourage the imitation of symbolic actions. As a child becomes more able to sequence actions, new meanings will emerge.

2. *Join in at a child's developmental level and build on his natural interests.* Treat whatever the child is doing as intentional and purposeful. Use exaggerated affect and action to woo the child into interacting. By giving every move the utmost attention, interest, and energy, adults convey that actions are meaningful and can elicit a response.

3. *Open and close circles of communication.* Build upon the child's natural interests, always focusing on maintaining a continuous flow of interaction. If adult involvement triggers anger, avoidance, whining, or tantrums, continue anyway. Anger is an acceptable response and often precedes the ability to express pleasure. Be indirect without imposing upon or overwhelming a child while opening and closing circles of communication.

4. *Help the child do what he wants to do.* Motor planning difficulties, low muscle tone, and poor "self-other differentiation" may cause a child to take an adult's hand to do something. Guide by putting hand over hand. Work face-to-face or at a mirror so the child can see adult expressions.

5. *Create a play environment.* Use anything that piques a child's natural interests, motivation, and curiosity. Focus on creative interaction; avoid structured games.

6. *Extend the circles of communication.* Interact in ways that help a child reach individual goals, such as obtaining a toy. Interact playfully, sometimes playing dumb or obstructing avoidance behavior.

7. *Broaden the child's range of interactive experience.* Extend the child's desire to expand upon emotional, sensory, and motor responses. Help a passive child become more outgoing, even aggressive, or an impulsive child to move in slow motion.

8. *Tailor interactions to a child's unique sensory processing differences.* Add sound, touch, vision, and movement at the appropriate developmental levels to the play with sensory, wind-up, and simple cause-and-effect toys to entice a passive child's interest and attention. Use sensory toys such as whistles, bubbles, textured blocks, and beanbags to capitalize upon strengths and to remediate weaknesses.

9. *Mobilize the six developmental stages simultaneously.* Share attention, engage the child with gestures and pre-verbal problem-solving to encourage two-way purposeful interaction, emotions, ideas, and thinking. Build bridges between ideas and the development of abstract reasoning, with the ultimate objective of maintaining mutual attention and engagement.

Floortime enables the child and the adult to feel connected and to communicate with each other. Floortime helps the child see the value of nonverbal communication through facial expressions, gestures, and other cues, and encourages the child to use these tools to communicate with others.

Several randomized-controlled studies showed DIR/Floortime to be an evidence-based practice. Children with autism who used Floortime showed statistically significant improvement in behavior when compared to those receiving a mix of behavioral approaches.[8]

The Home Program

Unlike many in-office therapy programs, most DIR sessions take place as an intensive home program. Parents, caregivers, and therapists typically interact with children in Floortime activities for at least 20 minutes, eight or more times a day; it becomes a way of life. DIR teaches children to respond to every utterance or gesture, in an effort to spark a response. For school-age children, when the child is ready, the program can be integrated into the classroom, which allows interactions with typically developing children.

Once a child begins to be interactive, peer play becomes an important part of the program. Children on the autism spectrum need to learn how to communicate with peers, who may be less-forgiving than adults. Playdates with typical kids are opportunities for the skills developed with adults to generalize to other children. At first, adults must be available to orchestrate children's interactions. As peer interaction improves, less adult intervention is necessary.

A well-balanced DIR program includes both spontaneous and semi-structured activities designed to facilitate mastery of specific processing abilities and emotional, cognitive, language, and motor skills. The recipe for balance depends upon a child's developmental profile. Structured activities at least three times a day address the following areas:

- *Motor and sensory skills:* running, jumping on a trampoline, spinning, navigating obstacle courses

- *Balance, coordination, and left-right integration:* walking on a beam; standing on one leg with eyes open and closed; throwing, catching, and kicking balls with each and both hands; drawing; standing and sitting with hands alone and together

- *Rhythm:* games such as patty-cake, dancing to music, clapping, playing percussion instruments

- *Modulation:* sessions that require the child to move at different rates of speed (a drum or special music can facilitate these games)

- *Visual-spatial skills:* activities such as treasure hunts, based on the work of Harry Wachs, OD, a longtime Greenspan collaborator (read more about vision and Wachs in chapter 11)

Prior to his death in 2010, Greenspan began consulting with the Rebecca School in New York City. The school institutionalizes Dr. Greenspan's Floortime methods, and its educators work to extend students' circles of communication using the DIR model. The clinical director, Gil Tippy, PsyD, collaborated with Greenspan on *Respecting Autism*, published in 2011, describing the successes of 16 students at the Rebecca School.[9] Several other schools in the United States and abroad are based on DIR.

The official organization of DIR/Floortime is the Interdisciplinary Council on Development and Learning (ICDL). Since Dr. Greenspan's death, ICDL has been under the leadership of some of his disciples, including his wife. Greenspan's son Jake carries on his legacy as a DIR therapist in Bethesda, Maryland. Those interested in ongoing training institutes should go to www.icdl.com.

Profectum and FCD™

In 2011 a new organization emerged, founded by over 60 DIR-trained therapists and professionals. Called Profectum, it embraces a new developmental model that is an outgrowth of DIR/Floortime. The new model, Foundational Capacities for Development (FCD), is the result of further recognition and elaboration of the significant role of vision, space, and movement in emotional and symbolic development, as well as in anxiety and behavior in the sequential and organizational capacities needed for functional competence. Affect and cognition are two sides of the same coin.[10]

In the 1970s Wachs combined optometry with Piagetian psychology in his groundbreaking book, *Thinking Goes to School.*[11] Greenspan, Wieder, and Wachs came from the fields of psychiatry, psychology, and optometry, respectively. As they examined the relationship between the DIR model and Wachs' unique model of vision therapy, they eventually concluded that their seemingly different approaches were congruent—they were all going down developmental paths to cognition.

Emotions are an inherent part of cognition; emotional interactions lead the way in virtually every stage of development. As typically developing children learn where they are in space, their understanding is accompanied by an emotional need for safety. For those who are "lost in space," like many on the autism spectrum, their poor visual-spatial thinking undermines their sense of safety, resulting in anxiety.

After Greenspan's death, Wieder and Wachs expanded on the intersection of their fields. In their book *Spatial Portals to Thinking, Feeling and Movement,* they describe the developmental processes that activate, organize, and integrate all experiences.[12] Exposure to experiences is insufficient for competence. The letter *C* is used as a guideline to capture the components of experience that advance development: comprehension, competence, confidence, control, caring, connection, creativity, conditions, coping, and community. Each child's uniqueness holds true in emotional development, as well, as each one's experiences has a unique developmental progression.

An example of how therapists can apply these principles is the "Bear Walk," described in depth in *Spatial Portals*. In this exercise, the adult goes through the following steps while walking on all fours, like a bear. Note that it follows the six stages of development of DIR with the exception of the final stage, which is hybridized from "emotional thinking" to "logical/abstract thinking." The six stages could take anywhere from a week to a year, depending upon the beginning developmental level of the child.

- *Bear Walk—Shared Attention:* Move around the room, trying to get a child's attention with words, gestures, and sounds.
- *Bear Walk—Attachment and Engagement:* Entice the child to follow you, using provocative gestures, sounds, and words.
- *Bear Walk—Purposeful Two-Way Communication:* Interact further, pointing and asking questions about directions and purpose.
- *Bear Walk—Shared Social Problem Solving:* Expand circles of communication by adding another person or playing tag or chase.
- *Bear Walk—Creating Emotional Ideas:* Suggest the child choose to be a different animal. Create a story and reasons for movement.
- *Animal Walks—Abstract and Logical Thinking:* Challenge the child, asking "wh-" questions. Negotiate. Challenge the child to make sense.

Profectum welcomes collaboration among DIR therapists, as well as related treatment approaches and service providers described in this book. For more information about this growing organization, go to www.profectum.org.

The Affect-Based Language Curriculum (ABLC)

For many years, Dr. Greenspan collaborated with speech-language pathologist Diane Lewis, MA, CCC/SLP, to develop the Affect-Based Language Curriculum (ABLC), which embraces the premise that emotion is critical for many elements of language acquisition and use. Without affect and engagement, a child will encounter difficulty developing purposeful and meaningful language. The ABLC is a home program.

The ABLC includes a series of structured and semi-structured activities undertaken with high affect and motivation so that they generalize quickly. In implementing the ABLC, caretakers first create a supportive environment in which a child is engaged in a pleasurable activity. While adhering to the DIR principles of attention, engagement, and closing circles, the adult introduces activities to enhance specific skills such as oral motor capacities and imitation, as well as receptive, expressive, and pragmatic language.

The ABLC moves through five developmental levels from Level A (0–9 months) to Level D2 (36–48 months). Sequential skills and activities make up the program. Caregivers use comprehensive checklists to chart progress and plan an individual child's program.

The ABLC focuses on traditional elements of language, such as phonology, syntax, grammar, and semantics, while also addressing reflective and abstract thinking. Those interested in learning more about the ABLC should refer to *The Affect-Based Language Curriculum (ABLC): An Intensive Program for Families, Therapists and Teachers.*[13]

Solving the Relationship Puzzle: Relationship Development Intervention© (RDI)

"I knew each child with autism could not make the same progress or reach the same goals. But, regardless of his or her abilities and limits, I wanted to give each of them something." So began the journey in 1995 of psychologist Steven E. Gutstein, PhD, the innovator of Relationship Development Intervention or RDI©. Gutstein describes RDI in his book, *Autism Asperger's: Solving the Relationship Puzzle.*[14] This synopsis of RDI is taken from that book and from Gutstein's website, www.rdiconnect.com.

RDI shares many features with other treatment approaches. Like DIR, RDI educates and coaches adults to interact and work with children on the spectrum. Its goal is the remediation of specific deficits that define autism spectrum disorders by creating numerous daily opportunities for the child to respond in flexible, thoughtful ways.

In addition, it helps children capture and stockpile critical memories that build a repository of competence, in gradually more complex environments.

RDI is not wedded to any series of techniques, but rather to developing effective methods to remediate those specific deficits which impede people on the autism spectrum from productive employment, independent living, marriage and intimate social relationships. RDI's goals are for those with autism to:

- Understand and appreciate the many levels of experience sharing;
- Become an equal partner in co-regulating experience sharing interactions;
- Value the uniqueness of others' perspectives, ideas, and feelings;
- Work to maintain enduring relationships;
- Become adaptable and flexible in both social and non-social problem solving; and
- Recognize that their own unique identity can continue to grow and develop.

RDI applies the ways in which typical children become socially competent, by steering children on the autism spectrum down a path of self discovery and social awareness to a world of meaningful friendships, shared emotions, and heartfelt connection with people in their lives. The Connections Center in Houston, Texas, the home of RDI Program©, now serves as an international consultation and training center for professionals and families. Hundreds of professionals in child development are certified as RDI Program Consultants.

Experience Sharing

Gutstein has named the innate pleasure derived from a variety of social encounters "experience sharing." For typically developing children, experience sharing takes place in levels, each with four distinct stages, starting at birth. He has systematically analyzed and labeled many levels of experience sharing, starting with "emotional attunement" and "social referencing," among others, at the early months, to "fluid transitions" in the second year of life, "unique selves" in the fifth year, and "enduring friendships" by age 11 or 12.

While this model is clearly a gross oversimplification of the millions of situations children experience, it provides a useful framework for understanding emotional development.

Autism: Life without Experiencing Sharing

According to Gutstein's model, individuals with autism have deficits in the understanding and appreciation of experience sharing. Gutstein believes that sometime during the first year of life, children with autism go down a developmental road that does not include the endless hours a typical child spends with social referencing, or "you-me" thinking and emotional attunement.

By the end of the first year of life, when objects begin to compete with people for a child's attention, the typical child enters the object world looking for enhancement, while the child with autism chooses objects over the people, and departs from the world of experience sharing. Typical children already know that adults are good reference points for safety, meaning, excitement, and resolving, while those with autism have not made that connection.

The Three Cardinal Principles of RDI

RDI recognizes that learning to be proficient in even the simplest forms of experience sharing requires many different abilities, and it is thus far more complex than most social skills programs. RDI provides a special therapeutic setting which amplifies critical information, minimizes distractions, and slows down the pace of interaction. Continued change and unpredictability, rather than scripted or discrete learning, are inherent aspects of experience sharing.

Gutstein has classified the three major principles that lay the foundation for RDI as "social referencing," "functions precede means," and "co-regulation."

- *Social Referencing:* The desire and capacity for social referencing is the foundation of experience sharing. Gutstein defines "social referencing" as a highly specialized form of perception and information processing that allows a person to evaluate the state of a relationship. In the process, a child is constantly reading the degree of similarity between something he is doing, feeling, perceiving, or thinking in order to interpret the relationship with social partners.

• *Functions Precede Means:* At each developmental level of experience sharing, RDI introduces the child to new aspects of experiences to be shared, thus establishing greater emotional connections. Eventually, children with autism, like their typical peers, develop a desire for deeper emotional experiences, leading them to pursue and spend many hours mastering new skills. They then learn to interact for the sole purpose of sharing their world with others, and become eager to apply newly learned skills both in and out of treatment settings.

• *Co-Regulation:* Once children have mastered "social referencing," and "functions precede means," RDI introduces "co-regulation," the ability to understand how one partner's actions impact the actions of another, in order to maintain the relationship. Co-regulation requires constant referencing of a partner. Give-and-take interaction produces curiosity about the other person. As co-regulation becomes more and more proficient, it provides the foundation for moving into exploring another person's mind. What will he do next? What is he thinking? How is he feeling?

The most crucial part of co-regulation for children with autism is learning how to observe when coordination has been lost or is in jeopardy. In early work on co-regulation, RDI, like DIR, recommends exaggerating non-coordination. For example, adults should deliberately and playfully impede a child's desired goal.

The RDI Program Protocol
Nine essential elements must be in place for the intervention to be classified as an RDI Program:

1. *Diagnostic evaluation:* The first step is for the child to undergo comprehensive language, cognitive, neurological, perceptual, motor, and medical evaluations called a "Relationship Development Assessment™" (RDA).

2. *Parent education:* Prior to beginning a program, all parents must attend a series of workshops, or, if impossible, view a comprehensive DVD about how to incorporate RDI into their daily lives.

3. *RDI program planning:* A certified RDI consultant reviews the results of the RDA, and provides a customized intervention plan with lengthy recommendations.

4. *Consultation:* Intervention is guided by a certified RDI Program consultant, or by someone who is currently receiving supervision from staff or designees of the Connections Center.

5. *Parents use RDI as a lifestyle and function as facilitators:* Parents are encouraged to spend three to six hours per week interacting with the child using RDI methods.

6. *Children work individually with adults, and then in therapeutic peer dyads or groups when developmentally ready:* The consultant monitors the stage at which a child is functioning. Eventually, children are matched by stage to work together.

7. *Episodic memory:* Intervention plans include specific methods designed to strengthen episodic memories. This includes regular addition to and review of Memory Journals that are constructed to be developmentally appropriate for the child.

8. *Emphasis on self-development:* Self- and social-development objectives are clearly balanced and sufficient time is spent working on objectives in both areas. Primary emphasis is given to development of relative thinking and executive functioning skills.

9. *The RDI Program is a primary intervention:* The RDI Program is carried out as a primary (but not necessarily the only) intervention. The RDI Program is not treated or considered adjunctive or secondary to any other intervention. Most participants in RDI Programs receive other interventions such as dietary modification, occupational therapy, vision therapy, and/or speech and language intervention.

The Relationship Curriculum

In developing his intervention program, Gutstein has painstakingly analyzed how each stage of experience sharing develops at six different levels, and applies this knowledge to facilitating emotional growth for the child with autism. The RDI curriculum consists of hundreds of step-by-step treatment objectives and customized activities developed after a child undergoes the RDA. Activities and objectives at each of six levels represent a dramatic developmental shift in the central focus of relationships. As a reference, Gutstein has labeled the six levels in the curriculum as Novice, Apprentice, Challenger, Voyager, Explorer, and Partner.

In summary, RDI provides a structured path for people on the autism spectrum to learn friendship, empathy, and a love of sharing their world with others. The program begins at an individual's level of capability and carefully, systematically teaches them the skills they need for competence and fulfillment in a complex world. Eventually, they learn not only to tolerate, but to enjoy change, transition, and going with the flow.

The Son-Rise Program®

Like other parents and professionals in this book, Barry Neil Kaufman and Samahria Lyte Kaufman refused to listen in the 1970s, when, at 18 months old, their son, Raun, was diagnosed as severely and incurably autistic. Experts advised the Kaufmans to institutionalize Raun because of his "hopeless, lifelong condition." Instead, they designed an innovative, unique, home-based, child-centered program to reach their son. It transformed Raun from a mute, withdrawn child with a very low IQ into a highly verbal, socially interactive youngster with a near-genius IQ. Bearing no traces of his former condition, Raun graduated from an Ivy League college and is working to help families like his today.

Responding to the demand to teach others their program, The Kaufman family established The Option Institute and the Autism Treatment Center of America™, where they have been offering The Son-Rise Program® since 1983. Raun is now CEO, and following the publication of his story, *Son-Rise*, now updated to *Son-Rise: The Miracle Continues*, and the award-winning NBC-TV movie *Son-Rise: A Miracle of Love*, lectures internationally.

Principles of the Son-Rise Program

The Son-Rise Program is based on the idea that adults must enter the world of autism instead of asking the child with autism to enter the "real" world. By mirroring repetitive and ritualistic behaviors and interacting with the child through play, accompanied by an optimistic, trusting, respectful, and nonjudgmental attitude of love and enthusiasm, adults can gradually lead a child toward a more normal life.

Son-Rise encourages parents to follow the child's lead or actions while simultaneously directing him or her into an expanded world. The unique feature of this program is the commitment to happiness. Parents are encouraged to explore their own belief systems and to question judgments that limit them.

The guiding principles of the Son-Rise Program are:

- *Autism is a relational, not a behavioral disorder.* Son-Rise views autism as an interactional disorder in which children have difficulty relating and connecting to those around them. Most of the so-called "behavioral challenges" stem from this relational deficit. That's why dynamic, enthusiastic, play-oriented methods focus so extensively on socialization and rapport-building. The goal is for parents to enjoy their child and for the child to enjoy interacting with adults.

- *Motivation, not repetition, holds the key to all learning.* Son-Rise strives to uncover each child's unique motivations, and use these to teach children the skills they need to learn.

The Son-Rise Program does not provide the child with information, or teach the child predetermined skills. Instead, it views the child's current level of performance as being the best that the child can do. The child thus participates willingly, demonstrating an increasingly long attention span, better retention, and the generalization of skills. The Son-Rise Program emphasizes total acceptance of the child and encourages the child to become a more motivated and participating individual.

• *"Stimming" behaviors have important meaning and value.* Son-Rise accepts and respects children's behaviors. The program thus encourages joining, rather than stopping, a child's repetitive, ritualistic behaviors. Doing so builds rapport and connection, the platform for all future education and development.

• *Parents are a child's best resource.* Nothing equals the power of parents. No one else can match the unparalleled love, deep dedication, long-term commitment, and day-in, day-out experiences with their children that parents possess. Son-Rise empowers parents to be confident directors and teachers by listening to them and providing them with skills training.

• *Parents and professionals are most effective when they feel comfortable with a child, optimistic about a child's capabilities, and hopeful about a child's future.* Son-Rise offers parents and professionals the resources, guidance, and support they need to re-energize and arm them with the tools they need.

• *All children can progress in the right environment.* Most children on the autism spectrum are over-stimulated by a plethora of distractions that others do not even notice. Son-Rise eliminates environmental distractions, thus creating an optimal work/playroom that facilitates positive interactions and reduces control battles.

- *A child's potential is limitless.* Son-Rise believes that no one has the right to predict what a child can and cannot achieve. It thus focuses parents on their own attitudes, striving to help them reclaim their optimism and see the potential in their children.

The Son-Rise Program is customized to each child's needs. Families come and stay at the Option Institute for a week or more at a time, and are trained to use skills that allow them to accept their child and become his or her teacher. Son-Rise begins with a five-day start-up program, a group seminar that outlines the basic components of the home-based program. Next is an intensive one-week seminar, which provides 40 hours of one-on-one work with a trained facilitator and the child. The advanced training seminar is a follow-up program after the implementation of a home-based program.

Son-Rise is an intensive program requiring an enormous commitment of time and money. While I am aware of no studies of the Son-Rise Program's effectiveness, many families who use it, swear by it, and report recovery from autism. For more information, go to www.autismtreatmentcenter.org.

Social Stories™

Carol Gray, a former consultant to students with autism spectrum disorders in and director of The Gray Center for Social Learning and Understanding in Michigan, became interested in the difficulty autistic individuals have assuming the perspective of another person. In 1991 she devised a technique, called "Social Stories™," to help them learn how to understand others' behaviors.

Social Stories help individuals with autism learn to "read" and understand social situations by answering "who," "what," "when," "where," and "why" questions to a variety of situations presented in the form of a stories. Each story describes a scenario, skill, or concept in terms of relevant social cues, perspectives, and common responses in a specifically defined style and format.

The goal of a Social Story™ is to impart accurate social information in a patient and reassuring manner, not to change an individual's behavior. However, heightened understanding of social events and expectations often leads to more mature behavior. A therapist can use a book of sample Social Stories Gray has devised for common issues such as going to a new place. They can also be individualized to the needs of the person with autism to teach routines, instructions for a specific activity, how to ask for assistance, and socially appropriate emotional responses to feelings such as anger and frustration.

Social Stories use four types of sentences: descriptive, directive, perspective, and control. *Descriptive and directive sentences* often occur together, in what Gray calls the Social Story ratio. She suggests that for every directive sentence, a story should have two to five descriptive sentences. This proportion minimally limits an individual's choices. The greater the number of descriptive statements, the greater the opportunity for the individual to supply his or her own responses to the social situation. The greater the number of directive statements, the more specific the cues for how the individual should respond.

Perspective sentences present others' reactions to a situation so that the individual can learn how others' perceive various events. Perspective sentences are combined with descriptive sentences in the same ratio as directive sentences.

The final type of sentence is the *control sentence*. This sentence identifies strategies the person can use to facilitate memory and comprehension of the Social Story. Directive or control sentences may be omitted entirely as the functioning level of the person with autism increases.

Although Gray developed Social Stories for use with children with ASDs, her approach has also been successful with adolescents, adults, and others who have social and communication delays. Social Stories are applicable for both readers and non-readers.

Implementing Social Stories

For a person who can read, the author introduces the story by reading it aloud twice. The person with autism then reads it independently once a day. For a person who cannot read, the author records the story on a tape or CD with a verbal cue or bell indicating when to turn the page. The person listens to the story and follows along daily.

Once an individual with autism successfully enacts the skills or appropriately responds in a particular type of social situation, the number of times a story is read per week can be reduced, or the story can be reviewed once a month or as necessary. Fading can also be accomplished by rewriting the story and gradually removing directive sentences.

Carol Gray and her associates have written two books with collections of Social Stories. *My Social Stories Book* includes topics such as grooming, dealing with unexpected noises such as barking dogs and ringing telephones, and going places like the movies and the grocery store.[15] The *New Social Story Book* was revised and expanded in 2010 to celebrate the tenth anniversary of Social Stories.[16] It covers topics such as learning how to chew gum, giving a gift and a hug, using the telephone, sharing, knowing when to say "thank you" and "excuse me," pets, personal care, cooking, helping around the house, picking flowers, school issues such as fire drills, recess and homework, escalators, seat belts, going to church, getting a haircut, shopping, new shoes, understanding the weather, holidays, vacations, and others. Gray also teaches the reader how to construct a Social Story.

The Gray Center offers workshops, support groups, DVDs, movies, and other educational materials. Carol Gray travels extensively to teach her method. A single study over 10 years ago concluded that Social Stories are a promising method for improving the social behaviors of autistic individuals.[17] For additional information about Social Stories, go to www.thegraycenter.org.

The Miller Method®

Arnold Miller, PhD, a Boston psychologist, and his wife, Eileen Eller-Miller, MA, CCC, a speech and language pathologist, now both deceased, developed the Miller Method® in the 1960s. They describe this hybrid approach as a cognitive-developmental approach for children with body organization, social, and communication issues.

The Miller Method is based on the belief that every child, no matter how withdrawn or disorganized, is trying to find ways to cope with the world. The ability to assess and respond to the outside world is essential for survival. The Millers believed that children learn most effectively when their whole bodies are physically and repetitively involved in the learning process. While the reader may argue that this therapy should rightfully be included along with those that integrate sensory processing, its place in this chapter is due to the fact that the founders are a psychologist and speech-language therapist who emphasize the end-product skills of social interaction and communication.

Miller theorized that children with autism become stalled at early stages of development, and progress to more advanced stages in an incomplete or distorted fashion. Lacking a sense of where they are in space, external stimuli drive them into scattered or stereotypic behavior from which, unassisted, they cannot extricate themselves. This results in aberrant systems involving people or objects, as well as a "hardening" of transitory formations seen in typical development, such as hand inspection, twiddling, or intense object preoccupation.[18]

All activities take place with children elevated 2 ½ feet off the ground on a special structure. Elevation enhances body awareness, focus, motor-planning, and social-emotional contact, thus increasing the ability to cope with obstacles and demands. Children with autism transition from one object or event to another, and from object involvement to representational play when placed on elevated boards.

Miller developed some unique methods for teaching communication through videotapes of signed and spoken language. The approach uses "narratives" accompanied by manual signs and words that guide children's actions. His little patients thus quickly learn to communicate as signs, spoken words, and related objects are presented simultaneously.

When obstacles are placed in the their paths, and a therapist narrates what a child is doing as he or she moves over, in, through, and across obstacles, the child develops a repertoire of meaning which can readily be transferred to the ground. Eventually, children begin to respond to spoken words and express themselves for the first time, without signing or object accompaniment.

Training films teach receptive and expressive communication of four clusters of concepts using manual signs adapted from the American Sign Language (ASL) for the deaf. Signs and their objects are associated with spoken words designed to establish certain linguistic functions, such as action meanings (come, go, stop, get up, sit down, etc.), eating words (knife, fork, pour, drink, etc.), familiar objects and events in their immediate surroundings (comb, toothbrush, sleep, wash, etc.), and two-word verb/noun combinations such as "eat cookie."

The Miller Method gradually transforms a child's limited reality systems by expanding his or her repertoire of activities. As a child with autism gradually tolerates and accepts new reality systems through repetitive activity, and can makes transitions from event to event without distress, the ability to cope with different life situations improves dramatically.

The Miller Method was first described in the book *From Ritual to Repertoire*.[19] A more recent book on the Miller Method by Dr. Miller with Kristina Chretien, a long time LCDC staff member, came out in 2007.[20] Chapters outline the underlying principles of the Miller Method and its practical application for parents and teachers to develop communication skills and social play. The book also addresses such behavioral issues as temper tantrums, aggression, and toilet training. A chapter on research outcomes demonstrates the efficacy of the method in practice.

For more information, go to www.millermethod.org.

The SCERTS® Model

SCERTS® is a comprehensive, multidisciplinary, integrative team approach that was developed out of 25 years of research and clinical/educational practice by speech-language pathologist Barry Prizant, PhD, CCC-SLP, and a multidisciplinary team of professionals trained in communication disorders, special education, occupational therapy, and psychology. SCERTS is an acronym for **S**ocial **C**ommunication, **E**motional **R**egulation, and **T**ransactional **S**upport.

SCERTS promotes social communication and emotional competence by building meaning into daily experiences from the preverbal to conversational level. The strength of this program is in its ability to recognize individual differences and to focus on the family. It capitalizes on forming a solid foundation of mutual respect, meaning, logic, and predictability for the individual with autism.

All activities and strategies are designed to enhance the development of emotional self- and mutual-regulatory capacities, and to modify attentional, arousal, and emotional states. SCERTS borrows from other sensory, motor, vision, and language models, always looking at an individual child's strengths and needs. Prizant may thus recommend that one child jump on a trampoline for arousal, and that another listen to soothing music for calming.

SCERTS provides support to ensure that behaviors generalize across settings, thus fostering successful interpersonal interactions, relationships, and productive learning experiences at school, in the community, and elsewhere.[21] The SCERTS Model encourages professionals from different disciplines to collaborate with each other, and is thus totally compatible with other treatment approaches in this book. Families measure progress by noting the number of functional activities a child with autism can do with a variety of partners.

For a complete overview of SCERTS, watch the three video or DVD set, *The SCERTS™ Model: A Comprehensive Educational Approach for Children with Autism Spectrum Disorders*,[22] or read *Autism Spectrum Disorders: A Transactional Developmental Perspective*.[23] Prizant has developed workshops and seminars of various lengths in many cities. Go to www.barryprizant.com for a complete schedule of presentations and to order materials.

Porges's Polyvagal Theory

Stephen W. Porges, PhD, director of the Brain-Body Center in the College of Medicine at the University of Illinois at Chicago, has developed a multidimensional intervention model for socio-emotional and communication disorders, termed the Polyvagal Theory. It derives from over 40 years of neuroanatomical, neurophysiological, and behavioral research,[24] and some consider it to be one of the most important links between the nervous system and behavior in the past 100 years.

Porges proposes that connections between our autonomic nervous system, the vagus nerve, and the middle ear provide the neurophysiological basis for emotions and behavior. The theory states that the vagus nerve and two muscles in the middle ear — the tensor tympani and the stapedius — control vocalization, facial expression, heart rate, and breathing.[25] By improving the communication among these physical parts, he shows benefits in language, social skills, and general well-being.

The Polyvagal Theory posits that the above brain structures regulating social behaviors are compromised in individuals with autism and other developmental disabilities.[26] This puts them in a constant state of high anxiety, in which they attend to all sounds in their environment, not only to the higher-frequency sounds that are human speech.

His intervention, similar to the Tomatis® Method described in chapter 10, provides acoustic stimulation during a quiet free-play session. The patient dons headphones and listens to specific sounds or music within a narrow frequency range, similar to that of human speech. Gradually, the therapist widens the frequency range, thus vigorously exercising the two muscles in the middle ear.

Dr. Porges believes that improvement in communication and social-emotional interaction is a result of an improvement in middle ear function. Gains in social and communication skills will in turn make the child more available to other forms of treatment. Since the middle ear muscles share the same neural connection with facial expression and vocalization, stimulating the middle ear allows a child to sort sound frequencies, regulate listening, reduce anxiety, and be more available socially and emotionally.[27]

This theory is in its infancy and is extremely complex. Those wishing to learn more about it should read Porges's book[28] or go to his website at www.stephenporges.com.

Building Socialization and Language through Animals

Animals were introduced as sensory integration therapy tools in chapter 10. Whomever the human, and whatever the animal, research shows that both normally developing children[29] and children with autism[30] benefit from interaction with animals. In the study referenced above, children with autism engaged in 55% more social behaviors when they were with animals, compared to toys.

Dolphin-Assisted Therapy (DAT)

Speech-language pathologist Janet Flowers, CCC-SLP, EdD, works with children in dolphin assisted therapy (DAT) sessions at Florida's Gulf World Marine Park in Panama City, Florida. Flowers's aim is to achieve greater results than traditional therapy in decreasing response time and increasing expressive communication skills. She looks at participants' attention span, communication, speech, language, gross and fine motor skills, and academics.

Children in her studies exhibit
- increases from 25% to 250% in time on-task,
- significant increases in mean length of utterance as well as in the complexity of expressive skills, and
- greater long-term retention than six months of conventional therapy.

DAT is also more cost effective than conventional therapy.[31]

Flowers believes that having a positive emotional experience during therapy increases motivation and confidence, and also enhances a child's long-term memory. Her experience is that a dolphin's unconditional acceptance of a child with a disability in a safe environment provides exceptional motivation to overcome obstacles and increase confidence.

The program motivates and jumpstarts a child, complements and reinforces therapy, and provides a stimulating reward. The achievements a child makes with DAT also assists other professionals who may be working with the child. She concludes that human-dolphin therapy is a cost-efficient program that achieves long-term retention of learned skills by qualified students. For more information, go to http://www.gulfworldmarinepark.com.

Service Dogs

Service dogs can provide a physical and emotional anchor for children with autism, thus enhancing opportunities for those on the spectrum to access a variety of environments safely. With their child tethered to a service dog, families feel they are newly freed to engage in activities as simple as going out to eat. When out in the community, a service dog can increase safety and make families feel secure.

In many cases, the service dog accompanies the child to school, where its calming presence can minimize and often eliminate emotional outbursts, enabling the child to more fully participate in his or her school day. Transitioning among school day activities is easier, and the service dog provides a focus through which the child can interact with other children. These opportunities increase a child's ability to develop better social and language skills, mobility, independence, and autonomy.

Research on this modality is scarce, although most studies emphasize increasing social behaviors and language use. A review of six published reports was encouraging. However, the authors recommended further research with better designs and larger samples to strengthen translation to clinical settings.[32]

Take-Home Points

The emergence of appropriate interpersonal interaction is typically the final step on the path to resolving autism spectrum disorders. While it is tempting to address deficient communication and interpersonal skills aggressively at a young age, that is probably not the best plan. Consulting with an optometrist, occupational therapist, biomedical doctor, or audiologist should usually take precedence over making an appointment with a speech-language pathologist or mental health professional. Even though some of the therapies in this chapter can begin in the first year of life, language and social skills therapies should almost always wait until a child's immune system is working efficiently, and motor and sensory skills are sound.

For adults, especially parents, trying to interact with a young child who doesn't look at, laugh with, talk to, or imitate them can be very frustrating. Observing a child in his "own" world can be heartbreaking. Watching a child botch an interaction can be most embarrassing. Acknowledging that a child has few friends can be extremely painful. Imagining how a teenager's social awkwardness might affect personal relationships and job performance in the future is downright frightening.

This chapter summarizes some extremely innovative programs based on a solid understanding of sensory processing. Most importantly, they respect a child's inefficient sensory systems, and view "aberrant" behaviors as attempts at coping with a confusing world. Joining a child in what appears to be purposeless play while following DIR, RDI, the Son-Rise Program, or Miller Method guidelines, often yields remarkable results. While intensive, demanding, and costly, these models can initially be the core of the therapy for an unresponsive child, and then adjuncts to a transdisciplinary program. Parents are the key to their success. Social Stories can be utilized by educators or parents, while principles of SCERTS and the Polyvagal Theory combine well with almost any communication-based model.

According to Daniel Goleman, author of *Emotional Intelligence*,[33] social intelligence is a better predictor of success than SAT scores. Most people with disabilities lose jobs because of social-emotional, rather than skill, deficits. Applying some of the brilliant methodologies described in this chapter empowers children on the autism spectrum to develop those skills necessary to join others, interact in socially acceptable ways, have friends, and eventually marry and hold a good job. Best of all, they can realize whatever potential they have to become confident, happy, productive individuals in a demanding society.

---

[1] Klaw R. Thoughtful response to agitation, escalation and meltdowns in individuals with autism spectrum disorders. DVD. Pittsburgh, PA: Autism Services by Klaw, 2007.

[2] Kranowitz CS. The Out-of-Sync Child, rev ed. New York; Perigee: 2006.

[3] Siegel DJ. Mindsight: The New Science of Personal Transformation. New York: Bantam Books, 2011, 60–61.

[4] Oberman LM, Hubbard EM, McCleery JP, Altschuler EL, Ramachandran VS, Pineda JA. EEG evidence for mirror neuron dysfunction in autism spectral disorders. Cognitive Brain Research, 2005, 24:2, 190–98.

[5] Bellini S, Peters JK, Benner L, Hopf A. A Meta-Analysis of School-Based Social Skills Interventions for Children With Autism Spectrum Disorders. Remedial and Special Education, May/Jun 2007, 28:3, 153–62.

[6] Greenspan SI, Wieder S. The child with special needs: Encouraging intellectual and emotional growth. Cambridge, MA: Perseus Books, 1998.

[7] Greenspan SI, Wieder S. Engaging autism: Using the floortime approach to help children relate, communicate and think. Cambridge, MA: Perseus Books, 2006.

[8] Pajareya K. A pilot randomized controlled trial of DIR/Floortime™ parent training intervention for pre-school children with autism spectrum disorders. Autism, Sep 2011, 15:5, 563–77; Casenhiser DM, Shanker SG, Stieben J. Learning through interaction in children with autism: Preliminary data from a social communication-based intervention. Autism, Mar 2013, 17:2, 220–41; Soloman RJ, Necheles J, Ferch C, Bruckman D. Pilot study of parent training program for young children with autism. The PLAY project home consultation program. Autism, 2007, 11:3, 205–24.

[9] Greenspan SI, Tippy G. Respecting Autism. New York: Vantage Press, 2011.

[10] Wieder S. Wachs H. Visual-Spatial Portals to Thinking, Feeling and Movement: Advancing Competencies and Emotional Development in Children with Learning and Autism Spectrum Disorders. Mendham, NJ: Profectum Foundation, 2012, 4–5.

[11] Furth H, Wachs H. Thinking goes to school. New York, NY: Oxford Univ. Press, 1974.

[12] Wieder and Wachs, Spatial Portals to Thinking.

[13] Greenspan SI, Lewis D. The affect-based language curriculum (ABLC): An intensive program for families, therapists and teachers. Bethesda, MD: Interdisciplinary Council on Developmental and Learning Disorders (ICDL), 2005.

[14] Gutstein S. Autism Asperger's: Solving the Relationship Puzzle. Arlington, TX: Future Horizons, 2000.

[15] Gray C. My Social Stories Book. Philadelphia: Jessica Kingsley, 2001.

[16] Gray C. The New Social Stories Book. Arlington, Texas: Future Horizons, 2010.

[17] Scattone D, Wilczynski SM, Edwards RP, Rabian B. Decreasing Disruptive Behaviors of Children with Autism Using Social Stories. Journal Autism and Developmental Disorders, Dec 2002, 32:6, 535–543.

[18] www.millermethod.org. Accessed Apr 9, 2013.

[19] Miller A, Eller-Miller E. From ritual to repertoire. Boston, MA: John Wiley & Sons, 1989.

[20] Miller A. Chretien K. The Miller Method®: Developing the capacities of children on the autism spectrum. New York: Jessica Kingsley, 2007.

[21] Gray C. Jenison Autism Journal, Winter 2002, 1–19.

[22] Prizant BM, Wetherby AM, Rubin E, Laurent AC, et al. The SCERTS™ Model: A comprehensive educational approach for children with autism spectrum disorders. Baltimore, MD: Brookes Pub, 2005.

[23] Prizant BM, Wetherby AM. Autism spectrum disorders: A transactional developmental perspective. Baltimore, MD: Brookes Publishing, 2000.

[24] Porges SW. The polyvagal theory: Phylogenetic contributions to social behavior. Physiology & Behavior, 2003, 79, 503–51.

[25] Porges SW. Orienting in a defensive world: Mammalian modifications of our evolutionary heritage. A Polyvagal Theory. Psychophysiology, 1995, 32, 301–18.

[26] Porges SW. The Vagus: A mediator of behavioral and physiologic features associated with autism. In Bauman and Kemper, The Neurobiology of Autism, 2nd ed. Baltimore, MD: Johns Hopkins Press, 2005, 65–78.

[27] Edelson S. Dr. Stephen Porges' research may support Berard's and Tomatis' Theory on middle ear muscle dysfunction. The Sound Connection, 2003, 9:4, 1–2.

[28] Porges SW. The Polyvagal Theory: Neurophysiological Foundations of Emotions, Attachment, Communication, and Self-regulation. New York: Norton Books, 2011.

[29] Melson GF. Child development and the human-companion animal bond. American Behavioral Scientist, 2003, 47:1, 31–9.

[30] O'Haire ME, McKenzie SJ, Beck AM, Slaughter V. Social Behaviors Increase in Children with Autism in the Presence of Animals Compared to Toys. PLoS ONE, 2013, 8:2.

[31] Nathanson DE, de Castro D, Friend H, McMahon M. Effectiveness of short-term dolphin assisted therapy for children with severe disabilities. Anthrozoos, 1997, 10:2/3, 90–100.

[32] Berry A, Borgi M, Francia N, Alleva E, Cirulli F. Use of Assistance and Therapy Dogs for Children with Autism Spectrum Disorders. A Critical Review of the Current Evidence. Journal of Alternative and Complementary Medicine, Feb 2013, 19:2, 73–80.

[33] Goleman, D. Emotional Intelligence. New York: Bantam, 2005.

CHAPTER 13

Behavioral Therapies, Neurofeedback, and Assistive Technology

This chapter focuses on a variety of topics which, at first glance, appear to have little to do with each other. Take a second look. They are all approaches that model and train behavior with the goal of more positive and rewarding personal interactions.

Behavioral approaches for those with autism spectrum disorders all use carefully designed programs of prompting, modeling, and rewarding. This chapter includes the following behavioral and cognitive-behavioral therapies:

- Applied Behavioral Analysis (ABA)
- Cognitive Affective Training
- The Social Skills Training Project

Neurofeedback, sometimes called neurotherapy or neurotechnology, is a painless, non-invasive procedure that has recently emerged as a powerful therapy for teaching the brains of those on the autism spectrum to function more efficiently. It beautifully complements biomedical and sensory approaches; that's why so many professionals from a variety of disciplines have embraced it.

If an individual with autism does not speak, assistive technology offers some other exciting methods to increase positive and more frequent interactions. Included under the umbrella of "assistive technology" are augmentative and alternative communication devices, computer programs, and apps for the iPad.

Behavioral Therapies

The use of consequences to modify behavior, also known as operant conditioning, is a tried-and-true training method. Modern-day clinicians are applying this approach, popularized by B. F. Skinner in the mid-20th century, to those with ASDs. If a teacher wishes a child to ask for a treat, initially she may give it to him if he grunts. Gradually, he must make the sound more intelligible to receive a reward. Finally, he must say an approximation of "please" to be rewarded. ABA is one popular form of operant conditioning used for individuals with autism.

Applied Behavior Analysis (ABA)

"Behavior analysis" is the systematic study of variables that influence the behavior of an organism.[1] "Applied behavior analysis" (ABA) is the process of systematically applying what scientists have learned in the laboratory to significant behaviors in real-life situations, such as home, school, and work.[2] ABA traces its roots back to the principles of operant conditioning described above. A comprehensive understanding of ABA requires many years of practice and study.[3]

The umbrella term "ABA" includes many interventions based on direct observations of behavior that make up a "functional behavioral assessment" or a "functional analysis of behavior." All ABA programs utilize the manipulation of antecedents and consequences of behavior to

- reduce inappropriate, self-injurious, and stereotypical behaviors;
- modify conditions under which interfering behaviors occur;
- teach new skills; and
- transfer and generalize behavior from one situation to another.

Clinical psychologist Ivar Lovaas, PhD, is considered the father of ABA therapy for autism. Today the term "Lovaas therapy," or simply "Lovaas," is often used synonymously with "applied behavior analysis"; however, Lovaas, also known as Discrete Trial Training (DTT), is a specific one-on-one intensive behavioral ABA teaching strategy that breaks down a complex skill set of behaviors into small, manageable tasks. Basic communication, play, motor, and daily living skills complement and build upon each other. Some consider DTT or Lovaas to be the only true ABA.

In 1987, as a Professor of Psychology at the University of California at Los Angeles (UCLA), Lovaas demonstrated scientifically what no one believed possible: the behavior of children with autism could be modified through teaching. Working intensively with 19 seven-year-old children with autism and 19 controls, 90% of the children in his study substantially improved, compared to the control group. In this study, 40 hours of therapy per week for three years with the original Lovaas method of behavioral analysis, was necessary for close to one-half (47%) to attain normal IQs and test within the normal range on adaptive and social skills.[4]

A follow-up study on these same children four years later, at an average age of 11½, showed that eight of nine were indistinguishable from average children on tests of intelligence and adaptive behavior.[5] A later study with 28 children receiving intensive ABA therapy for four years found the same results, with 48% being able to succeed in regular classroom settings.[6]

Between 1985 and 2010, over 500 articles were published about ABA and autism. A 2010 review of the research found that outcomes for the behavioral intervention group were consistently significantly better than those for the control and comparison groups.[7] Success of intervention was strongly correlated to the intensity of intervention (35 or more hours per week for more than a year is necessary), and to higher intelligence.

Studies documented the effectiveness of ABA for treating autism across a wide range of

- *behaviors*, including those that are self-injurious,[8] stereotypical,[9] communicative,[10] social, academic, leisurely, and functional;

- *populations*, including children and adults with a variety of behavioral, learning, and developmental disorders, as well as ADHD[11];

- *therapists and educators*, including parents, teachers, and remedial specialists; and

- *settings*, including schools,[12] homes, institutions, residential placements, hospitals,[13] and businesses.[14]

ABA therapy became the therapy of choice in the 1990s. In 1999, the late Bernard Rimland, PhD, founder and director of the Autism Research Institute (ARI), wrote a passionate letter in his newsletter that he entitled "The ABA Controversy."[15] He believed that it was a major mistake to think of ABA as being competitive with, rather than complementary to, many other interventions, and urged therapists, schools, and others recommending ABA as the *only* scientifically based therapy for autism to consider biomedical treatments as well. By that point in time, much research on the benefits of vitamin B-6, magnesium, and DMG had been published.

Centers where patients with autism could receive a biomedical approach combined with ABA was one of Dr. Rimland's dying wishes. The Rimland Center for Integrative Medicine, the multidisciplinary practice of Elizabeth Mumper, MD, FAAP, in Lynchburg, Virginia, is named in his honor.

The Language of ABA. Behaviorists define *learning* as a change of behavior resulting from experience. *Target behaviors* are anything observable and measurable, and can include receptive and expressive communication, adaptive living skills such as toileting and grooming, learning academics, and social skills such as sharing and taking turns. An example of a target behavior is, "When given the direction 'Touch your nose,' the child will do so independently."

Behaviors have definable and measurable frequency rates, durations, and intensities, and they consist of specific actions that can be maintained, increased, or decreased. Feelings, such as happy, sad, and angry, are not used in ABA because they cannot be accurately measured by any of the above criteria.

ABA is not a specific program, but rather many programs that follow a set of principles and guidelines. It uses some very specific terms to describe actions therapists take with their clients:[16]

- *Task analysis:* Breaking skills down into small, attainable parts.

- *Reinforcement:* A consequence that increases the probability of a desired response.

- *Positive reinforcement:* Receiving a reward of something viewed as pleasurable as a consequence of doing something new or in a different way. Example: Getting to jump on a trampoline for matching colors.

- *Negative reinforcement:* Getting a reward of something viewed as pleasurable for *not* doing something the adult wants to diminish. Example: Getting an M&M for not flapping arms when excited.

- *Punishment:* A consequence that decreases the probability of a desired response.

- *Errorless learning:* A process that presents information in a way that reduces trial and error and avoids mistakes.

- *Prompting:* A technique used to help the child get a correct response to ensure errorless learning. Therapists use several types of prompts: physical (touching), verbal (providing the answer for the student to repeat), gestural (pointing with exaggerated facial expressions), and modeling (showing how to do something) are just a few.

- *Fading a prompt:* Getting a child to give the correct response with less assistance or without a prompt.

- *Discrete trials:* Instructions or questions, a child's response, reinforcement, consequences, and prompting, followed by fading prompts, as necessary.[17]

- *Redirection:* A non-intrusive method of interrupting self-stimulatory or repetitive behaviors, and diverting attention toward an acceptable behavior. Example: When a child exhibits self-stimulatory behavior, put something interesting in his hand to redirect the behavior.

- *Shaping:* A way of adding a new behavior to a person's repertoire by reinforcing a successful approximation of the target behavior. Shaping is like playing "hot and cold" — the closer the person comes to the behavior, the closer he is to the reward.

- *Chaining:* The combining of simple, sequenced component behaviors into a more complex, composite behavior. Example: Putting on pants, shirt, socks, and shoes to the request, "get dressed."

- *Expansion Activities:* Generalizing and combining skill sets to new materials and a variety of conditions. Example: If a child masters turn taking and matching colors, use a game such as Candyland to maintain both skills with a functional application. Or, if a child learns to independently complete a jigsaw puzzle at a table, provide opportunities to do different types of puzzle in different settings.

The delivery of ABA techniques includes all of the above. While treatment is always based on the principles of ABA, its implementation varies based on a child's unique needs. Educators have the responsibility to offer experiences that are appropriate for each learner. The "magic "of ABA comes from a good fit between the teacher's methodology and the student's learning style.

ABA and Autism

Currently, many individuals, clinics, and even entire school systems are applying programs grounded in ABA for the assessment and therapeutic/educational intervention of children, teens, and adults with autism. ABA focuses on the reduction of maladaptive behaviors and on the development of adaptive, socially significant behaviors.

ABA, like many other therapies, is most effective with children diagnosed with autism at a young age. While therapists originally used this method only with children under five, with some modifications, it is now in programs for older children. With preteens, high school students, and adults, collaboration with educators and other professionals at school and in the community is essential.

Treatment typically begins with 10–15 hours per week and gradually increases to 35–40 hours per week by the age of three. Instructors use any opportunity to take advantage of situations occurring in the natural environment to teach new behaviors. This is called "incidental teaching." Different settings provide variety.

Therapy intensifies as the child gets older, and interactions become more elaborate. Language advances from one-word responses to simple questions to speaking in complete sentences. Children learn turn taking, how to learn in groups, and how to make and keep friends.

Typically, a child and instructor work one-on-one on a specific task for 2–5 minutes and then take a 1–2 minute break. Lengthier play breaks of 10–20 minutes occur every hour or so, during which a child and instructor might swing, play a game, or eat a snack. Breaks offer opportunities for a child to generalize newfound skills.

ABA is certainly compatible with other therapies. Integrating it with biomedical interventions can be quite effective. However, some practitioners have reservations about using it with "inside-out" therapies, such as sensory integration based occupational therapy and other sensory approaches (see chapter 10). Critics believe that *all* behaviors are meaningful, and that the ABA approach to extinguishing socially unacceptable behaviors is disrespectful of the body's attempts to self-regulate.

Incorporating Sensory Integration into ABA

Some ABA therapists and other professionals are finding ways of accommodating a child with sensory issues by incorporating sensory integration (SI) theory into ABA.[18] Accommodations include the following:

• *Modify environmental stimuli.* Be aware of sounds and sights that may distract a child. Use a quiet voice for the hypersensitive child. Organize or limit the use of visual materials that are too exciting or distracting. Use light or heavy touch, depending on the child's level of sensitivity.

• *Encourage proper posture during seated activities to enhance attention.* Stabilize a child's feet on the ground for maximum sensory feedback and support. Use a cushion or wedge to help the child with low muscle tone or inadequate postural stability to keep the pelvis in a position that will facilitate muscular activation and arousal.

• *Provide opportunities for individualized sensory input.* Children need different sensory inputs at different moments throughout the day, depending upon their physiological state. Sometimes touch will help a child focus, while at other times movement is more helpful. Each child has a unique sensory profile and requires an individualized sensory diet. (See chapter 10.)

• *Allow a child to choose, rather than prescribe input in a standardized manner.* This small step can greatly enhance regulation; however, some children with motor planning difficulties may be unable to initiate or sequence the steps. It may be necessary to prompt them to obtain the input their bodies need to be calm and attentive.

• *Use imitation, and pair actions with objects to increase social interest and eye contact.* If a child has difficulty imitating, play patty-cake and peek-a-boo. Form dyads of children, using two identical objects to enhance imitation and turn taking.

• *Use reciprocal social praise to enhance self-regulation, attention, and social responsivity.* Wait both for a child to give a response, and to give praise. Ample wait time gives a child with autism the experience of natural conversation.

Recent Innovations in ABA Therapy

Initially, ABA programs for children with autism included any and all forms of behavioral therapy. In recent years, the strict DTT approach has given way to more flexible treatments that are still based on the science of ABA. While discrete trials are an essential element of ABA-based interventions, they are not the whole program. These programs alleviate some of the issues that caused criticism of DTT: that target skills are limited, DTT is primarily adult- not child-initiated, and that edible reinforcers often contain dyes, sugars, gluten, or casein, to which many autistic children react negatively.

Good programs utilize many teaching approaches, all based on the principles of applied behavior analysis. Programs continue to evolve as children progress and develop more complex social skills. Many of the newer ones place greater emphasis on the generalization and spontaneity of skills. Sometimes, therapists set up a specific environment in the clinic, so that learning in a given situation can generalize. They may also take therapy out of a clinical setting to more familiar environments, such as the playground, where a child is already interacting. Most importantly, GF/CF treats, playtime with a favorite toy, or watching a video have replaced M&Ms, Cheerios, and gummy worms as reinforcers.

Each of the following ABA methodologies identifies and focuses upon different behaviors and applies a unique system of instruction:

- *The Center for Autism and Related Disorders, Inc. (CARD)* is one of the largest organizations in the world providing treatment for those on the autism spectrum. Doreen Granpeesheh, PhD, who studied with Dr. Lovaas at UCLA, is the founder and executive director. She has dedicated over 25 years to the study and treatment of ASDs using ABA techniques.

  CARD employs hundreds of therapists worldwide, and has provided services to tens of thousands of children since opening its doors in 1990. At CARD, therapists develop unique and individualized behavioral programs based on each child's particular strengths and weaknesses. The goal is to teach all children the functional skills necessary to replace previously learned maladaptive behaviors, enabling them to live independent and productive lives.

Initially, one-on-one behavioral therapy takes place in the home, and then generalizes to other settings such as school. Instruction covers the following skills: speech and language, gross and fine motor, academic, self-care, and, most importantly, socialization. Basic skills are taught in the first years and advanced social and language skills are taught in the final years. CARD treatment starts between 20–59 months old, and is intensive: 20–40 hours per week for at least two years. It focuses on the flexible, individualized treatment of each child, and inclusion of parents as an integral part of the treatment team.

For more information, go to www.centerforautism.com.

• *Pivotal Response Treatment (PRT)* is a variation of ABA that is the product of 20 years of research from Robert and Lynn Koegel, PhD, cofounders of the Koegel Autism Research Center at the University of California, Santa Barbara. PRT emerged to address the acquisition of complex skills that go beyond the basics.

By working with each child's natural motivations in natural learning opportunities, PRT stresses functional communication over rote learning. It targets and modifies communication and language, behavior, and social skills by capitalizing upon an individual child's idiosyncratic interests and obsessions.

PRT rewards children by creating less-structured, playful opportunities to do more of what they already enjoy. For instance, in one study, therapists played a game of tag on a huge map. Because the child was a geography expert, he was motivated to move from place to place in the game. Increased social interactions he learned during the game of tag continued after the game ended.[19] In another study, children used more appropriate conversation following PRT training than with DTT.[20]

For more information on PRT, read *The PRT Pocket Guide: Pivotal Response Treatment for Autism Spectrum Disorders* by the Koegels,[21] and go to http://www.education.ucsb.edu/autism/index.html.

• **TEACCH** is a result of the work of the late Eric Schopler, PhD, psychology professor at the University of North Carolina, Chapel Hill. The acronym stands for **T**reatment and **E**ducation of **A**utistic and Related **C**ommunication Handicapped **Ch**ildren. Schopler's heir and director of UNC's Division TEACCH today is Gary Mesibov, PhD.

A less-intensive form of ABA, the TEACCH philosophy embraces and accommodates, rather than remediates the "culture of autism," which it denotes as:

1. *Relative strengths in and preferences for processing visual information* (compared to difficulties with auditory processing, particularly of language)
2. *Strong attention to details* with difficulty understanding the meaning of how those details fit together
3. *Difficulty combining and organizing* ideas, materials, and activities
4. *Difficulties with maintaining and shifting attention*
5. *Problems with pragmatic language*
6. *Difficulty with concepts of time*
7. *Routine-driven*, with the result that disruptions in routines are upsetting
8. *Strong and rigid interests* in favored activities
9. *Marked sensory preferences and dislikes*[22]

With TEACCH, children sit at workstations, and therapists reward them for completing activities such as matching tasks. The TEACCH program relies on small laminated squares with picture symbols on them depicting everything from locations in the classroom to curriculum materials and self-help skills.

These "prompts" guide students through their days. The long-term goals of the TEACCH approach are both skill development and fulfillment of fundamental human needs such as dignity, engagement in productive and personally meaningful activities, and feelings of security, self-efficacy, and self-confidence.

Because those on the autism spectrum do well with these visual materials, the TEACCH conclusion is that vision is a strength for those with ASD. This profound misunderstanding of vision frequently prevents students working in a TEACCH environment from receiving the vital visual intervention that many require (see chapter 11).

For more information on TEACCH, read *The TEACCH Approach to Autism Spectrum Disorders*,[23] and go to www. teacch.com.

• *Verbal Behavior* is a methodology designed by Vincent Carbone, EdD, that places an emphasis on day-to-day activities and learning information in context. In Verbal Behavior, learning is functional; the methodology utilizes a systematic, highly structured teaching approach that moves away from the traditional ABA and DTT by combining behavioral principles with the functionality and generalization of Floortime® (see chapter 12) to emphasize language development. Like Floortime, Verbal Behavior uses children's own motivations for reinforcement by encouraging therapists to probe a child's skill level and fade prompts as quickly as possible.

Verbal behavior relies on a fast tempo and is peppered with many questions from both the adult and child. To increase spontaneous language and encourage conversational skills, Carbone uses prompting and fading procedures along with his version of discrete trial training in both natural environments and during intensive teaching sessions. Videotaping is a technique upon which he relies heavily.

The principles of Verbal Behavior are as follows:

1. All learners have the potential to develop skills beyond current levels and should be free of behaviors and activities that cause injury, pain, or limit opportunities for full social interaction and community involvement.

2. Communication and other skills that lead to rewarding personal relationships, well-being, vocational productivity, and self-determined daily activities should be targeted.

3. Reliance on the evidenced-based literature of the science of applied behavior analysis and its underlying assumptions lead to the best possible learner outcomes.

4. Functional communication is the foundation that supports the development of skills in all areas.

5. Reliable data, gathered and analyzed on a schedule sufficient to make informed decisions, is necessary to achieve the best outcomes for learners.[24]

Visit www.carboneclinic.com for more information.

Cognitive-Behavioral Therapies

Another class of therapies that applies operant conditioning techniques is cognitive-behavioral therapies. These therapies differ from behavioral therapies like ABA in that they also take an individual's feelings into account. Many view the approaches included in this section as a more humane form of ABA. The use of words such as "affective" and "fun" to describe cognitive-behavioral approaches hints that these approaches are also somewhat less mechanical than those using stricter operant conditioning.

Cognitive Affective Training (CAT)

British psychologist and professional autistic adult Tony Attwood, PhD, is the best known cognitive behaviorist applying a cognitive-behavioral approach exclusively to those with autism and other developmental disabilities. He calls his version Cognitive Affective Training or CAT. CAT is available as a kit consisting of visual, interactive, and customizable communication elements for children and young adults. It is designed to help students become aware of how their thoughts, feelings, and actions all interact, and, in the process of using the various visual components, they share their insights with others.

CAT teaches about nine feeling categories: joy, sorrow, fear, love, anger, pride, shame, surprise, and safety, with 10 sub-groups under each, making 90 emotions available for students to choose from. The CAT-kit includes a word piece and a face piece for each of the 90 emotions, which can be rated according to intensity and frequency. Blank pieces are available for customization.

A simplified body figure allows students to identify where emotions affect them physically, such as a stomachache. Role-playing exercises concretize a student's relationships, friendships, and interests with people both within and outside the family, including with strangers.

Special tools help develop and support the concept of time, over a day, week, or as long as a year. Students can place events in order and associate different emotions to those events, assisting in the understanding of how a person can be very happy and feel comfortable in one situation and then a second later become angry or sad.

Four different types of behavior are presented within four colors: red (outright aggressive), yellow (passive aggressive), grey (submissive), and green (assertive). These tools promote understanding and help develop the student's ability to self-regulate. To learn more go to www.catkit-us.com.

The Social Skills Training Project

Clinical psychologist Jeb Baker, PhD, represents the next generation of cognitive-behavioral training. Entertaining and irreverent, Baker has developed a unique, practical, and very popular approach to social-communication difficulties. Three principal goals guide Baker's method:

- To provide social skill instruction that generalizes into daily routines
- To make socializing fun
- To help "typical" peers and professionals become more understanding, accepting, and engaging of those with social difficulties

Baker's approach is a flexible five-part model involving the student, parents, and teachers as a team:

1. *Assessment:* First, the team prioritizes three or four relevant skill goals to work on for a specified time period. Focus is on actions that a student might and might not take that could interfere with social interactions in specific settings.

2. *Motivation:* Next they establish a good reason for the student to learn and use these skills.

3. *Initial skill acquisition:* Then, adults use strategies in the classroom and home that match the student's language, cognitive, and attention abilities to the targeted goals, making sure that the strategies are appropriate for the student's developmental levels. Some will require modeling and prompts; those with higher-level skills can use discussion.

4. *Generalization:* Adults coach students to use their newfound skills in natural settings and to broaden their interests and preferences.

5. *Peer sensitivity training:* Students interact with carefully chosen typical peers to increase generalization, reduce isolation, increase opportunities for friendship, and decrease bullying. Typical peers can be coached to protect and support those with disabilities in natural settings.

For more information on Baker and his approach, go to www.jedbaker.com and www.socialskillstrainingproject.com.

EEG Neurofeedback

What if it were possible for individuals on the autism spectrum to learn how to control their brainwaves to sustain attention, increase concentration, improve sleep, and decrease anxiety? Due to the advent of super-fast computers, which are capable of handling real-time data from the brain, it is!

Researchers have been trying to unlock the mysteries of the brain since ancient times. In Egypt, France, and Peru, anthropologists have discovered century-old skulls with carefully drilled holes, suggesting that curious scientists have been looking into the relationship between brains and behavior in ancient cultures for many years.[25]

In the early-20th century, scientists were able to show signals from an intact skull for the first time. Furthermore, they could measure electrical nerve impulses and demonstrate differences in brainwave frequencies depending upon the emotional state of an individual.[26]

Eventually, scientists began mapping the brain, and learned that specific centers of the brain controlled specific functions. By stimulating or disabling various parts of the cortex, they were able to increase and decrease abilities in motor, language, sensory, and emotional abilities.[27]

EEG Neurofeedback is a technique with origins in biofeedback training, developed in the 1970s. Biofeedback is a method by which electronic or mechanical instruments relay information to an individual about some aspect of physiological activity, such as heart rate, temperature changes, sweat gland functions, muscle tone, or electrical action in the brain.

Neurofeedback therapy is based on the premise that a mind-body connection to disease and disability exists. The body is like a city—an interdependent information communication system. When a single system breaks down in a city or human body, other systems dysfunction.

The brain is the center of the body, and reflects its health. A healthy brain is flexible and has the ability to change its arousal and attention in response to the demands of the environment. An unhealthy, dysregulated (and autistic) brain is inflexible and "out-of-sync" with itself. Its inability to process information at the right speed produces a discontinuity in communication and inappropriate responses to its surroundings.[28]

Brain dysregulation produces systemic mind-body effects, clearly demonstrated in patients on the autism spectrum who show symptoms in virtually every system. Almost no one would argue today about dysregulation in the gut. Dysregulated gut function ultimately degrades brain function in autism, and the reverse can be true, as well.

Siegfried Othmer, PhD, Chief Scientist of EEG Spectrum International, has been monitoring results of EEG biofeedback for ADHD, Tourette syndrome, autism, learning problems, and, most recently, post-traumatic stress disorder (PTSD) in veterans, for many years. He believes that one way the dysregulated brain can dysregulate the gut is by shifting the balance between the sympathetic and parasympathetic nervous system. As neurofeedback gradually decreases arousal levels and restores a healthier balance between the two parts of the autonomic nervous system, gut dysbiosis alleviates. Neurofeedback training can potentially affect every bodily system by regulating the central rhythmic activity of the brain. Go to his website at www.eeginfo.com to learn more.

It was not until the 1950s that researchers proposed using the power of the brain's own electricity to treat undesirable behaviors. When doctors stimulated specific centers in the brains of schizophrenics, the patients reported general feelings of well-being and a reduction in symptoms, such as anxiety, palpitations, and rage. In the 1970s, Dr. Joel Lubar and his associates first applied this treatment to attention deficits.[29] Now research is showing that neurofeedback is an evidence-based treatment for ADHD.[30]

Neurofeedback uses computer technology to turn brainwave signals into meaningful information in the form of a visual display with auditory signals, and occasional tactile feedback. The visual display serves the dual purpose of entertainment and feedback about what the brain is doing, making it possible for the training to proceed even with nonverbal individuals with autism. The brain continuously does its best, primarily at an unconscious level, to adjust to the demands of its environment, regardless of the cognitive level of the patient.

Neurofeedback, unlike many medications, has long-lasting gains without any negative side effects. Many practitioners are optimistic about neurofeedback being an efficacious treatment for those on the whole continuum of autism spectrum disorders.

Brainwaves and Their Frequencies

The EEG is an instrument similar to a car's tachometer; both show how fast the machinery is working. The car's engine revs slowly when idle and more quickly when the car is in motion. The revolutions increase the faster the car goes. Likewise, the EEG shows the brain, an extraordinarily complex communication system, at work. When the body is sleeping, brainwaves are slow; when a person is actively alert, they are faster.

Brainwaves are measured in frequencies of cycles per second (cps) or hertz (Hz) units, which equal one cycle per second. Brainwave frequencies reflect what a person's brain is doing at any given moment. An EEG's signals are composed of many different frequencies, which are organized in frequency bands. Table 13.1 shows these bands and the mental states of interest to those interested in doing neurofeedback as therapy. The boundaries of bands may differ slightly from practitioner to practitioner.

Table 13.1
Brainwave Bands and Their Mental States

Frequency Name	Cycles per Second (Hertz)	Mental State
Delta	<4	Sleep
Theta	4–7	Drowsy
Alpha	8–11	Inattentive
SMR (Sensori-motor rhythm)	12–15	Calm
Beta	16–20	Focused
High Beta	>20	Excited

Brainwave patterns and behavioral issues differ at the different parts of the autism spectrum. Table 13.2 shows typical brainwave patterns at the mild, moderate, and severe ends and areas of deficit that neurofeedback training addresses.

Table 13.2.
Brainwave differences in Autism Spectrum Disorders

Diagnosis	Neurofeedback Patterns	Goals
ADD & ADHD	Too much Theta; too little Beta	Improve focus
LD & Asperger's	Too much Theta; too little Alpha	Visual retention
		Mathematics skills
		Spatial reasoning
		Language processing
PDD/Autism		Decrease over-arousal

The brains of those with attention deficits demonstrate a dominance of low-frequency theta waves, which produce a drowsy mental state, resulting in symptoms such as lethargy, poor focus, and compromised memory.[31] While an abundance of theta waves are appropriate before sleep, they are inappropriate for the classroom. It may seem paradoxical that kids with ADHD are in a state of under-arousal; however, their hyperactive behavior is actually compensatory, as it functions to keep their brains awake.

Too many theta waves can also disturb sleep. In order to sleep, the brain must slow down and produce delta waves. Too much theta can cause trouble falling asleep, staying asleep, and having restless sleep, symptoms that are very familiar to parents of children on the spectrum.

A study comparing brainwaves in 18 adults with autism to 18 typical controls found that the autism group exhibited a significantly greater number of brainwaves in the 3–6 Hz and 13–17 Hz ranges, and significantly fewer in the 9–12 Hz range. The conclusion was that those with autism experience both over- and under-connectivity.[32]

Neurofeedback Training for Autistic Spectrum Disorders

Neurofeedback, like most therapies in this book, treats underlying dysfunction; in this case, the dysfunction is in the patient's brain, the body's central processing mechanism. If balance, memory, or emotional status is dysfunctional, the reason could be that the system as a whole, not an individual part, is malfunctioning. Brain training enhances an individual's regulatory function broadly, with favorable outcomes resulting across the board. This broad impact is traceable to the central role of the brain in the expression of many autistic features.

Dr. Barry Sterman is considered the father of modern neurofeedback training. The new EEG neurofeedback is showing positive outcomes with those diagnosed with not only attention deficits, but also reading disabilities,[33] Asperger syndrome,[34] and autism. A pilot study done by Jarusiewicz in 2007 showed promise.[35] Later research confirms positive outcomes in key areas of social, emotional, and cognitive function.[36]

Neurofeedback practitioners have a choice of using standard training protocols that address different common brain wave patterns, or formulating individualized training programs specifically designed to treat a patient's unique needs. One way they can develop a program is by using a new EEG called a quantitative electro-encephalograph, or qEEG, which aids in the diagnostic process and guides the neurofeedback treatment program.

Neurofeedback itself is simple and painless. First the patient sits in a comfortable chair, like a recliner, in a small, dimly lit, well-insulated room. The neurofeedback equipment consists of two computer monitors on a desktop, one for the patient to watch the visual display, and the other to show brainwave activity to the therapist.

The therapist applies conductive paste to the sensors, which are wired to an amplifier and then to the computer. The number of sensors attached to areas of the scalp are dependent on the individual needs of the patient and the therapist's therapeutic plan. As the patient relaxes, the sensors act like tiny receivers conducting electricity produced by the brain through the wires.

The purpose of each session is to train the brain to communicate more efficiently by regulating specific brain regions. Many patients on the autism spectrum need to train their brains to calm down; others need to make their brains more active. Training always starts with the parts of the brain that are the most troublesome, as a "trickle down affect" results that can improve less-problematic issues. If, for instance, a child's brain is producing too many low-frequency waves, a therapist rewards him with points or a desirable tone each time the brain makes some high-frequency waves.

As activity in a desirable frequency band increases, the display moves faster, or the patient receives more rewards. As activity in an adverse band increases, no reward materializes. The client receives immediate visual and auditory feedback on both a video monitor and through headphones. Gradually, the brain learns to respond to the sensory cues, and new brain wave patterns emerge. Through practice, individuals become familiar with their bodies' unique patterns and responses, and learn to alter them to improve function.

The following generalized benefits are often seen with neurofeedback training:

- progression toward calming
- normalization of sleep patterns
- increased flexibility, resilience, and emotional well-being
- improvement in ability to interact with others
- reduction in self-stimulating behaviors
- improvement in attention

Sessions for those on the autism spectrum last from 30 to 50 minutes, depending upon the functioning level of the subject. At least 20 sessions are usually required to achieve results. The cost of diagnostic testing and treatment sessions are about the same as for academic tutoring. Many insurance companies are now covering neurofeedback for conditions like anxiety disorders and chronic pain, though only a few recognize neurotherapy as an acceptable treatment for autism. However, patients are finding ways around this problem in the same way they are finding ways to pay for vision therapy, using methods such as a medical savings account.

In general, individuals on the autism spectrum often appear calmer after just the first few minutes of training. As sessions continue, many demonstrate the ability to focus and concentrate for longer periods of time, exhibit fewer or no self-stimulatory behaviors, and respond with appropriate reactions.

New forms of neurofeedback are emerging quickly, and each practitioner has his or her favorites. Many show promise for those with autism, so shop around to find a good fit between the therapist and the individual requesting treatment. Two of the most exciting are the following:

- *Hemoencephalography (blood-brain-image) or HEG*, where the goal of treatment is to increase either blood perfusion or oxygenation at specific sites, such as the frontal cortex. This form of neurofeedback allegedly improves frustration, tolerance, sleep, and cognitive, social-emotional, behavioral, and mental functioning.[37] For more information, go to http://www.biocompresearch.org.

- *Low Energy Neurofeedback System or LENS,* which uses very low-power electromagnetic fields (EMFs), such as those that surround digital watches and electrical wiring, to carry feedback to the subject. Although the feedback signal is weak, it produces measurable changes in brainwave frequencies without conscious effort from the subject. For more information on LENS, go to www.ochslabs.com

Who are Candidates for Neurofeedback?

While nearly everyone, with or without a disability, is capable of responding positively to neurofeedback, among the disabled, high-functioning individuals at the less-severe end of the spectrum, who enjoy computer tasks, are the best candidates. Other excellent responders include some who are nonverbal and may have higher potential than is evident superficially, and those who are facile with and attracted to computers and other gadgets.

Children adopted from orphanages in foreign countries, who have had early sensory and other deprivation and are now in loving, sensory-rich homes, are also a particularly interesting and very promising group. In some cases, neurofeedback wakes up their brains and is showing much success in eliciting sociability and language processing as their brains become better organized.

Impediments to Success with Neurofeedback

The following are the most common reasons for failure of neurofeedback training with those on the autism spectrum:

- *Sensory defensiveness:* Individuals with autism may dislike various aspects of the sensors—how they feel on the scalp, the smell of the paste, or even the sound made by the machine. However, just like the optometrist can gradually overcome sensory issues to allow the use of lenses, so can the neurotherapist who is intent upon working with autistic patients.

- *Poor sustained attention:* Being able to pay attention to a screen for lengthy periods of time is a function of progressive training. A graded program to improve attention by increasing time in training enables many autistic children to gain skill and improve flexibility without frustration.

- *Medications:* Some neurofeedback practitioners refuse to work with patients on medication because it can interfere with the ability to sustain attention, as described above. Others inform patients that as the brain learns how to control itself more efficiently, medication dosages may be able to be lowered, or may no longer be necessary. Collaboration with the patient's physician is key in this process.

- *Attitude:* People who question whether neurofeedback has efficacy or is worth their money, especially if it is not covered by insurance, can sabotage training. Their belief system simply interferes psychologically with the brain's willingness to accept the challenges that neurofeedback training presents.

Collaboration with Other Professions

Professional collaboration between neurofeedback practitioners and others can be an extremely successful two-way street when both professionals recognize the potential of the others' services. Clues of issues that require a referral and result in collaboration can present themselves both in the initial intake interview and during neurofeedback training.

The largest gains occur when neurofeedback is combined with biomedical and sensory therapies. Changes resulting from the normalization of the neuronal networks' communication pathways favorably impact not only cortical function directly, but also autonomic, endocrine, and immune system regulation. The neurofeedback practitioner can observe obvious visually-based behaviors, such as a head tilt, squinting or postural issues that signal a need for a vision consult, or motor planning issues that suggest a referral to an occupational therapist.

The response to brain training can be both profound and relatively quick. Devotees of EEG neurofeedback believe it to be one of the best pathways toward an improved quality of life for an autistic child and the family. It also has the potential to rend other therapies more effective. Any child on the autistic spectrum is a candidate for a trial of neurofeedback. The challenge to future researchers will be to determine the longevity of neurofeedback training. Does this intervention hold over time, or are occasional "booster shots" necessary?

Several books extol the virtues of neurofeedback for attention deficits and autism. The classic, which put this intervention on the map is *A Symphony in the Brain*, revised and updated in 2008.[38] Since then an explosion of books has occurred. Websites with current research, courses, certification, and directories of neurofeedback therapists all over the world are www.eegspectrum.com, www.brianothmerfoundation.org, www.bcia.org, www.eegoinfo.com, and www.aapb.org.

Assistive Technology

In the past, those who were nonverbal, non-interactive or otherwise locked into their bodies could communicate only with those who could understand the meaning of their behavior and gestures. Friends were few, and opportunities to socialize negligible. Fewer than 10 years ago, all that changed with technology, as engineers have developed some amazing devices and programs that can allow those with autism to communicate at home and school as well as outside their small circle of family and friends. Most require significant training to use properly.

Augmentative and Alternative Communication (AAC) Devices

Augmentative and alternative communication (AAC) is an umbrella term for any strategy used to express thoughts, needs, wants, and ideas. Early "low-tech" AAC devices included laminated pictures for exchange, the Mercury system, and other tablet devices based on the Microsoft XP Home edition. These allowed anyone to use common word processing programs, the Internet, and e-mail, as well as talk on the telephone, listen to CDs, watch DVDs, change channels on the television, and turn lights on and off. Mercury had ports for switches, head pointers, joysticks, and other access methods. Originally a miracle product, today it is an anachronism.

Software developers quickly recognized that computers were not just for word processing and video games. Hundreds of programs emerged in the 1990s aimed at teaching everything from reading, writing, and arithmetic to skiing and tennis, and, of course, remediation for language and social skills.

In just the past five years many people have abandoned their PCs, Macs, and augmentative devices in favor of tablets and phones for communicating. Now tens of thousands of apps for phones and tablets can be downloaded in seconds, and many of them are free!

Thanks to assistive technology, we have been able to get inside the brains of nonverbal individuals like Carly Fleischmann and Ido Kedar, just two of the many amazing individuals on the spectrum who have struggled to make themselves understood.

Doctors predicted not only that Carly would never communicate, but that her brain would never develop intellectually beyond age two. At ten, she had a breakthrough when she typed, "Help! Teeth hurt," on her therapist's laptop! Today she has lengthy electronic conversations with her supporters online, and she attends regular education classes. Read her story in *Carly's Voice: Breaking Through Autism*.[39]

Kedar spent his early years trapped in silence, misunderstood by adults who presumed that he lacked understanding because he could not reply verbally. First using a communication board, and now an iPad, Ido was finally able to explain what was going on in his mind. He is advocating for thousands of others with autism who are locked in, as he was, and thus unable to show their true capacities. Read his story in *Ido in Autismland: Climbing Out of Autism's Silent Prison*.[40]

At age nine, Elizabeth Bonker explained her world by tediously typing the following poem:

Me

I sometimes fear

That people cannot understand

That I hear

And I know

That they don't believe I go

To every extreme

To try to express

My need to talk

If only they could walk

In my shoes

They would share my news:

I AM HERE

And trying to speak every day

In some kind of way.[41]

The change has been profound for those with autism and other disabilities because the technology of tablets and phones has given them a voice. Today, a person with autism or another disability can use any part of the body, a pointer attached to a body part, an adapted computer mouse, or even eye tracking or scanning to select target pictures or symbols and thus communicate.

Computer Programs and Video Modeling

Watching other people tie their shoes, color, play, and interact, and then mimicking what they do is the basis for many of the social skills and communication programs. Do you think you could ski after watching a skiing video? Doubtful. Give a speech after watching a graduation address? Probably not!

Kids with motor planning problems, oral motor issues, and unintegrated reflexes are not going to be able to copy the gestures they see on videos easily, yet programs promoting this approach persist. A better option is to remediate the foundations for these coveted abilities first, and watch these higher-level skills emerge spontaneously.

That said, some social training software such as "Social Skill Builder" and "DT [for discrete trial] Trainer," which use video modeling to teach key social thinking, language, and appropriate behavior, are still popular. Motivating interactive games that depict social scenarios challenge the player(s) to determine appropriate responses, thus learning the rules of social communication in a variety of unstructured environments, such as in the grocery store and at school. For instance, "School Rules!" allows the child to practice everything from the right amount of social touch in the locker room to appropriate lunchtime interaction.

Rapid Prompting Method (RPM)

Soma Mukhopadhyay, a highly educated chemist from India, was convinced that her nonverbal son Tito, diagnosed at age three with severe autism, had strong intellectual aptitude despite his limited motor abilities. She tutored him tirelessly, prompting him to point to numbers and letters in books, while physically assisting his body through the motions.

By working with her son, Soma developed what she calls the Rapid Prompting Method (RPM). RPM is included in this section because it is a behavior modification program, albeit a low-tech approach that requires only an instructor, student, paper, and pencil.

This method is a "Teach-Ask" paradigm for eliciting responses through intensive verbal, auditory, visual, and/or tactile prompts, which compete with a student's self-stimulatory behavior. In RPM, the teacher matches her pace to the student's speed of self-stimulatory behavior, while continually speaking and requesting student responses in order to keep the student focused on the lesson at hand.

At first, Soma starts a lesson with a few sentences, and she asks a question based on what she has just said. Soma writes two possible answers on separate pieces of paper and encourages the student to pick up the correct answer. Soma moves quickly from two choices to three or more, from picking up pieces of paper to having the student point to the answer, and then to pointing to letters to spell the answer.

Because shifting the arm side to side is easier than lifting it up and down, Soma's students first learn to make choices from a horizontal field, and they progress to choices presented vertically.

Despite not speaking, Tito communicates. His book, *How Can I Talk if my Lips Don't Move?*, which he wrote as a preteen using the Rapid Prompting Method, eloquently describes how his autistic mind works: "One day I happened to realize that when people moved their lips, they made a talking sound known as a voice. For the next few days I would go upstairs, and stand in front of the mirror in the hope of seeing my lips move . . . And why wouldn't the mirror talk? It would not talk, simply because it had no lips to move."[42]

In 1999, experts from the National Autistic Society in Great Britain determined that Soma was correct: Tito was intellectually gifted. Soma and Tito came to the United States under a grant from the now-defunct nonprofit Cure Autism Now! to apply her teaching method on nine children with autism in Los Angeles.

Since then, Soma has worked with hundreds of students throughout the United States using the RPM, which she continually refines. The family has now settled in Austin, Texas. To learn more about this controversial approach, read *Developing Communication for Autism Using Rapid Prompting Method: Guide for Effective Language*[43] and *A Curriculum Guide to Autism using Rapid Prompting Method.*[44]

Tito was one of the first in a wave of people with autism who have since found their voices. Another was Jeremy Sicile-Kira, who wrote, "Autism is an important influence in my life. The hardest part is not being able to talk. God must have been out of voices when he made me. Having autism has hindered my ability to speak, but not my ability to communicate."[45]

When Jeremy's mother, Chantal, one of the most respected voices in the autism community, heard about Soma and Tito in 2002, she was impressed by her method and her high expectations for these severely autistic, nonverbal students. Having tried different well-known strategies with limited success for her son born in 1989, she decided to try RPM. It worked!

Jeremy now uses assistive technology to make friends. His extraordinary attempts to communicate landed him a prize from MTV as the second-most inspirational moment out of nearly 300 entries in 2007. Jeremy and Chantal now lecture together, giving hope and a voice to those who have neither. Learn more about Jeremy on his website, www.jeremysicilekira.com.

DynaVox

DynaVox, the grandfather of assistive technology devices, has kept up with the times, especially for nonverbal individuals with autism; the company is now in its fifth generation of computer-based communication. Founded in Pittsburgh, Pennsylvania, in 1983 on the belief that technology's greatest benefits are realized when it empowers individuals with disabilities, the company is now teamed with Mayer-Johnson, publically traded and global.

Its signature product is a sleek, lightweight, portable, programmable computer that can be customized for individual use. In many cases, school systems can include this device in the Individualized Education Plan (IEP), and the high cost of about $7,000 does not fall on the family. For many children on the spectrum it gives a voice with which to communicate to friends, family, and teachers. For more information about this complex system, go to www.dynavoxtech.com.

The iPad

In June 2007 the first iPhone hit the market, and in January 2010 Apple introduced the iPad. With those inventions, the way people communicate has forever changed. Our preferred method of communication is no longer a telephone—rather we e-mail or text.

Many families now have one or more iPads; most are used for entertainment. Playing games, watching and making movies, listening to music, and taking pictures are just a few of its features that provide hours of fun. However, the iPad can also be a powerful communication tool. Loading it with some special apps turn it into an AAC device that makes the lives of those with autism much easier.

If a student with autism is used to the iPad as an entertainment device, learning to use it as a communication tool may be tricky. Jonathan Campbell, an expert in assistive technology at the Simon Technology Center in Minneapolis suggests using a different iPad to communicate than to play games, music, and movies. It's like having two pairs of shoes: one for hiking and one for dancing. The color of the cover or the size of the iPad can allow individuals to identify its function easily.

Simply owning an iPad, like owning a telephone or a computer, is not enough. The ultimate goal is to use it consistently, regularly, and eventually automatically as a communication tool instead of grunting, pointing, dragging an adult toward the desired object, or guessing.

That is what happened with Jason. He was working at a local grocery store, and the adults supervising him thought he could learn how to travel by public bus by himself from his home to his job. Using one of the apps below, his parents took photos of each step required to get Jason from home to work. Jason learned how to view the procedure step-by-step on his iPad and follow the sequence of events from standing at the bus stop to getting off at the proper stop and walking to the store. After following the 15-step sequence for almost a month, Jason was able to travel alone without using the iPad.

Obviously, in order to be successful at using an iPad app, not only must the individual with autism learn its many functions and how to access them, but so must all those in his world: his family members, teachers, friends, and anyone else he has regular contact with. That takes time and training, but boy, is it worth it!

Communication apps. Thousands of apps appropriate for individuals with autism are available for the iPad, other tablets, phones, and other handheld devices. Apps cost anywhere from nothing to over $200. Generally, you get what you pay for. The free ones are limited in vocabulary and customization. The more costly ones are flexible in the number of pictures per page, voices to choose from, languages, accents, and the ability to upload your own pictures. Here are some of the most popular:

- **AutisMate** combines visual modeling, picture schedules and social stories in an easy-to-use format that covers communication needs from pre-school to the workplace. Developed in early 2013 after 18 months of intense research, Jonathan Izak joined with a business partner Ankit Agarwal and put his new degree in Computer Science to a very good use: helping his younger brother with autism communicate. Under the New York City-based company, SpecialNeedsWare, they have knocked the socks off the autism apps market.

While an off-the-shelf product, anyone can customize an individual's home, school, and work environments quickly using AutisMate's extensive content library. Interlinked screens minimize the number of clicks to go from one environment to another. While presently available only for the iPad, plans are in the works to have an Android-based version soon. Another planned exciting upgrade is for teachers to be able to access the tablets of their students remotely. For more on this cutting edge product, go to www.autismate.com.

• **Proloquo2Go™** is an app that provides a full-featured communication solution for people who have difficulty speaking. It brings natural sounding text-to-speech voices, up-to-date symbols, powerful automatic constructions, a default vocabulary of over 7,000 items, and full expandability and extreme ease of use to the iPhone and iPod Touch. While expensive for an app (about $200), it is quite a bargain compared to the DynaVox. See www.assistiveware.com.

• **Tap-to-Talk** is one of the most popular, customizable AAC devices available. It works on PCs, Macs, the iPad, and other tablets as well. For a one-time payment of about $180, you can choose pictures from a library of almost 3,000 items, a language, a voice, and an accent, and organize them in albums for different purposes. Training is available online and from special courses. To learn more, go to www.TapToTalk.com.

• **TouchChat** is similar to Tap-to-Talk, and a little less expensive at $150. It includes words, phrases, and messages spoken with a built-in voice synthesizer or a recorded message. Text from other applications can be copied to TouchChat so it can be spoken out loud. Also, text generated in TouchChat can be copied to other applications. It is available in three versions varying amounts of features. Learn more at www. TouchChatApp.com.

Determining Which Device Is Best

The best way to choose a communication app is to work with an assistive technology professional who knows many options and can evaluate which is best for an individual. Some speech-language pathologists, by necessity, have become experts in sorting out augmentative and alternative communication devices.

Generally, a professional assesses an individual's needs and the various settings in which a communication device might be used, and for what purpose. Can the individual use a finger to point, the eye to focus, or a finger to move to the next page? Is focus consistent enough for the individual with autism to be dependable after some practice? Is the school, workplace, or home conducive to the use of a communication device? Who are the key players in making sure that the device is used properly?

Some parents go into an IEP meeting and demand an iPad for their son or daughter. That approach is backwards. First, the school must determine if the student is capable of using *any* AAC, and if it would facilitate learning. Only after completing an assistive technology assessment, which considers the student, the school environment, and the tasks necessary to be accomplished, is an appropriate device chosen. Sometimes it will be a computer or a DynaVox; iPads aren't for everyone!

Two-Dimensional vs. Three-Dimensional Learning

While most applaud the extraordinary opportunities these electronic wonders offer, some are concerned that, for our youngest children on the spectrum, three-dimensional sensory experiences are being replaced with two-dimensional activities. Instead of feeling blocks, puzzles, dolls, and game pieces, they are manipulating virtual blocks, dragging puzzle pieces, clicking on games, and moving make-believe dolls and flat letters and numbers by touching a screen or by pointing and clicking.

One psychologist who is particularly worried about what effect screens have on the developing minds of all children is Jane Healy, PhD. In her book *Failure to Connect How Computers Affect Our Children's Minds — and What We Can Do About It*,[46] she argues convincingly for limiting screen time of all types until age seven, at least.

Take-Home Points

Applied behavior analysis and EEG Neurofeedback, two therapies based upon the science of operant conditioning, are very popular for children and adults of all ages and on both ends of the autism spectrum. Using the brain's ability to process and change its behavior, those with attention deficits, learning difficulties, social skills problems, and inappropriate behaviors are fitting in better. When these therapies are adjuncts to reducing Total Load factors, including toxicity, dietary issues, and sensory problems including visual dysfunction, "recovery" may be a word that will be appropriate with increased frequency for those on the autism spectrum.

Therapies that stress communication and social skills are using both a cognitive-behavioral approach and technology. Experts in psychology, language therapy, and other fields have used behavioral models to assist those on the spectrum in communicating more effectively, learning social skills, and adapting to their environments at home, school, and work.

Technology has remarkably increased opportunities for those with autism to be more fully integrated into society. Many who do not speak, and who previously had no voice, can now communicate using augmentative and alternative devices to make friends, interact, and learn. Synthesized voices on computers, tablets, and the iPad express their needs, feelings, and desires. Now is an amazing time to be a person with a disability. Many doors previously shut tight have opened to allow integration into society should they so desire. Socialization online has allowed them to make friends and stay in touch. Who knows what lies ahead?

[1] Sulzer-Azaroff B, Mayer R. Behavior analysis for lasting change. Fort Worth, TX: Holt, Reinhart & Winston, 1991.

[2] Baer D, Wolf M, Risley R. Some current dimensions of applied behavior analysis. Jrl Applied Behavior Analysis, 1968, 1, 91–97.

[3] This overview of ABA is a compilation from many sources. The author is grateful to Susan Varsames, MA Ed, of the Holistic Learning Center in White Plains, NY, (www.holisticlc.com) for her contributions.

[4] Lovaas OI. Behavioral treatment and normal educational and intellectual functioning in young autistic children. Jrl Consulting and Clinical Psychology, 1987, 55, 3–9.

[5] McEachin JJ, Smith T, Lovaas OI. Long-term outcome for children with autism who received early intensive behavioral treatment. American Journal on Mental Retardation, 1993, 97:4, 359–72.

[6] Sallows GO, Graupner TD. Intensive behavioral treatment for children with autism: Four-year outcome and predictors. American jrl on mental retardation, 2005, 110:6, 417–28.

[7] Eldevik S, Hastings RP, Hughes JC, Jahr E, Eikeseth S, Cross S. Using participant data to extend the evidence base for Intensive Behavioral Intervention for children with autism. American Journal on Intellectual and Developmental Disabilities, 2010, 115, 381–405.

[8] Rojahn J, Schroeder SR, Hoch TA, ed. Self-Injurious Behavior in Intellectual Disabilities. Elsevier, Amsterdam, The Netherlands, 2007.

[9] Ahearn WH, Clark KM, DeBar R, Florentino CJ. On the role of preference in response competition. Appl Behav Anal, 2005, 38:2, 247–50.

[10] Lambert JM, Bloom SE, Irvin J. Trial-based functional analysis and functional communication training in an early childhood setting. Jrl Applied Beh Anal, 2012, 45, 579–83.

[11] Hupp SD, Reitman D, Northup J, O'Callaghan P, et al. The effects of delayed rewards, tokens, and stimulant medication on sportsmanlike behavior with ADHD-diagnosed children. Behavior Modification, 2002, 26:2, 148–62.

[12] Bradshaw CP, Mitchell MM, Leaf PJ. Examining the Effects of School-wide Positive Behavioral Interventions and Supports on Student Outcomes: Results From a Randomized Controlled Effectiveness Trial in Elementary Schools. Journal of Positive Behavior Interventions, Jul 2010, 12:3, 133–48.

[13] Horner RH, Carr EG, Strain PS, Todd AW, et al. Problem behavior interventions for young children with autism: A research synthesis. Jrl autism developmental disorders, 2002, 32:5, 423–46.

[14] www.centerforautism.com. Accessed Apr 11, 2013.

[15] Rimland B. The ABA Controversy. Autism Research Review International, 1999, 13:3, 3.

[16] Newman B, Reeve KF, Reeve SA, Ryan CS. Behaviorspeak: A Glossary of Terms in Applied Behavior Analysis. New York: Dove and Orca, 2003.

[17] www.lovaas.com. Accessed Apr 13, 2013.

[18] Zier A, Hoehne K. Bridging Sensory Processing Theory and Practice with Discrete Trial Teaching. New Developments Newsletter, 1998, 6:3, 4.

[19] Baker M, Koegel RL, Koegel LK. Increasing social behavior of young children with autism using their obsessive behaviors. Jrl Assoc persons severe handicaps, 1998, 23:1, 300–8.

[20] Koegel RL, Camarta S, Koegel L, Ben-Tall A, et al. Increasing speech intelligibility in children with autism. Jrl Autism Dev Dis, 1998, 28:3, 241–51.

[21] Koegel LK, Koegel RL. The PRT Pocket Guide: Pivotal Response Treatment for Autism Spectrum Disorders. Baltimore, MD: Paul H. Brookes Publishing Co, 2012.

[22] www.teacch.com. Accessed Apr 13, 2013.

[23] Mesibov G, Shea V, Schopler E. The TEACCH Approach to Autism Spectrum Disorders. New York: Springer, 2004.

[24] www.carboneclinic.com. Accessed Jun 30, 2013.

[25] Robbins JA. Symphony in the Brain. New York: Grove Press, 1990, 9.

[26] Hill RW, Castro E. Getting rid of Ritalin: How neurofeedback can successfully treat attention deficit disorder without drugs. Charlottesville, VA: Hampton Roads Pub. Co., 2002, 16–20.

[27] Hill and Castro, Getting rid of Ritalin, 17–23.

[28] Hill and Castro, Getting rid of Ritalin, 74–76.

[29] Lubar JF, Shouse MN. EEG and behavioral changes in a hyperactive child concurrent training of the sensorimotor rhythm (SMR), a preliminary report. Biofeedback and Self-Regulation, 1976, 1, 293–306.

[30] Moriyama TS, Polanczyk G, Caye A, Banaschewski T, et al. Evidence-based information on the clinical use of neurofeedback for ADHD. Neurotherapeutics, 2012, 9, 588–98.

[31] Mann CA, Lubar JF, Zimmerman AW, Miller CA, Muenchen RA. Quantitative analysis of EEG in boys with attention-deficit/hyperactivity disorder: Controlled study with clinical implications. Pediatric neurology, 1992, 8:26, 30–36.

[32] Murias M, Webb SJ, Greenson J, Dawson G. Resting state cortical connectivity reflected in EEG coherence in individuals with autism. Biol Psychiatry, Mar 2007, 62:3, 270–73.

[33] Nazari MA, Mosanezhad E, Hashemi T, Jahan A. The effectiveness of neurofeedback training on EEG coherence and neuropsychological functions in children with reading disability. Clinical EEG and Neuroscience, 2012, 43, 315–22.

[34] Thompson L, Thompson M, Reid A. Neurofeedback outcomes in clients with Asperger's syndrome. Appl Psychophysiol Biofeedback, Mar 2010, 35:1, 63–81.

[35] Jarusiewicz G. Use of neurofeedback with autistic spectrum disorders. In Evans JR, ed., Handbook of Neurofeedback. Binghampton, NY: Haworth Medical Press, 2007, 321–39.

[36] Coben R, Padolsky I. Assessment-Guided Neurofeedback for Autistic Spectrum Disorder. Journal of Neurotherapy, 2007, 11:1.

[37] Ames G. Biofeedback and autism. New Visions Magazine, Nov/Dec 2006.

[38] Robbins, J. A Symphony in the Brain, rev ed. New York: Grove Press, 2008.

[39] Fleischmann A, Fleischmann C. Carly's Voice: Breaking Through Autism. New York: Touchstone Books, 2012.

[40] Kedar I. Ido in Autismland: Climbing Out of Autism's Silent Prison. 2012.

[41] Bonker E, Breen VB. I Am in Here: The Journey of a Child with Autism Who Cannot Speak but Finds Her Voice. Amazon: Kindle Books, 2011.

[42] Mukhopadhyay T. How Can I Talk if my Lips Don't Move? New York: Arcade Publishing, 2008, 17.

[43] Mukhopadhyay S. Developing Communication for Autism Using Rapid Prompting Method: Guide for Effective Language. Parker, CO: Outskirts Press, 2013.

[44] Mukhopadhyay S. A Curriculum Guide to Autism using Rapid Prompting Method. 2011.

[45] www.jeremysvision.com. Accessed Apr 10, 2014.

[46] Healy J. Failure to Connect: How Computers Affect Our Children's Minds — and What We Can Do About It. New York: Simon and Schuster, 1999.

CHAPTER 14

Academics: Finally Learning to Read, Write, Spell, and Calculate

When *are* children with autism really ready to read, write, and do mathematics? When they have strong sensory and motor foundations, and show interest in and begin to participate in those activities spontaneously. Reading specialist Debra Em Wilson targets six specific supporting foundations for academics:

- good postural control,
- efficient tactile, proprioceptive, and kinesthetic processing,
- solid midline skills,
- appropriate vision and visual processing,
- normal hearing and processing of sound, and
- strong motivation and focus.[1]

Previous chapters cover the importance of these skills, how to recognize skill deficits, and remedial procedures for alleviating them. Emphasizing academics before a majority of these skills are present can result in compensatory strategies, frustration, and failure. In order to outsmart autism, patience about acquiring academics is a must!

Preparation for Academics

Visual Readiness

Ready readers and writers use their eyes together as a team, can change focus easily from the book or paper to the teacher, and can perceive just-noticeable differences among visually similar objects and words. They can move their eyes across the page[2] without upper body or head movements using saccades — rapid, small, simultaneous movements of both eyes in the same direction from one point of fixation to the next.[3] They can recognize whole words by sight, sound out words phonetically, and read with understanding.

Refer back to chapter 11 for some of the ways that vision affects reading and writing. As a review, be aware of the following:

- *Visual acuity at near point:* Readers must be able to see the printed page clearly. If the page is not clear, the use of lenses for magnification or correction of an astigmatism might be indicated.

- *Convergence:* If the eyes do not converge with ease, they may drift out, causing blurring, headaches, and the tendency to get sleepy when reading.

- *Eye turn or strabismus:* If either eye turns in, out, up, or down, a student may demonstrate a head or upper body turn to compensate and use only one eye. This condition could slow down reading and writing speed and possibly affect comprehension.

- *Holding the breath:* If reading or writing is stressful, a student may hold his or her breath. This symptom could be present with almost any visual stress.

- *Visual thinking:* The ability to run pictures or movies in the mind's eye is an essential skill for reading with comprehension and writing with clarity and description. Those with poor visualization often need more body-in-space experiences to become good visual thinkers.

Auditory Readiness

English words are made up of sounds, or phonemes, the components in a word that affect its meaning. Readiness for language on paper includes the ability to hear, identify, discriminate, blend, and sequence phonemes in words, a skill called "phonemic awareness."

Just as eyesight and vision are different, with the former related to clarity and the latter a result of the brain processing what it sees, so do hearing and listening differ. Hearing refers to clarity of sound, while good listening skills require the brain to give meaning to what it hears. Specialists in both of these key areas may be members of the team working with a student on the autism spectrum.

Because English is not a fully phonetic language, however, phonemic awareness and the associated skill of using phonics to sound out unknown words is somewhat limited in its usefulness. Furthermore, the ability to blend sounds requires good visualization, as a student must keep the sounds and associated symbols in the mind's eye to blend the sounds in the right order successfully.

Some signs that a student lacks auditory readiness are mispronunciation of words, such as "pasketti" for "spaghetti," difficulties following sequential directions, such as "go upstairs and bring me a roll of toilet paper from the hall closet," and frequent interruptions during conversations or reading.

Vision and Audition Must Integrate

While visual and auditory readiness share many components, such as sequencing, reversals, directionality, and figure-ground, Harry Wachs, OD, notes some important differences. In his landmark book, *Thinking Goes to School*,[4] his goal is to integrate vision with every sense, which he does with more than 150 games and activities. While written more than 20 years ago, this resource is still a gem!

For visual-auditory integration he starts with sequencing concrete objects such as colored tokens, each representing a sound. For instance, the nonsense word "pap" could be represented by red-green-red. To change "pap" to "pip," a child replaces the green token with any other color, say blue, to show that the middle vowel sound has changed. The next stage is to change "pip" into "pit" by replacing the ending red token with yet another color, say black. So, red-blue-red is "pip" and red-blue-black is "pit." The final stage is to change "pit" into "tip." Yes! Black-blue-red represents "tip."

Eventually, printed letters replace colored tokens. Letters introduce laterality concepts, as a child must be able to distinguish a *b* from a *d* and *p* from *q*, concepts that are bypassed by using colors alone.

Finally, Wachs removes the visual clues, asking a child to say a word such as "carpenter" without the "pen." In order to do this correctly, the student must visualize the whole word and remove the targeted part to get "carter." Not easy is it?

Wachs's book is full of activities that connect vision to audition. Integrating what is seen and what one hears is foundational to so many aspects of learning and life. That is exactly what we do when we follow directions, watch a play, and listen to someone telling us about his or her vacation!

Reflexes Must Integrate

Chapter 9 elaborates upon the role of infant and postural reflexes in the emergence of foundational skills for development. Reviewing and understanding this very important chapter is essential before applying reflex integration techniques to academics. Integration of lower-level reflexes, such as the Moro and Tonic Labyrinthine Reflex (TLR) are key to the integration of higher-level reflexes, such as the Symmetrical Tonic Neck Reflex (STNR).

Integrating reflexes in developmental order is mandatory! Programs that bypass lower-level reflexes and focus on higher ones, such as the STNR, end up spending an excessive amount of time because remedial exercises could be fighting against lower-level reflexes. The best reflex integration programs and academic readiness programs understand the importance of integrating reflexes in order.

That being said, recall from chapter 9 how important the STNR is for learning. In a 1976 study, Miriam Bender, PT, PhD, found that 75% of those diagnosed with learning disabilities had a retained STNR.[5] O'Dell and Cook, psychologists who cofounded and directed a center in Indianapolis continuing Dr. Bender's work, found a retained STNR (a reflex that should not be active after the toddler years) to be a significant factor in a group of children with ADD and ADHD. All improved markedly when STNR reactivity diminished as a result of a specific movement program. O'Dell and Cook's book focuses on STNR integration to remediate reading problems.[6]

Bein-Wierzbinski used an infrared computerized eye tracking machine to show that the STNR was a factor in a group of children with eye tracking problems.[7] Later, Pavlides found that a high percentage of children with learning disabilities omitted stages of crawling and creeping in infancy, which is consistent with a retained STNR.[8]

Programs for Enhancing Academic Readiness

For teachers and parents who want to use a variety of academic readiness materials, many prepackaged programs are available. Designed and developed by seasoned educators and clinicians, they are inexpensive and appealing to students of all ages. They work well in schools for whole classes, in small groups of students in need of extra help, and for one-on-one intensive tutoring. Strongly consider using them before going directly to the alphabet, reading, and writing.

Growing Brains

For over 10 years, educational consultant Kathy Johnson has specialized in helping people struggling with learning academics to achieve individual success by focusing on the foundations. Her *Growing Brains* program combines specialized auditory, visual, reflex, motor, and cognitive activities in 10-minute-a-day intensives over 150 days. *Growing Brains* is divided into five sections of 30 days apiece, with each module comprising only minutes.

Growing Brains includes six reflexes: Moro, Spinal Galant, Tonic Labyrinthine, Symmetric Tonic Neck, Asymmetric Tonic Neck, and the Palmer. The program comes with instructional videos, worksheets for duplication, and very clear day-by-day instructions. Repetition is the key! Parents and teachers can purchase the DVD-based program from www.pyramidofpotential.com.

S'Cool Moves™ for Learning

Reading specialist Debra Em Wilson and occupational therapist Margot Heiniger-White recognized that many children with special needs still lack the motor, visual, and auditory foundations necessary for success in reading and writing. So they developed a program that includes some engaging pre-reading and pre-writing warm-ups for the classroom, called "S'Cool Moves™." These activities, which include reflex integration and vision therapy exercises, transition students from therapy to reading and writing by continuing to focus on improving motor planning, rhythm, timing, core posture, vestibular activation, brain integration, and sensory-motor integration in a group setting.

S'Cool Moves for the classroom includes large posters, a DVD, and an instruction booklet. Teachers can select either Level 1 (developmentally preschool to second grade) or Level 2 (third grade and up). A therapy and home version is also available. Movement routines are set to music as warm ups for using the eyes together in order to read fluently, write legibly, and focus overall. To learn more, go to www.schoolmoves.com.

Brain Gym® for Academics

Chapter 8 includes a discussion of Educational Kinesiology or Brain Gym®, a program developed by educators Paul and Gail Dennison. Teachers often use PACE, a group of four Brain Gym activities, as a quick warm-up for reading, writing, and mathematics. Refer back for a detailed description of this powerful tool.

In addition to PACE, additional Brain Gym activities can prep the body for reading, spelling, writing, and math. In their book *Hands On: How to Use Brain Gym® in the Classroom*,[9] an occupational therapist and special educator target Wilson's key foundational areas with the following movements

- *Reading:* "Positive Points" for motivation and comprehension, "The Thinking Cap" for phonics and listening, "The Rainbow" for visual tracking, and "The Owl" for increasing reading speed and fluency
- *Spelling:* "The Elephant" and "The Owl"

- *Handwriting:* "Neck Rolls," "Arm Activation," and "The Calf Pump"
- *Mathematics and Number Concepts:* "Cross Crawl"

Copyright laws prohibit including instructions here, so readers are encouraged to consult a Brain Gym specialist or purchase *The Brain Gym Teachers Edition*[10] to learn these simple exercises.

Figure Eights

For years, occupational therapists, developmental optometrists, and others have recognized the value of the "lazy eight:" the number eight lying on its side instead of standing on end: ∞. Its formal name is a lemniscate; mathematicians will also recognize this figure as the sign for infinity.

Using the lemniscate as a tool for improving perception in those with challenges is attributed to learning disability pioneer Newell Kephart, who collaborated with others, including optometrist G. N. Getman.[11] Today, therapists of many disciplines believe that moving the whole body, or one or more of its parts, in the shape of a lazy eight integrates the left and right sides of the brain, leading to increased focus and attention, spatial awareness, lateralization, and bilateral integration of eyes, ears, and limbs.

Bottom line: improvement in all of these foundational skills benefits a student's ability to read fluently and with comprehension, write legibly with good expression, and calculate with precision. Debra Em Wilson claims to have improved students' reading fluency rates 20–30 words per minute by having them do figure eights before testing.[12]

Lemniscate exercises. Working from control over the larger body down to smaller components, begin with **Walking Eights**. A student simply walks around a three-to-four foot lemniscate drawn on the floor. Follow this exercise with **Drawing Eights**, first standing at a chalkboard and then sitting, while drawing it on paper. Use both the dominant and non-dominant hands. Next try **Ribbon Eights** with a foot-long ribbon tied onto a short stick, like a child's fishing rod. Move the ribbon in the pattern of an eight, first with one hand, then the other. End with both hands on the rod together.

Pair students or an adult and child to do **Partner Eights**. Mirror each others' movements, as if you are two sets of windshield wipers. Next do **Air Eights**: a student follows thumb movements with the eyes in the lemniscate pattern while either sitting or standing. The eyes should follow the thumb with little to no head movement; the neck should be relaxed. Do three rotations in each direction. The highest level is **Nose Eights**. Pretend you have a pen at the end of your nose, and "draw" around the ∞.

Most therapists start at the midline, moving down and counterclockwise. Repeat in the opposite direction. Most important is to keep the exercise fun and relaxed, and not to correct the student. Believe it or not, performance will self-improve!

Australian movement expert Brendan O'Hara has created several Figure Eights exercises using beanbags.[13] His materials are available in the United States at www.braingym.org .

TLR 8s—foot goes out and in, in time with the hand. TLR 8s integrate the upper and lower halves, and the left and right sides of the body, for the integration of movement and vision.

1. Stand straight, holding beanbag in the left hand at the navel. Move beanbag up and to the left as if tracing the ∞, while moving the left foot out and in, in time with the beanbag as it sweeps one half of the ∞.
2. Left hand passes beanbag to the right hand at navel.
3. Complete the ∞ by moving the beanbag up and out to the right side, and back to home base at the navel. The right foot moves out and in, in time with the beanbag.
4. Repeat many times.
5. **Malkuth 8s—do standing, squatting slightly, and with knees slightly bent.** This exercise integrates the spinal galant reflex and stabilizes the spine.

In Front:

1. Hold a beanbag in both hands in front of the pubic bone.
2. The right hand takes the beanbag and begins tracing an imaginary lemniscate by sweeping up and out to the right, down and around, and back up to the pubic bone;

3. Pass the beanbag from the right hand to the left hand, which continues the sweep up and out to the left, down and around, and back to the pubic bone. One cycle is completed.
4. Do many cycles.

Out Back: Repeat the activity behind the body with the sacrum as the center point of the lemniscate. Repeat for three cycles. Focus on the breath and the legs while moving.

Do this activity in multiple ways: (a) with hips still, (b) with hips gently swaying with the flow of the leminscate, and (c) with hips swaying opposite to the flow of the lemniscate.

Eights are part of Brain Gym, as well. A slanted *Lazy 8* helps kids transition from printing to cursive writing. Instructions for *Alphabet Eights* and *Double Doodles* (doing the same movement pattern at the same time with both hands, either in the same or opposite directions) are available in many Brain Gym publications.

Infinity Walk. In the late 1980s psychologist Deborah Sunbeck, PhD, developed a variation on the figure-eight pattern that she calls Infinity Walk. Occupational therapists and developmental optometrists learned about Infinity Walk through parents, special educators, and early education teachers. The program was a good fit for their work in sensory integration and visual-motor training.

The Infinity Walk is both very simple and quite profound. Sunbeck elaborates upon moving through the simple lemniscate pattern by adding multitasking skills to the basic movements. For instance, she has the walker visually focus on a stationary target, track a target in motion, or practice visual search of numerous targets while continuing to walk forward along the figure-eight pathway. By adding the visual component during the walk, the eyes constantly cross the midline. This action stimulates the vestibulo-oculo-cervical (VOC) triad described in chapter 10. Refer back for more information.

The unique way in which the Infinity Walk combines the figure-eight movement pattern with sensory, perceptual, language, cognitive, and relational skills can produce lasting positive changes in attention, torso rotation, eye tracking, and neck reflex action. Veteran occupational therapist Mary Kawar has become an expert in the Infinity Walk and incorporates it into several of her courses on visual processing.

One of Sunbeck's contributions is the discovery that many of the above skills improve even when experienced passively. Sunbeck calls these actions "Infinity Ride," as an adult pushes a student in a scooter, golf cart, wheelchair, or stroller, or the student rides the pattern on a lawn mower or even on a horse!

For more information about this interesting tool and how to use it to develop the foundations for academics, go to www.infinitywalk. org.

Cognitive Enhancement Programs

Several remediation programs focus on "brain training," an umbrella term that targets various components of "executive function," including, but not limited to, attention, memory, logic, reasoning, problem-solving, and processing speed. Cognitive enhancement programs rely on neuroplasticity, the brain's ability to grow new neuronal connections and change when given specific learning tasks. Therapists apply this concept when working with stroke or accident patients to rehabilitate their speech, language, and gross- and fine-motor skills, and it is now accepted by some as applicable to those with autism.[14]

While a few of these packages include activities that mimic vision and listening therapies, occupational and physical therapies, and reflex integration, most do not work on coordinating the brain with the eyes, ears, or other body parts, but rather with end-product skills. Before embarking on these costly alternatives, read the previous chapters and ensure that a student has properly working sensory integration.

- *Learning Rx* is a franchise founded in the 1980s by optometrist Ken Gibson, OD. Learning Rx targets sustained, selective, and divided attention; long-, short-term, and working memory; auditory and visual processing; and logic, reasoning, and processing speed. Activities, such as quickly reading color words printed in a different color ink than the word itself, require the brain to be flexible and pay close attention.

In 1994, Learning Rx launched PACE, for **P**rocessing **a**nd **C**ognitive Enhancement (not to be confused with Brain Gym's PACE warm-ups), which certifies educators to use their materials. Based in Colorado Springs, today the company has over 80 sites nationwide and is a tool used by professionals of many disciplines. Go to www.learningrx.com.

• *Audiblox* is a similar system of cognitive exercises aimed at foundational learning skills, including visual and auditory perception, processing, and memory. Home kits are available as tangible, hands-on materials and as software for a computer. Exercises cover skills necessary for students from elementary through high-school level reading, writing, and mathematics. See www.audiblox2000.com.

• *Brain Highways* is unique in that it combines "brain training" with academics, including content areas such as science. Available in just two physical centers, in San Diego and Denver, it is primarily an online program for earnest parents of both typical kids and those with special needs.

After an assessment, everyone starts with the "Pons course," followed by the "Midbrain course" to improve brain organization with reflex, motor, and sensory activities. Enrichment courses for reading, writing, and mathematics are available only in San Diego and Denver. The website is clear that this is a supplemental program and does not take the place of therapy. For more information, as well as informative videos, go to www.brainhighways.com.

• *BrainWare Safari* is video game published by the Learning Enhancement Corporation. Through increasingly difficult challenges, it develops 41 cognitive skills through 20 different exercises in six areas: attention, memory, visual and auditory processing, sensory integration, and thinking. Experts recommend 3–5 times per week for 30–60 minutes over 12 weeks for improvement. In addition to Safari, the publisher offers two new programs that target pre-reading and reading skills. Ramps to Reading™ is for ages four to seven, and SkateKids™ for ages seven to twelve.

In 2007 an Ohio-based group tested this software on a mixed age and gender group of students diagnosed with autism. The highest functioning students were the most likely to benefit from the program. For more information, visit www. mybrainware.com.

Academic Skills

Reading

Many parents introduce storytelling and reading beginning almost at the day of birth. When listening to oral language, whether spoken or read, children naturally become aware of sounds. Rhyming games further enrich their vocabularies by pairing letters with sounds, words with pictures, and objects with concepts.

Children who have strong visual memories can recall whole-word configurations and develop a sight vocabulary. Others learn through phonemic awareness and instruction using phonics. As the eyes move across the page, fluency increases, and children increase their vocabularies.

In the early elementary grades, students learn how to read by combining visual, auditory, and language skills. By third grade, when they have "broken the code," they read to learn subjects such as science and social studies. When we read, many pieces come together as the visual, auditory, language, and memory centers integrate, and comprehension takes place automatically. Eventually, pictures and tangibles are no longer necessary because students derive meaning by running movies in their minds' eye.

A few students with autism read very young, some as early as two. Extremely early reading, called "hyperlexia," is a sign of uneven development, especially in the area of vision. Early reading is not a sign of a budding genius, and, believe it or not, should be discouraged. The pre-school child needs to develop control over the body first, and when the body is "still," the mind is ready to learn without moving.

The best reading programs for those on the autism spectrum contain subject matter that is developmentally appropriate. Just as kindergarten and first grade readers focus on content of interest to five and six year olds, the "just right" reading program for older children who are slow to read should include their interests and not be too difficult to decode. Many publishers specialize in "high interest, low level" readers.

In addition to these programs are some series that are both therapeutic and of interest to the quirky obsessions of those on the spectrum. A few favorites are listed here.

Fast ForWord® is a family of interactive computer-based listening programs developed in the mid-1990s by four research scientists: Michael Merzenich, PhD, William Jenkins, PhD, Paula Tallal, PhD, and Steven L. Miller, PhD. Their collaboration resulted in the formation of Scientific Learning®, a publically traded international corporation, now offering services in over 40 countries worldwide.

Fast ForWord is designed to improve language, reading, and learning skills from preschool through adulthood by listening through headphones. Based on over 25 years of brain research, it includes many different levels.[15]

Using an intensive series of adaptive, interactive exercises of acoustically modified speech and speech sounds, six different training programs target temporal sequencing, sound discrimination, phonological awareness, decoding, sustained focus, attention and listening comprehension, vocabulary development, word recognition, and other important reading skills. An individual plays a series of appealing computer games that automatically adjust to a student's improving competence level. Progress is charted daily.

The newest program is BrainPro® Autism, which combines Fast ForWord educational software with individualized consultant services online to improve oral and written receptive and expressive language. Its market is verbal students who are on the high end of the spectrum and can work on a computer for at least 30 minutes a day. To find a Fast ForWord practitioner, and for more information, go to www.scilearn.com.

Earobics® consists of multimedia computer games using acoustic enhancement of speech signals and adaptive training. It is aimed at developing many specific auditory processing and phonological skills, including auditory attention, discrimination, figure ground, identification, memory, and vigilance, and also targets reading vocabulary, fluency, and comprehension.

Earobics has multilevel programs for ages four to adult. Its format allows students to progress at their own pace. Individuals can use Earobics games at home or in a clinic at least once a week. Length of sessions depends on the level. The more extended the program, the greater the benefit. In a research study, students with learning disabilities or attention deficits, who worked with Earobics software for eight weeks, showed measurable improvement in auditory processing and exhibited positive changes to speech stimuli in quiet and in noise.[16]

Earobics is now in use in thousands of schools and in many foreign countries. To learn more and to find a practitioner, go to www. earobics.com.

Lindamood-Bell® Learning Processes has been developing reading programs that improve sensory-cognitive processing of language for students for over 25 years. The programs target students in the middle elementary grades with all types of learning issues, including those on the autism spectrum. *Seeing Stars® for Symbol Imagery (SI™)* develops phonemic awareness for reading, spelling, and fluency, while *Visualizing and Verbalizing® (V/V®)* develops concept imagery for language comprehension, vocabulary, and critical thinking. Read more about this program in this chapter under "Written Language."

Lindamood-Bell also has a mathematics remediation program called *On Cloud Nine® (OCN™)* which applies symbol and concept imagery to arithmetic and mathematical reasoning, with the goal to improve computational skills and the ability to solve word problems.

About 50 Lindamood-Bell® centers are located throughout the United States, the United Kingdom, and Australia. To learn more and find a location near you, go to www.lindamoodbell.com.

Symbol Accentuation™ Reading Program is an extension of the Miller Method discussed in chapter 12. Once children can speak or sign two- and three-word sentences, the Miller Method introduces the reading program to teach the symbolic function of printed words by acting out the meaning of a group of familiar words. An adult facilitates interplay between a student and animated sequences, combining video with flashcards and workbook materials to encourage a child to compose sentences. First children develop a sight vocabulary; they then learn to sound out unfamiliar words using phonetics. Finally they combine the two methods for reading and writing.

Handwriting

According to handwriting expert Nan Jay Barchowsky, the history of handwriting goes back thousands of years. The alphabet we use is based on the Greek letters that were adapted by the Romans. Italic handwriting, developed in the 14th century, came to the Americas primarily through Spanish conquests and has been the method of choice since the Renaissance.

Beginning in the 16th century, handwriting included fancy swirls and flourishes, but these gradually disappeared. In the latter part of the 19th century, the Palmer and Zaner-Bloser methods became the most popular approaches to teaching handwriting to American students.

By the turn of the 20th century, educators had concluded that handwriting would be easier for children to learn if the characters looked the same as ones that were in the books they used for reading. A few years later they reversed their thinking, deciding that print script was not suitable for grown-up writing, so they looked back to the conventional cursive of the 19th century.

Now many children are taught print script first. Then, in second or third grades, educators ignore the complications of retraining young hands, and introduce conventional cursive, the script that joins every letter in words with loops. Today, some schools teach conventional cursive only.[17] Others are ignoring cursive altogether.

With the trend toward tablets, touch screens, and voice activation, many educators fear that handwriting may be on its way to becoming extinct. Neuroscientists hope not. Forming letters is a bilateral integration task that prepares the brain for lateralization and specialization, according to a recent Indiana University study.[18] Cursive writing activates areas of the brain that do not light up when keyboarding or touching a screen.

Handwriting is a complex process that requires the integration of touch, proprioception, kinesthesia, vision, motor coordination, and language. Subtle feedback from the muscles to the brain, called proprioception, monitors the pressure and speed of writing. Eventually, the muscles develop memory, and writing becomes an automatic skill, like walking. The brain actually depends more on tactile and proprioception feedback than on vision to write.

Recall that good postural control is one of the key foundations for academics. To write without stress, a student must have good control of core muscles so that sitting posture is stable and relaxed. A balanced trunk, in which the muscles in front of the spine are as strong as those in the back, allows easy arm movement across the body's midline. The arm must be able to rotate, so the wrist can move freely and change position to form various strokes. As the trunk, shoulder, forearm, and wrist move in concert, the hand muscles can support finger movements.

Handwriting and Autism

Surprise! Individuals with autism have difficulty with letter formation in handwriting. According to a 2009 study at Kennedy Krieger published in the esteemed journal *Neurology*, motor skills were significantly predictive of handwriting performance, whereas age, gender, IQ, and visual-spatial abilities were not.[19] How researchers measured these visual-spatial abilities is unclear, and probably did not include the type of comprehensive vision exam described in chapter 11.

Children having difficulty with handwriting should have developmental evaluations by both an occupational therapist and a developmental optometrist. Specific remediation delivered as occupational or vision therapy can result in improved letter formation. Difficulties could be based in weakness in motor and/or visual functions, or possibly in the lack of integration of key reflexes. One or both professionals should thus be knowledgeable about and trained in reflex remediation.

For children who are struggling with any aspect of handwriting, occupational therapists can provide aids such as special papers, grippers, slant boards, cushions, and writing implements. The need for these, however, usually means that the demands exceed a child's physical maturity levels. A better approach is to fall back and work at a level at which a child is comfortable, while remediating visual and motor weaknesses and reflex issues.

Unfortunately, most schools demand writing before many students with autism have a strong core. The bodies and vision of even some of our older students on the spectrum show symptoms of stress, such as slumped posture, a poor or awkward pencil grip, wrist movement, trouble staying inside the lines, unusual letter formation, or poor legibility.

Handwriting warm-ups. Debra Wilson, the developer of S'Cool Moves (see above), recommends the following *"One-Minute Moves"* developed by physical therapist Freddie Ann Chandler to improve foundational handwriting skills. These include the following:

- *Deep pressure stimulation:* Press the thumb deeply and firmly into all parts of the palm of the opposite hand, about 10 pushes. Next, cross the arms over each other, and squeeze the forearm, upper arm and shoulder of the opposite side five or six times.

- *Skin sensation:* Rub the palms, then the backs of the hands together. Next, rub in between the fingers. Clap the hands together five times. Lastly, pat the forearms, the shoulders, and give the back a pat.

- *Muscle sensation:* Pretend to put a long glove on the writing hand, using the non-dominant hand. Pull the glove all the way up to the shoulder, using firm pressure. Repeat several times.

- *Resistive pressure:* Push the palms together with fingers straight. Then bend and grasp fingers together at chest level while continuing to rub the palms together. While grasping tightly, try to pull the palms apart.

- *Joint compression:* Press both hands onto the desk and rub the desk several times. Then press the hands into the thighs as if to push the feet into the floor.

- *Strengthen core postural muscles:* Get in position to write. Sit up tall, planting both feet firmly onto the floor. Place the paper at a slight angle to the midline of the body. For right-handed students, tilt the paper and head to the left; left-handed students tilt to the right.

Remedial Programs for Handwriting

A number of programs for handwriting focus on helping those with developmental delays, including autism spectrum disorders, to write legibly.

Handwriting Repair. No one understands the complexities of writing for individuals with autism better than Kate Gladstone, a woman diagnosed with Asperger syndrome who created a program called "Handwriting Repair" out of her own efforts to remedy her (then) dysfunctional handwriting. Kate is the only known handwriting service provider who has actually experienced the handwriting production and decipherment issues common to those with ASDs.

Kate offers an iPhone trainer app called "Better Letters." She also teaches a five-session webinar for parents and teachers, called "Improve Your Handwriting," through Pyramid of Potential. It includes sections on handwriting competence, as well as how and why we teach handwriting and what we can do to improve the state of handwriting today.

Handwriting Without Tears, the granddaddy of handwriting programs, is the most comprehensive of all the programs, addressing handwriting challenges from preschool through cursive with manipulatives, music, writing tools, and remediation strategies. Developed over 30 years ago by Maryland occupational therapist Jan Olsen, it is developmentally based and incorporates visual, auditory, manipulative, tactile, and kinesthetic teaching strategies. This classic is available in its original paper-and-pencil form, as well as in an electronic version as an app.

Jan emphasizes that technology should never replace multisensory writing activities. Materials move from a pre-kindergarten through elementary school age, and include cursive writing. Training workshops are available for teachers and schools to adapt the program to all levels. To learn more, go to www.hwtears.com.

Callirobics (from CALLIgraphy and aeROBICS) is a series of simple exercises set to music. This self-guided, creative approach, devised by handwriting expert Liora Laufer, is for home or school use. The multisensory exercises are designed to improve eye-hand coordination, fine-motor skills, self-esteem, and work habits. Many children succeed with Callirobics because the activities are brief (one to three minutes apiece), and the task of tracing abstract shapes is easy to grasp. Exercises are set to "old-fashioned" music such as *Danny Boy* and *London Bridge*, as well as to original melodies. Each program comes with a workbook and audiocassette. Five levels of Callirobics are available, from Pre-Writing Skills with Music (ages four to seven) to handwriting skills for adults who are in need of relearning writing skills. To learn more, go to www.callirobics.com.

Let's Do It—Write! is a series of workbooks designed to teach children how to write legibly and quickly. The goal of author Gail Kushnir, an occupational therapist and special educator, is for children to enjoy acquiring the skills that are precursors to writing. In her workbooks, "much of the 'work' is really child's play . . . which is how it should be."

First in the series is "Writing Readiness Workbook," suitable for children developmentally five to seven. Easy instructions are provided for the parent, teacher, or therapist. Following the antics of Benjy Bear, the prewriting exercises are designed to improve the child's sitting posture, sensory awareness, cutting skills, pencil grasp, spatial orientation, shape formation, and problem-solving skills. Next is "Copying from the Board," geared to develop children's actual handwriting skills. A friendly kangaroo entices the child to copy accurately. Order from www.therapro.com.

Getting it Write, by occupational therapists LouAnne Audette and Anne Karson, is a remedial program for clinical or classroom use. This six-week program is designed for groups of four to ten children, ages six to twelve. Already knowing how to form alphabet letters is a prerequisite for this program.

An occupational therapist and at least one other trained adult are present throughout each one-hour class. A gym or movement area is also necessary, as the exercises concentrate on gross-motor skills that affect a child's handwriting ability. Based on a blend of sensory integration and cognitive theory, as well as various handwriting approaches, the program covers areas such as body awareness, motor planning, kinesthesia, tactile discrimination, coordinating both sides of the body, memory, visual perception, ocular control, fine-motor coordination, and hand strengthening. To order go to www.gettingitwrite2.com.

Loops & Other Groups: A Kinesthetic Writing System, by Mary D. Benbow, MS, OTR/L, is a widely used handwriting curriculum based on studies of neurology and developmental hand anatomy. It is targeted to students with disabilities from second grade through high school. Students learn to form letters in groups that share common movement patterns. Memory and motor cues help them visualize and verbalize while experiencing the "feel" of the letter. "Clock Climbers," for instance, are the letters *a, d, g, q,* and *c,* which a child can visualize on a clock face. "Hills and Valleys" are *n, m, v, y, x,* and *z.* This program is readily available from occupational therapy distributors.

Barchowsky Fluent Handwriting (**BFH**) is an inexpensive app for the iPad geared to all ages. Start with "Letters Make Words" to learn letter formation and the sounds of letters in words. Move to "Beginners' Handwriting," which introduces students to prewriting activities using rhythmic gross-motor movements. Finally "Fluent Handwriting" takes the student through four levels, from lowercase letters, capitals, and numerals in a large size to smaller characters, spacing, posture, and direction. To learn more, go to www.bfhhandwriting.com.

Handwriting for Lefties

The incidence of left-handedness is slightly above 10% in the general population, and as high as 65% in those with ASDs.[20] "Left-handedness is connected to a lot of neurodevelopmental disorders," says Daniel Geschwind, MD, a UCLA expert in neurobehavioral genetics. "People with autism and schizophrenia are more likely to be left-handed," he adds.[21] Many with autism are ambidextrous, preferring one hand for strength-related tasks and the other for fine-motor skills. This is often thought to indicate poor brain lateralization,[22] and could also be due to vision issues.

Being a "southpaw" in a right-handed world is challenging enough. But for students with ASD, it is a double whammy. Without proper instruction, left-handers often develop unusual pencil grasps and body postures, which hide and smudge what they've just written. Their motor systems can tire easily as a result of their compensatory efforts. With the early introduction of correct fine-motor skills, experts believe that left-handers can write just as well as their right-handed friends.

A British company has a subspecialty in handwriting for lefties. *The Left-hander's Handbook* by Diane G. Paul has endless helpful suggestions. Exercises from their *Left Hand Writing Skills* series can be used at school or at home to replace incorrect fine-motor skills with more appropriate skills. The printed books are spiral-bound at the top to give free left-handed movement from the left side and across the page. Every page carries icons reminding users exactly how to hold their writing implements and how to position their paper in front of them on their work surface. Go to www.robinswoodpress.com to learn more.

Written Language

Putting one's thoughts down on paper is the most complex form of communication. Yet, as early as kindergarten, students are being asked to write about their experiences.

Written language is to academics as social skills are to communication. For success, all the senses, especially audition, vision, and proprioception, must be well-developed and integrated with each other, the brain, and the body. This arduous task requires memory, motor coordination, perception, visualization, and attention. Coherent writing, along with social skills, are among the last areas to develop.

Today communicating in writing is complicated by texting, where we abbreviate and use shorthand such as LOL ("laugh out loud" or "lots of laughs") to express ourselves. No doubt electronics have complicated written language so much that many students do not know what proper English is and what is not!

The ability to visualize is the highest form of visual thinking. This skill allows us to read with understanding, write with clarity, and organize our lives. Refer back to chapter 11 in the section entitled "Visual Thinking" for more on this important subject, and resources for developing this skill.

Several of the programs mentioned above, such as Lindamood-Bell, include writing as natural extensions of reading. According to Nanci Bell, the cofounder of Lindamood-Bell, "You must be able to think before you can write. Without the ability to think—rational, organized, lucid thoughts—writing is unorganized, disjointed, non-specific, and rambling."[23]

Bell thinks that schools put too much emphasis on the mechanics of writing and pay too little attention to the content. The Visualizing and Verbalizing program (V/V) is a much-needed bridge between oral and written language for students on the autism spectrum, who typically have general language weaknesses. It develops foundations for writing by helping students create images in their minds' eye. It encourages them to write, edit, write, edit, write, and edit some more.

Here is a summary of the steps Bell uses in her V/V program:
1. Stimulate gestalt (big picture) processing.
2. Teach sentence structure, basic punctuation, and spelling.
3. Move to paragraph writing, sequencing from copying to editing and finally writing from cue cards.
4. Write expository paragraphs following a specific organizational format.
5. Write narrative paragraphs.

Consistent with the V/V model is the request from many teachers to draw a picture to accompany a child's writing, if time permits. For struggling students, completing the picture first, rather than as an afterthought, is a better way to go. Drawing a specific scene or object forces visualization of color, size, setting, and more.

The ability to write a sentence with a subject, verb, and object with correct grammar, correct spelling, and appropriate punctuation and capitalization is still a reasonable goal. Despite the use of electronics, students *must* learn this essential skill.

Spelling

Have you ever watched the televised National Spelling Bee? How do the best spellers recall words? Some look up or close their eyes, as if searching their brain for the word. Others write the word with their finger in the air or on their palm or forearm. All are using their visualization skills to recall the "look" of the whole word gestalt.

Yes, spelling is a visual memory skill, and because vision is so intimately tied to our motor system, pairing a spelling word with a motor activity is a good way to seal it into our memories. Vision therapist Donna Wendelburg created this program using balls to teach spelling:

Table 14.1.
Spelling and Movement

GRADE	TYPE OF BALL	BOUNCE/DRIBBLE	SPELLING OUT LOUD
		IX for EACH LETTER	
K	Playground ball	Bounce and catch ball with 2 hands.	(Parent writes the word on large piece of paper.)
			Spell word forward. Spell word backward.
			Ask, "What letter comes before/after the letter _?"
1	Tennis ball	Bounce ball with right hand, catch ball with left hand. Bounce ball with left hand, catch ball with right hand.	(Parent writes the word on large piece of paper.) Spell word forward. Spell word backward.
			Ask,"What letter comes before/after the letter_?"
2	Tennis ball	Dribble ball with alternating hands.	Visualize the word.
			Spell word forward. Spell word backward.
			Ask, "What letter comes before/after the letter _?"
3	Tennis ball	Dribble ball in pattern: 2x with right hand, Ix with left hand.	Visualize the word. Spell word forward. Spell word backward. Ask, "What letter comes before/after the letter _?"
4	1 1/2" diameter	Dribble ball in pattern: 3x with left hand, 2x with right hand.	Visualize the word. Spell word forward. Spell word backward. Ask, "What letter comes before/after the letter _?"
5–6	1" super bouncer	Dribble in patterns of 3s: Ix right, 2x left, 3x right. 1x left, 2x right, 3x left.	Visualize the word. Spell word forward. Spell word backward. Ask, "What letter comes before/after the letter _?"
7–8	1" super bouncer	Dribble in patterns of 3s, USING ONLY TWO FINGERS.	Visualize the word. Spell word forward. Spell word backward. Ask, "What letter comes before/after the letter _?"

Even though we usually have an automatic spell check available, and often text without regard to correct spelling, knowing how to spell is a life skill that serves a student well. This especially includes the commonly confused homonyms, such as "two," "to," and "too."

As far as I am concerned, teaching spelling to those with ASD is no different than teaching it to anyone else. Thus few "special" programs are listed here.

Mathematics

Like language, the foundation for understanding numbers is based in sensory experiences. According to optometrist Harry Wachs, mentioned above, a child learns concepts such as same/different, greater/smaller, and first/last through touch, movement, pressure, vision, and even taste and smell, by creating images in his mind's eye. Rote learning of number facts or rote counting is not the same.

Wachs cites three foundational skills based on Piagetian conservation principles, all essential for successful understanding of mathematics:

1. *Visual Thinking concepts*, such as part-whole, figure-ground, perspective, and time perception. Activities using parquetry blocks and pegboards can enhance visual thinking.

2. *Numerical literacy* includes the ability to read numerals, position commas, and understand place value. Base ten blocks, available commercially, can assist in building skills in this area.

3. *Visual logic* adds the component of logical reasoning to visual thinking. A child needs to understand one-to-one correspondence, order, conservation of mass, weight, volume, number, and linear length, as well as classification, seriation, and probability to learn traditional academic arithmetic or geometry. Children with poorly developed visual logic might master basic computations but will struggle to solve word problems.[24]

Good programs focusing on teaching mathematics adhere to these constructs for children with and without issues to fully comprehend number concepts. Using manipulative materials, number lines, and concrete materials are the best choices. Activities that include estimation of time, money, and measurement are preferable to drill with paper and pencil. The Lindamood-Bell program, "On Cloud Nine," mentioned above, is an example.

Organizational and Study Skills

If good organizational and study skills are goals for a secondary school aged child with attention deficits or autism, then working with mathematics concepts is the way to go. Comprehending mathematics is closely aligned with the understanding of time and space, both visual concepts.

Students who are well organized are usually good in math and are able to develop their own study methods. While courses in study skills can offer some kids a few tools to help them get organized, most disorganized students have underlying visual-spatial issues, and thus cannot conform to someone else's timelines and structuring of space. Provide students with the tools to organize themselves, such as a wristwatch with a built-in stopwatch, alarm clock, calendar (weekly and monthly), organizer, measuring tape, allowance (in a denomination that is easily broken down, such as one dollar), and pedometer.

Other Considerations

Tutoring

In the same way that parents are very concerned when their young children are not talking, they become anxious about late readers and writers. The chosen panacea is often hiring a tutor. In a developmental model of autism and related disorders, tutoring is inappropriate until at least age eight, or when foundational skills are at a five to six year level. Spend the time and money on foundational therapies instead. For older children, find a tutor who uses a combination of methods, rather than one who recommends only one approach.

Positioning and Lighting

Schools and families need to take into account both positioning and lighting for all academics. Ensure that desks and chairs are the right size for every body; one size does not fit all. Each should be adjustable, so that a child's feet are fully on the floor at right angles to the waist, and the desk meets the student's body slightly above the waist. Desks and chairs that do not match in size, and that are too high or low, can make learning more difficult.

Use of ergonomically validated lighting systems can increase the speed with which students perform reading and writing tasks.[25] Lights must not have glare or buzz. Refer back to chapter 3 for more on this subject.

Take-Home Points

Teaching students with autism spectrum disorders how to read, write, and understand number concepts occurs in chapter 15, not earlier, because many sensory, motor, language, and cognitive foundations are necessary for success. *No*, we are not "dumbing down" our special kids; we are protecting them from undue failure. Until those with ASD master control over and become competent in visual, auditory, language, gross- and fine-motor skills, academics will be challenging and frustrating for them. And we know they need no more frustration in their lives!

That said, many programs exist that focus on the building and strengthening of foundations, thus allowing the natural progression of reading, writing, and counting to take place spontaneously. These programs are well-conceived, fun, and readily available both as tangible materials and electronically. Therapists of many types can access them and supplement their remedial programs. Furthermore, schools using some of the programs described in this chapter will find that students with various severities of autism take to them easily and happily.

If, in your impatience to outsmart autism, you are reading this chapter out of sequence, and have skipped earlier ones on more foundational skills, please refer back and ensure that all systems are "go" before proceeding onward, no matter what age the student.

Even those teens with visual and auditory processing deficits can benefit from a review of the basics. Our older students and young adults are the subject of the next chapter. Keep reading if your child is ready for transitioning.

---

[1] Allington R. The Five Pillars of Reading Instruction. Reading Today, Jun/Jul 2005.

[2] Suppes P. Eye-movement models for arithmetic and reading. In Kowler, ed. Eye movements and their role in visual and cognitive processes. Elsevier, 1990.

[3] Carpenter PA, Just MA. What your eyes do while your mind is reading. In Rayner, ed. Eye Movements in Reading: Perceptual and Language Processes. New York: Academic Press, 1983, 275–307.

[4] Furth HG, Wachs H. Thinking goes to School. New York, Oxford Univ Press, 1972.

[5] Bender ML. Bender-Perdue reflex test. San Rafael, CA: Academic Therapy Publications, 1976.

[6] O'Dell N, Cook P. Stopping Hyperactivit— A new solution. Garden City Park, NY: Avery Publishing Co, 1996.

[7] Bein-Wierzbinski W. Persistent primitive reflexes in elementary school children: Effects on oculomotor function and visual perception. Paper presented at the 13th European conference on Neurodevelopmental delay in children with specific learning difficulties, Chester, England, 2001.

[8] Pavlides O, Miles T. Dyslexia research and its application to education. Chichester, England: Wiley Publications, 1987.

[9] Cohen I, Goldsmith M. Hands On: How to Use Brain Gym in the Classroom. Ventura, CA: Edu-Kinesthetics, 2003.

[10] Dennsion PE, Dennison GE. Brain Gym Teacher's Edition. Ventura, CA: Edu-Kinesthetics, 2010.

[11] Kephart NC. Slow Learner in the Classroom. Columbus, OH: Charles E. Merrill, 1960.

[12] Wilson DE. School Moves Poster PE DVD. Shasta, CA: School Moves, 2002.

[13] O'Hara B. Beanbag Ditties CD. Victoria, Australia: The F# Music Company, 2003.

[14] Just MA, Keller TA, Malave VL, Kana RK, Varma S. Autism as a neural systems disorder: A theory of frontal-posterior underconnectivity. Neuroscience and Biobehavioral Reviews, 2012, 36, 1292–313.

[15] What Works Clearinghouse. Beginning Reading intervention report: Fast ForWord. U.S. Department of Education, Institute of Education Sciences, Mar 2013.

[16] Hayes EA, Warrier CM, Nicol TG, Zecker SG, Kraus N. Neural plasticity following auditory training in children with learning problems. Clinical Neurophysiology, 2003, 114.

[17] Barchowsky NJ. The history of handwriting. http://www.bfhhandwriting.com/history.php. Accessed Jul 28, 2013.

[18] James KH, Atwood TP. The role of sensorimotor learning in the perception of letter-like forms: Tracking the causes of neural specialization for letters. Cognitive Neuropsychology, 2009, 26:1, 91–100.

[19] Fuentes CT, Stewart BS, Mostofsky H, Bastian AM. Children with autism show specific handwriting impairments. Neurology, Nov 2009, 73:19, 1532–37.

[20] Colby KM, Parkison C. Handedness in Autistic Children. Journal of Autism and Childhood Schizophrenia, 1977, 7:1.

[21] Flam F. What's so special about Left Handers? The Philadelphia Inquirer, Nov 3, 2007. Academy of Reading Publications, 1991, 177.

[22] Geschwind N, Galaburda AM. Cerebral lateralization: Biological mechanisms, associations, and pathology: A hypothesis and a program for research. Archives of neurology, May 1985, 42.

[23] Bell N. Visualizing and Verbalizing for Language Comprehension and Thinking. San Luis Obispo, CA: Gander Publications, 2007.

[24] Wieder S, Wachs H. Visual/Spatial Portals to Thinking/Feeling and Movement: Advancing Competencies and Emotional Development in Children with Learning and Autism Spectrum Disorders. New York: Profectum, 2012.

[25] Mumford RB. The Role of Lighting. Visual Impairment Research, 2004, 6:1, 29–33.

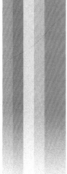

STEP 5

Plan for the Future

CHAPTER 15

Facing Adulthood:
Moving Toward Independence

In April 2012 I received an unexpected e-mail: "Hi Patricia. We are parents from Kuwait with an autistic son. We met you in 1996 in Washington, DC. Do you remember us? Our son was five at that time; he is 21 now. Awaiting your kind reply."

My correspondents were in the process establishing a center for young adults with disabilities and required a team of experts to advise them. Kuwait is no different from the rest of the world, where those babies born at the beginning of the autism epidemic are turning 21 this year. Like parents around the world, these and other Kuwaiti parents were frantic about what their son would do all day once he had no school, no program, and no reason to get up in the morning.

Six weeks later my team of three arrived in Kuwait, not knowing what awaited us. Our mission was multifaceted. First and foremost, we were to advise Kuwaiti officials, professionals, and parents on all aspects of the proposed center, including curriculum, architecture, and engineering. In addition, we were scheduled to meet and consult with a dozen families, put on a conference, and visit every government agency and nonprofit organization having anything to do with autism, cerebral palsy, Down syndrome, genetic disorders, and other developmental disabilities. All in a week, in 110-degree heat, with a mandatory siesta each afternoon!

Many think of Kuwait as a place where the streets are paved with gold and everyone wears Rolex watches; that's a myth. Yes, the *country* is rich and takes excellent care of its citizens, but the *people* are just like us. While they do not have to pay taxes or worry about the cost of gasoline, they work hard to make a living. They are lawyers, accountants, computer specialists, investment bankers, and business owners. If they decide to go out of the country to seek help for their children with disabilities, it's often on their own nickel.

Few parents have only one child with issues. Because they live as large, loving, extended families, many homes have several children with delays, including autism, Down's, and some rare genetic syndromes I had never heard of. Obviously the chemical soup from the Gulf Wars; unknown viruses and bacteria; and combinations of heavy metals including depleted uranium, mercury, and who-knows-what-else tweaked their genes in a unique way. I could not help but wonder if the deer tick that carries Lyme disease has a cousin who lives in date palms. Add an incomprehensible vaccination schedule that starts with tetanus shots for the pregnant mother at the fifth and seventh month, a hepatitis B shot at birth for the baby, and monthly boosters containing up to ten pathogens, and you have an immunological nightmare!

The pattern of autism within birth order defies everything we thought we knew about toxic load. The oldest children may be neurotypical, then one or more with autism, and then a couple more without delays. We saw as many females as males with disabilities.

Our conference attracted dozens of parents and professionals who carefully wrote out questions and waited over an hour to query us in person. "Will my child ever lead a 'normal' life?" "How can I calm my two nonverbal adult sons with autism sufficiently so they can fly out of the country?" "How can I stop my son from masturbating?" "Two of my five children have autism and my wife is pregnant. How can I prevent my new baby from becoming autistic?" "What will happen to my son when I am gone?" I really struggled to find quick solutions that were compatible with Kuwaiti culture, religious beliefs, and family values.

But Kuwaiti parents had taken the bull by the horns and petitioned the Kuwaiti government for help. Just before their e-mail to me, they had received government approval to forge ahead. After a year of hard work, Center 21 was born.

A small camp during the summer of 2013 comprising a dozen or so individuals with autism, cerebral palsy, and variety of other special needs is just the beginning. In 2014 the day program moved into a villa where 15 or so participants are being monitored by a half dozen bilingual Arabic-English-speaking mentors, including special educators, occupational therapists, and a physical therapist. Occupational therapy (OT) is an emerging field in Kuwait, with new degree programs now becoming available at Kuwait University. Until the first classes graduate, like almost all other commodities, including food, cars, and clothing, therapists are imported. Putting together teams of developmental movement, language, reflex, and vision experts is ongoing.

Setting up a testing program to evaluate, identify, and prescribe treatments for probable underlying biomedical issues is next. We have already started working with an American laboratory and supplement company. A Kuwaiti pharmacy is prepared to import whatever is necessary to treat underlying problems.

Some lenses, prisms and simple visual therapy activities can make a **huge** difference for these young adults. I believe we can "buy" 10–15 IQ points with visual measures that take stress off the nervous system and free up energy for other functions. Is it too late? Never!

A Universal Problem

The need for young adult programs is universal and prodigious. In the poignant Chinese film *Ocean Heaven*,[1] we see the universal nature of this problem. After discovering that he is dying of liver cancer, Wang—single father of a severely autistic, nonverbal, young-adult male—struggles to find a place for his son to go. Each place he calls and visits is inappropriate: his boy is too low-functioning for a post-secondary school and too old, or too "normal," for the asylum of the mentally ill. How many of today's parents are having this same experience?

In his desperation, Wang teaches his son to boil eggs, counting by rote until they are cooked. He trains him to take the bus to his beloved aquarium, where he swims with the dolphins, and he playfully teaches him how to dress and undress himself. Despite feeling deep sadness as the father passes away, the audience is gladdened that all of his efforts pay off as the boy becomes more independent.

No one knows the exact number of students with autism aging out of schools each year. According to a 2011 public television documentary film, *Autism: Coming of Age*, in the next decade close to 800,000 will enter adulthood needing support services:[2] a veritable "autism tsunami."

Grassroots organizations are popping up in Japan, the United Kingdom, Australia, and the United States. One of the largest of these is the Autistic Global Initiative (AGI), under the auspices of the Autism Research Institute (ARI). The mission of this group is twofold: to design and direct initiatives specific to adult concerns, and to provide support for adults on the spectrum.

Every member of the AGI is an adult with ASD. They come from all regions of the United States and represent a broad range of fields within the autism community, including education, psychology, social work, medicine, employment, fitness and wellness, rehabilitation counseling, and visual and graphic arts. To learn more about what AGI offers, go to www.autism.com.

Increasing awareness of the critical need for adult autism services is vital because after awareness come programs and support. This chapter provides an overview of presently available resources for transition, education, living, employment, finances, establishing relationships, and continuing treatment.

Transition

Preparing for Transition

From birth, parents around the world strive to support their children in becoming independent. The groundwork for transition actually starts before anyone has even thought about a transition plan. Can he toilet himself? Brush his own teeth? Can she make a sandwich? Swim without a life jacket? Does he have hobbies and leisure time activities he enjoys other than watching television and playing video games?

For children with special needs, a continuous "push-me/pull-you" occurs between the need to protect and the need to let go. If a child has had chronic medical or behavioral issues, the need to protect is so strong that letting go is even more difficult. Maybe he or she will get stung by a bee, unknowingly eat something with peanut oil, be bullied, or wander away. But as philosopher Friedrich Nietzsche so wisely noted, "What doesn't kill us makes us stronger."[3]

Most people can cite a mistake from which they learned a lesson that changed their lives. Since a majority of individuals on the autism spectrum learn best by doing, for them making mistakes is crucial. And, as with those without disabilities, we must start letting them make "little" mistakes like being late and missing an event, so they don't make "big" ones like having unprotected sex and getting pregnant. One of the most difficult parts of the developmental process for parents and caregivers is knowing when to let go. With proper planning, however, letting go becomes easier.

According to the 2004 reauthorization of the Individuals with Disabilities Education Act (IDEA),[4] by age 16 a student's Individualized Education Plan (IEP) must provide for "transition services" to move him or her from under the umbrella of the school system to the "real world." State laws vary markedly on transition services. Parents must learn what services are available in their resident state, as well as how to access them and how they are funded.

IDEA guarantees the right to an appropriate, free education for all students with disabilities from birth through age 21. Most, but not all, students on the autism spectrum continue in the school system until their 22nd birthdays, although some who are higher functioning leave earlier.

Preparation for transition begins early. During elementary and middle school, parents must be extremely vigilant to keep teachers and related service providers accountable for meeting IEP goals and objectives, thus ensuring that their child continues to move forward rather than fails to meet the same unreachable goals year after year. Sometimes this process can lead to irreversible decisions that put students on an educational "track" that is impossible to veer from.

Many experts are in a big hurry to prepare students for the workplace, and some schools start placing them outside the school as early as age 14. Successful transition is based on some degree of literacy, such as the ability to read signs; write name, address, and telephone number; and comprehend basic concepts of time, money, and measurement, as well as skills like maintaining schedules, budgeting, cooking, and building.

From the beginning of the IEP process, fighting for some degree of inclusion in the "least restrictive environment" that the law mandates is the best way to challenge seemingly low-functioning students. Early decisions that underestimate students' abilities and place them in too-restrictive environments can be extremely difficult to overcome, especially in an inflexible school system that offers only "academic" and "non-academic" tracks.

Even some minimal inclusion early on makes learning and gaining new skills easier during transition. For instance, if a nonverbal student with autism has been "dumbed down" and placed in a skills-based class rather than an academic one, by sixth grade, it may be very difficult for him to catch up academically. Transitioning to middle school, he may be too far behind to be placed in a mainstream class. He is now qualified to receive only a certificate of attendance and not a high school diploma. This possibility is especially relevant in mathematics where students are entering accelerated math classes earlier and earlier, and the requirements for high school graduation often include calculus, trigonometry, or both.

Personal life skills such as oral or facilitated communication, self-care, grooming, personal management, relationship-building, and merging home and work life are preparations for transition. The work required to develop other important abilities, including managing emotions, reading body language, taking criticism, suppressing reactions, and generally responding appropriately, is ongoing. All of these are vitally important to being successful in further education and to keeping a job at any level in the future.

Transition is a Team Sport

From the first multidisciplinary team evaluation that precedes diagnosis through adulthood, a host of professionals compose a decision-making group that plans for the future of an individual on the spectrum. Members of the transition team are as varied as that individual himself.

In addition to the transitioning teen, parents, and school system personnel, consider including advocates and experts in the following areas on the transition team:

- assistive technology
- community living
- employment
- exercise and physical health
- financial planning
- mental health
- nutrition
- sensory integration
- transportation training
- vision
- vocational rehabilitation

Transition Services

The late Andrew S. Halpern, Professor at the University of Oregon, is considered the grandfather of transition. His definition, written just 20 years ago, takes into account both the individual and his environment. At the time of his death in 2008, Halpern could not have imagined how important this well-conceived idea would be to so many millions of students today:

"Transition refers to a change in status from behaving primarily as a student to assuming emergent adult roles in the community. These roles include employment, participating in post-secondary education, maintaining a home, becoming appropriately involved in the community, and experiencing satisfactory personal and social relationships. The process of enhancing transition involves the participation and coordination of school programs, adult agency services, and natural supports within the community. The foundations for transition should be laid during the elementary and middle school years, guided by the broad concept of career development. Transition planning should begin no later than age 14, and students should be encouraged, to the full extent of their capabilities, to assume a maximum amount of responsibility for such planning."[5]

A common thread running through successful transition programs is a balance between an individual's personal sensory needs and his or her sensory environment. The area of sensory needs is an important one for self-advocacy (see below). Revisit chapter 10 for more information on a sensory diet. Only the individual can determine whether the environment is too loud, his clothes too tight, or his world too bright. Providing young adults with sensory barometers and ways to communicate discomfort ensures a more peaceful transition at home and in the workplace.

Transition services are based on all of an individual student's needs, taking into account many aspects of a student's future life in many environments. These include but are not limited to transportation training, diet, medical needs, recreation, leisure, friendships, and more. At some point, teachers and parents realize that they must change their primary focus from remediating weaknesses to capitalizing on strengths.

Examples of transition services are adult services, post-secondary education, continuing and adult education, vocational education, integrated employment (including supported employment), independent living, supported living, and any type of community participation. They might also involve specific types of instruction, related services, community experiences, the development of employment and other post-school adult living objectives, and, when appropriate, acquisition of daily living skills.

Assessment

Before writing a student's annual transition plan, school systems are required to perform a functional vocational evaluation. Transition assessment is an ongoing process that continues throughout the transition years. As young adults get closer to graduation, needs change and goals become more specific. Transition assessments are updated each year as part of the IEP process.

The assessment process includes anecdotal and formal observations in a variety of settings, on-the-job tryouts, classroom performance examples, formal and informal tests, work samples, inventories, and any other sources of information leading to an understanding of the following:

- aptitudes
- oral and written communication skills
- interests
- strengths
- weaknesses
- learning style
- medical issues
- work habits
- unusual behaviors
- hygiene
- social skills and
- values

Unlike diagnostic testing completed to categorize a student based on his or her deficits, functional assessments provide a description of what an individual with a disability *can* do, learn, and achieve. Unlike previous assessments, during which the student participates, sometimes passively, the functional assessment involves the student's active participation. Young adults with autism spectrum disorders, no matter how severe, are important members of the transition team; their interaction, to the best of their ability, is essential to increase their chances of achieving their dreams successfully. Parents and teachers are obviously also crucial, and their goals and objectives for their students must be "just right": neither too low nor unrealistic.

Students with autism who want to attend a post-secondary educational institution must be able to pass competency tests in reading, writing, and mathematics because most post-secondary schools provide accommodations but not curriculum modifications. This requirement limits the number of students with autism who are accepted. However, if a student graduates with an IEP diploma, indicating that the high school curriculum has been modified, he can still have a successful transition to further education and possible job opportunities if a focus is on life skills, functional reading, writing, and arithmetic.

Community-Based Instruction (CBI)

For those students with lower skills, most schools introduce Community-Based Instruction (CBI) at some point. Many private programs in the community, such as Goodwill Industries and Jewish Adult Services, are supported and funded by the school system, local universities, or technical schools. Programs outside the school system usually combine educational and academic components with job training and life-skills instruction. These on-the-job training programs provide opportunities for students with autism to learn what they like and do not like to do.

Starting as trips to local sites which offer job-training opportunities in real-life settings and moving on to assisted internships and "trial" jobs, each placement is crafted to meet the particular needs of a student on the spectrum and to utilize strengths while continuing to implement IEP goals and objectives. Focus is generally on communication and social goals, such as the following:

- advocating for oneself
- purchasing food
- balancing a checkbook
- doing laundry
- using the library
- locating, carrying and purchasing items in a store
- using public transportation

- attending community events
- ordering food in a restaurant
- identifying potential employers in the community

Despite everyone's best efforts, most students with autism are not prepared for the working world at age 22 or beyond. Premature transition to a "job" could result in placements that are hardly more than babysitting services, or settings for which they are neither cognitively nor emotionally ready. Waiting for a few more years of physical, social, and emotional maturation makes sense. Extra years to solidify skills can make the difference between restocking shelves in a grocery warehouse and keeping inventory at point-of-sale. While these two jobs may not seem too dissimilar, their contrasting demands may account for increased job satisfaction and moving from minimum wage to a decent salary.

The Americans with Disabilities Act (ADA)

The Americans with Disabilities Act of 1990 (ADA), extends services beyond secondary school into college and the workplace. The ADA requires publicly funded colleges and universities to remove barriers that keep out disabled students. Students with disabilities can arrange to take college entrance exams with accommodations. Once accepted, colleges must provide recorded books and lectures, an isolated area to take tests, and permission to record rather than write reports, depending upon a student's individual needs. Today most colleges have a Students' with Disabilities Office.

The ADA also applies to the workplace, where it guarantees equal employment opportunities for people with disabilities and protects disabled workers against job discrimination. Employers may not consider the disability when selecting among job applicants. They must also make "reasonable accommodations" to help workers who have handicaps do their job. Such accommodations may include shifting job responsibilities, modifying equipment, or adjusting work schedules. During transition, parents, educators, employers, and the individual with autism must be aware of the provisions ADA mandates so that everyone can advocate for and respect the rights of the employee or student with a disability.

Post-Secondary Education and Living Arrangements

When the school bus stops coming, life stops for many young adults with special needs. No school, no program, no life. Alternatives exist, and more are showing up each year as more and more students with special needs exit the only schools they have known.

Unlike their siblings who sometimes go off to college, 18-year-olds with special needs are stuck at home with Mommy and Daddy. Their parents, who could have become empty-nesters once their neurotypical children were launched, are at home tethered to their adult children with autism. Soon someone begins to wonder what will happen to these "special" kids when parents are gone. Many parents cannot imagine their offspring living anywhere but home. Others begin the transition to supported living while the child is still in high school. As with aging parents, experts recommend that you cannot start too soon.

In Kuwait, where families are large and extended, taking care of an adult with autism may not be so problematic. In countries where family members and their responsibilities are scattered, a time eventually comes to explore different living arrangement options: with parents, with another relative, with a friend, with a paid aide in a rental apartment, in a licensed home, in a group home, or alone. No matter the placement, a familiar, supportive, comfortable environment with the right sensory stimulation is key to success for many on the spectrum.

Day Programs

An emphasis on friendships, physical fitness, use of community resources, developing creative and personal interests, and medical and therapeutic monitoring are components of most day habilitation programs. States differ markedly in their offerings, and financial arrangements vary according to a child's special needs. Parents must take the time to investigate options along with specialists in the public school system who usually knows what is available.

Community Colleges have become increasingly flexible in programming for students on the autism spectrum. Some allow students to take courses pass/fail while others offer support, such as mentors, readers, and even tutors. Options change with the seasons, so parents are urged to check with their local programs to see what is available.

Not surprisingly, parents have been at the forefront of developing post-secondary programs for their offspring whose needs were unmet by available offerings. One of these is Chantal Sicle-Kira, whose son Jeremy is described in chapter 13. Although nonverbal, Jeremy graduated from high school in California with an academic diploma. In 2011 his mother founded Autism College to share with others what she had learned about advocating for him.

Autism College is not an actual college, but rather an online resource to educate parents and professionals so they can make important life decisions regarding education and therapy for young adults with autism. To utilize this service go to http://autismcollege.com.

The ultimate goals for individuals with autism are the same as for anyone: to have friends, to have something to get up for in the morning, and to lead a productive, meaningful life. That is the goal in the United States, Japan, Great Britain, and for the members of Center 21 in Kuwait; it is universal whether they live at home, in a supported residential setting, or at a post-secondary educational facility. The next section covers residential programs, some of which include an educational component, that help to meet this goal.

Camphill

Camphill is an international movement consisting of more than 100 communities in 22 countries. Inspired by the works of philosopher, educator, and Renaissance man Rudolf Steiner—collectively called "anthroposophy" —Camphill was founded in 1939 in Scotland by Austrian pediatrician and educator, Karl Koenig, MD, and others. At Camphill, children, youth, and adults with and without special needs live, learn, and work together.

Camphill's goals are:

1. Providing education, advocacy, therapeutic care, and other services to support people with disabilities and helping them participate fully in the world as contributing citizens;

2. Caring for and healing the earth through sustainable and healthy methods of consumption, agriculture, and natural resource use; and

3. Creating social arrangements designed to nurture the growth and development of individuals, so that all community members contribute their time and skills according to their capabilities.

Camphill was established in North America in 1959. Today, ten independent communities serve over 800 people. Camphill is interested in expanding its programs to include more individuals with ASDs. Two communities specifically serve young adults:

- **Soltane** houses approximately 90 people, about half of whom have disabilities, on a 50-acre site about an hour west of Philadelphia. "Learning for Life," is a five-year continuing education experience. Three years of continuing education is followed by a two-year transition program during which students have access to elective classes offered through the education program. For more information, go to www.camphillsoltane.org.

- *Triform*, located in the Berkshire Mountains near Hudson, New York, is a dynamic residential community of over 100 people spanning several generations, including 40 young adults with disabilities. Those with autism, Down syndrome, and other special needs live and work side-by-side with staff on a 410-acre biodynamic/organic farm. Go to www.triform.org to learn more.

For more information on Camphill programs throughout the world, go to www.camphill.org.

Other Unique Post-Secondary Programs

Chapel Haven, in Connecticut, was established in 1972, making it one of the oldest programs of its kind in the nation. It now offers several two-year residential programs for those ages 18 and older with Asperger syndrome and other learning and social disabilities that make them vulnerable in other settings. Four- and eight-week summer programs are also available in Connecticut, and in Tucson, Arizona. The Residential Education at Chapel Haven program provides life skills and functional academics along with social skills training, communication competency, and recreation opportunities. Participants prepare for supported employment and life outside the home.

The Asperger's Syndrome Adult Transition program is for higher functioning students and offers opportunities to attend college-level classes at local schools and work in appropriate internships. Students live in staffed apartments where they learn housekeeping, meal preparation, time management, and social skills.

This program is approved for funding in several New England states as well as Arizona. For more information, go to www. chapelhaven.org.

The College Internship Program (CIP) is a year-long, post-secondary transition program offering individualized academic, social, career, and life skills support for young adults with Asperger syndrome and other high-functioning autism spectrum disorders, attention deficits, and learning disabilities. Founded in 1984 by Michael McManmon, EdD, who was diagnosed with Asperger syndrome in his early 50s, CIP's mission is to help young people make successful transitions from adolescence to adulthood.

In this multidimensional residential program, students live in furnished apartments in California, Florida, Indiana, Massachusetts, and New York. They are monitored carefully to develop life skills such as organizing, cooking, cleaning, and living independently, while attending a local college or university. Well-trained staff provides whatever supports are necessary for a student to be successful socially, academically, and personally, including a personal fitness plan of nutrition, exercise, stress-reduction practices, sensory diet, and sleep regimens. All CIP students eventually develop appropriate employment skills through extensive training, counseling, community service, résumé development, and internship and job placements. For more information, go to http://www.cipworldwide.org/.

Center for Discovery in the Catskill Mountains, 90 minutes northwest of New York City, offers residential-living options to individuals over 21. The program emphasizes individual preferences and community participation by providing a wide variety of activities such as exercise, yoga, swimming, concerts, sporting events, and enrichment classes that enhance and support residents to achieve their full potential. A working farm, on-site bakery, and other venues provide options for vocational training and experience. For more information, go to www.centerfordiscovery.org.

The Autism Trust. Dynamo parent Polly Tommey founded the Autism Trust in the United Kingdom in 2007 after her middle son, Billy, was diagnosed with autism. Its objective is to create a future with purposeful employment and training opportunities for young adults with autism everywhere.

Tommey began with a small operation in Sunninghill, UK, that provided space for individuals with ASD to create art and crafts sold in a boutique called Polly's Place. Polly Tommey and her family have moved to Austin, Texas, from where she is supervising the building of residential and outreach centers both in the UK and in the US. These campuses will provide adults with autism and other related disabilities supported opportunities to develop vocational skills. Tommey also publishes the bimonthly magazine *The Autism File*. For more information, go to www.theautismtrust.com.

Bird's Nests. Julie Buckley, MD, developed a passionate interest in healing autism when her daughter regressed at four years of age. In 2012, she co-founded the HealthyUNow Foundation, a 501(c)(3) nonprofit dedicated to creating "green," nontoxic, healthy living treatment and residential facilities for individuals with autism and their families. These facilities, both virtual and physical, will integrate the local community with its residents. The physical communities will be called "Bird's Nests."

The Bird's Nest campuses will include healing centers with medical care and a variety of resources for developing social, physiological, and physical skills. Also included are respite care, education centers, and resident cottages. Plans are in the works for animal therapies, movement options, and non-allergenic foods. Initial locations are outside of Asheville, North Carolina, and in Northeast Florida. For more information and updates, go to www.HealthyUNow.org.

Careers and Employment

Parents and teachers must help teens turn their strong interests, talents, and obsessions into paid work and even into vocations. Love of computer technology, music videos, car parts, collecting, classifying, and categorizing can all be translated into meaningful careers.

That's what happened to John Elder Robison, a multitalented man who did not receive an autism spectrum diagnosis until well into adulthood. His love of tinkering with cars led to a very successful high-end automobile repair and detailing business, which he describes in the delightful book *Look Me in the Eye*.[6]

Mark Rimland — autistic son of Bernie Rimland, the late founder of the Autism Research Institute (ARI) and his wife, Gloria — is a professional artist whose paintings sell for large sums. He turned his love of painting into a vocation from which he derives great pleasure and an income.

Choosing a Career

Obviously, individuals with autism differ in career choices as in every other aspect of their being. Temple Grandin believes, however, that some jobs are particularly well-suited to individuals on the spectrum. In her book, *Developing Talents: Career Planning, Including Higher Education, for Students with Autism and Asperger Syndrome*[7] she describes many of these fields, which include:

- Animal handling
- Art
- Auto repair
- Computer programming or repair
- Crafts
- Drafting
- Engineering
- Graphic design
- Landscaping
- Theatre lighting and sound
- Music
- Web design

Looking ahead to a possible career for his son with autism, Dane Thorkil Sonne left his job of 15 years, refinanced his house, and founded Specialisterne (The Specialist People Foundation) aimed at creating jobs for adults with autism. Specialisterne offers a three-to-five-month individual assessment where participants identify their strengths, weaknesses, special aptitudes, capabilities, and interests.

This is followed by a training program during which they map out their needs for support, guidance, and environmental adjustments in order to perform successfully as Information Technology (IT) consultants. Specialisterne has dozens of consultants who solve computer problems for leading telecommunications companies around the world. The foundation also runs a school with a three-year program for young adults ages 16 to 24 with ASDs.

The Specialist People Foundation has set the ambitious goal of providing meaningful and productive jobs for one million people with autism and other invisible disorders. To do this, they will replicate Specialisterne operations around the world. Specialisterne USA hired its first group of consultants, all with diagnoses on the autism spectrum, in July 2013; they are now official Specialisterne USA employees. To learn more about this ambitious project, go to http://specialistpeople.com/.

Underemployment

Despite these mandates, only a small percentage of those with autism spectrum disorders hold full-time jobs. Why? Primarily because of their difficulties with the unwritten rules of the workplace, not their job skills. Many come late to work, have not had a daily shower, wear their favorite clothes day after day without washing them, are inflexible when demands or circumstances change, and a myriad of other reasons. In her frequent keynote addresses to autism groups, Temple Grandin is adamant that those with autism learn the "rules."

A guidebook that covers this topic is *The Hidden Curriculum of Getting and Keeping a Job: Navigating the Social Landscape of Employment: A Guide for Individuals With Autism Spectrum and Other Social-*

Cognitive Challenges.[8] Authored by two adults on the spectrum who have extensive experience in guiding others, it is a must for anyone helping those with ASD become and stay employed.

Finances

Who assumes the costs of care for an individual with autism? From day of diagnosis, this is one of the biggest concerns facing families. While their parents' insurance covers young adults up to the age of 26, when costs exceed insurance caps, this question looms large.

Guardianship

One option is guardianship; begin the process once your child is 17 ½. Delaying could cause a gap that could jeopardize an emergency medical situation. Parents are usually the legal guardians of all of their children until they turn 18, at which time they are legally considered adults and are held responsible for making their own decisions about money, healthcare, residence, and more. Many parents of children with autism choose to apply for guardianship because they recognize that at 18, their children are not able to make these decisions independently. Consult with an attorney specializing in this area before making this momentous decision.

Both "full" and "limited" guardianship are options. Obtaining full guardianship presumes that a child is "legally incompetent." Another adult takes complete responsibility for a child's welfare, stripping him of some legal rights, such as the right to choose a home, vote, or marry without consent.

Alternatives to full guardianship include

- Obtaining limited guardianship, which makes a parent or someone else responsible for money or medical care, and allows the individual with autism to retain his or her remaining rights;

- Obtaining power of attorney, which gives someone else authority to make legal, financial, and medical decisions in behalf of the person with autism; and

- Appointing a temporary guardian or conservator in an emergency situation when certain decisions must be made immediately and the individual with autism cannot make them independently.

The Guardianship Capacity Questionnaire, which can be obtained at http://www.nccourts.org/forms/Documents/846.pdf, can be helpful in deciding which option to choose. Whichever option works during parents' lifetimes, make arrangements for a replacement guardian after death, and put this in parents' wills.

Special Needs Trusts

Since 1993, the Federal government has authorized several specific trusts that can create a fund to supplement the care and quality of life for individuals with disabilities, including autism. The term "Special Needs Trust" usually refers to (d)(4)(A) trusts; the letters and number allude to where they can be found in the statute that authorizes them.

Special Needs Trusts are solely for the benefit of individuals who are under age 65 and disabled according to Social Security standards. Also called Disability Trusts or Supplemental Needs Trusts, these funds can be established by an individual's parent, grandparent, legal guardian, or the Court for the sole benefit of an individual with a disability.

Special Needs Trusts are irrevocable, meaning they cannot be altered. The idea is that the person with autism can earn or be gifted money, thus protecting him from losing certain government benefits that are denied people who have personal bank accounts that exceed $2,000 at any given point in time. Benefits may include Supplemental Security Income (SSI), Medicaid, vocational rehabilitation, subsidized housing, food stamps, and other benefits based upon need. A Special Needs Trust provides for supplemental and extra care over and above that which the government provides.

A properly-drafted trust includes provisions for termination or dissolution under certain circumstances and explicit directions for amendment when necessary. All assets in the trust belong to the beneficiary. Each Supplemental Needs Trust is its own "entity" with its own EIN issued by the Internal Revenue Service. Many types of trusts require legal help to understand and draft. Variations include

Third Party Irrevocable Trusts, Sole Party Trusts, First Party Trusts, and Pool Trusts. The Special Needs Alliance offers a handbook on this subject (see www.specialneedsalliance.org).

Special Needs Trusts are a tax benefit for a person with a disability and his family. Unlike a traditional trust, a properly drafted and administered Special Needs Trust is not counted as an asset, and trust disbursements are not included as income under the rules that apply to SSI and Medicaid.[9]

Families interested in establishing a Special Needs Trust must find an attorney with expertise in trusts and discuss the unique situation of their offspring on the spectrum. Some insurance companies and pro bono lawyers also provide such services.

Government Funding

Allocation of funds for those with disabilities varies markedly state to state and year to year. The law requires that schools put families in touch with local programs and benefits as part of the transition process. However, they do so with rather wide ranging success or lack thereof. Most school systems offer a free annual open house where all providers, lawyers, housing, etc., in the area exhibit. The school is only obligated to provide the information; whether a program is successful is up to the parent to discover.

Here are some of the revenue streams that are available to pay for housing, rehabilitation, nursing, medications, and other continuous needs once an individual with autism turns 21:

- **Supplemental Security Income (SSI) and Medicaid** are called "means-tested" benefits because to qualify, an applicant must both be disabled and have extremely limited assets and income. For SSI, an applicant can have no more than $2,000 in assets.

Those with autism generally qualify for Supplemental Security Income (SSI), a payment made jointly by the federal government and the state of residence to cover some of the living costs for individuals with disabilities. If a young adult lives at home and pays rent, he may qualify for higher-income SSI.

People who qualify for SSI and live outside their family home usually receive **Personal and Incidental Money (P&I)** every month as part of their SSI payment. This money is for clothing, entertainment, or other "incidental" expenses. If the person earns an income, then this money is deducted from the P&I and must be reported to Social Security.

• **Medicaid Waiver:** Home and Community Based Services Waiver is open to those with several specific disabilities, including autism. Waivers may allow for Medicaid and services such as a Personal Care Assistant, respite, transportation, etc. There are several types of waivers. A good source of information is http://www.familiesusa.org/issues/medicaid/other/waivers/waiver-faqs.html.

• **Social Security Disability Insurance (SSDI):** Some individuals may also be receiving Social Security Disability income under their own claim or Social Security Disabled Adult Child benefits under a parent's claim. The amount of money received by the adult child depends upon parental income and the number of years of contribution to Social Security paid by the disabled parent. After 24 months on SSDI, an individual is eligible for Medicare.

• **Health Insurance:** Obama's Affordable Care Act of 2010 has many provisions for autism. With it, families whose children are on the autism spectrum have expanded access to insurance options through the Health Insurance Marketplace and improvements in Medicaid and Medicare.

Also, new health plans sold in the individual and small group markets cover "essential health benefits" to help make sure that health insurance is comprehensive. Health insurers offer annual out-of-pocket limits to protect families' incomes against the high cost of health care services.

• **In-Home Supportive Services:** Money from this source can be used to pay for someone to come to the home to help with personal tasks such as cooking, shopping, cleaning, paramedical services, medical transportation, and protective supervision. Parents have the option of being the paid provider for an adult with disabilities.

• **Shift Nursing:** Several government programs offer funding for nursing, if needed, under the Nursing Facility Waiver for persons over age 21. Shift nursing may cover nursing expenses up to what it would cost if the individual were to be placed in residential care. This care is available for adults residing in their own homes, licensed homes, and foster homes, as well as for those in independent or supported living.

Relationships

The idea that individuals with autism don't like people is outdated. Everyone needs friends and companions with whom to share interests, activities, and even intimacy. The impetus for many adult programs targeted at those with ASDs is providing continual opportunities for the same types of relationship-building available to those going to college and interacting in the workplace. The other side of this coin is preventing isolation at home with aging parents.

While the Internet has opened the floodgates to global social networks, everyone realizes that having a "friend" on Facebook is not the same as having one with whom to go to the movies or to a party. Furthermore, those with disabilities, especially if cognitively challenged, are vulnerable and can be targets for abuse and bullying online.

An important value to local programs is that most offer workshops, recreational activities, and other social programs that build relationships. Some are for those with autism themselves, and others are for their caregivers. All provide the means for fostering friendships and relationships, creating a social life, and learning how to become more independent.

Dating and Marriage

Intimacy and autism are two words that one rarely sees together in the same sentence. A recent Canadian study comparing sexuality in adults with high functioning autism with neurotypical peers found that individuals with ASD showed no significant differences in breadth and strength of sexual behaviors and comprehension of sexual language when contrasted with non-ASD participants.[10]

With increasing frequency, experts are speaking out on sexual and intimacy issues in autism. Difficulties with language, social skills, sensory processing, and more make moving from friendship to dating to sexual contact especially challenging for those on the spectrum. For those who are lower functioning, parents and caretakers must deal with channeling the physical needs that arise with hormonal changes.

The Internet, while offering different types of "friendships," also offers the opportunity to get to know someone (assuming he or she is telling the truth!) without face time, reading social cues, and the awkwardness of making small talk, all skills those with autism find difficult. "Singles" sites, in fact, may be ideal places for those on the spectrum to experiment with dating, albeit with some vulnerability.

Two famous couples have taken on the subject of dating and marriage and written extensively about it. Sarah and Tony Attwood, living in Australia, have a number of books on dating, sexuality, and intimacy available from Jessica Kingsley Publishers. They often lecture in the United States and offer advice through various types of media. Americans Jerry and Mary Newport met at an Asperger support meeting, divorced, and then remarried each other. They are the subjects of the movie "Mozart and the Whale," which fictionalizes their relationship. Their knowledge is accessible through books and conferences from Future Horizons.

For those interested in more specifics, *The Asperger Love Guide: A Practical Guide for Adults with Asperger's Syndrome to Seeking, Establishing and Maintaining Successful Relationships*[11] is a free download online. It includes subjects such as assessing your readiness for a relationship, how and where to seek and find someone else, whether or not to disclose Asperger's, dating safely, maintaining a relationship, co-habiting, and marriage. Autism Victoria (based in

Australia), known also as Amaze (because life with autism is a maze in which our charges constantly amaze us!), has a brilliant piece called "Romantic Relationships and Autism Spectrum Disorder" by psychologist Kristy Kerr, which details the many aspects of dating and relationship-building.[12]

Gender Identity

The beginning of the autism epidemic in the late 1980s and early 1990s parallels the increase in more open discussion of gender differences and the increased visibility of the lesbian, gay, and transgender movement. While the media and academia have treated this phenomenon sociologically, is it possible that gender differences, like autism spectrum disorders, are biologically based? How? Maybe the same endocrine disruptors that interfere with detoxification, digestion, and development are also accountable for gender confusion.

Swedish researchers at the Karoninska Institutet think so. In a letter to the editor of the *International Journal of Andrology*[13] (andrology is the medical branch focused on male health), they cite endocrine disruptors as a hypothetical common contributor to both ASD and gender identity disorder. The authors refer to two papers that support this hypothesis.

In one paper, prenatal exposure to phthalates (see chapter 2) was associated with a less typical masculine play behavior in boys.[14] In the other, males with ASD were found to look younger than chronological age and to have sparse body hair and high-pitched voices. Many were androgynous, not only in appearance, but also in their self-concepts and sexual preferences.[15] Females with ASD were likewise androgynous and had elevated testosterone levels.[16]

According to a recent French study, gender identity clinics are now reporting an over-representation of individuals with ASD among their patients.[17] In a Dutch study, the prevalence of ASD was tenfold higher among patients with gender identity disorder (GID) than in the general population.[18] Another study in Japan found similar results.[19] However, few case reports or studies in English-speaking countries have dared to broach the subject of the co-occurrence of ASD and GID, even though they seem to be closely related.

In the Canadian study mentioned above despite similarities in sexual behaviors to their neurotypical peers, individuals with ASD showed a higher rate of asexuality. Temple Grandin is an example of this presentation, about which she is open and self-effacing. In addition, results indicated that females with ASD showed a significantly lower degree of heterosexuality when compared to males with ASD. The results also suggested a higher degree of homosexuality among females with ASD, although this effect was not statistically significant.[20]

Obviously, this subject is very loaded even though it has broad implications, especially regarding early intervention treatment options. Further research is clearly indicated.

Self-Advocacy

This chapter would be incomplete without a discussion of advocacy. For their entire lives, most individuals with ASD have depended upon parents, teachers, and others to advocate for them. No matter how disabled a person is, at some point during transition, he or she must learn some self-advocacy skills to survive. These may be as simple as indicating the need for help when lost, a more complex skill such as learning to use assistive technology to communicate, or as complicated as going to court to access desired services.

Learning how to stand up for yourself starts at a young age. We teach preschoolers to stand up for themselves on the playground and in the block corner. Likewise, we should work from the start with our students with special needs to ensure that their needs, hopes, and desires are being met. Many lack the language to stand up for and speak for themselves. We must use the latest techniques and programs·to give them an individual voice.

For those with special needs, self-advocacy starts with knowing what the law says about rights and responsibilities. Self-advocacy courses should be a part of every transition program. A student with autism who wants to be included in the mainstream, whether as a part of a sports team, a club member, or a participant in a dance contest must learn that inclusion is a right. After graduation, pamphlets, books, workshops, webinars, and seminars can help those with autism understand the various ways in which they can stand up for themselves.

Recognizing the need for learning self-advocacy, Valerie Paradiz, PhD, Director of the Autistic Global Initiative, and Andrew Nelson, MEd, a trainer at the West Virginia Autism Training Center at Marshall University, have joined with the Houlton Institute to create "Integrated Self-Advocacy," an online course for educators to use to teach self-advocacy as a part of the transition process. Each of two modules lasts 12 weeks and is self-paced. To learn more go to www.autismselfadvocacy.com.

Continued Treatment

As kids grow into adults, their needs change. As their bodies get bigger and heavier and hormones rage, be sure to work with health care practitioners and revisit dosages and frequencies of medications and supplements. Small adjustments can make a big difference in behaviors, focus, language, and learning.

Instead of discontinuing therapies, consider making them more pragmatic. For instance, the emphasis in vision therapy might move from tracking and eye teaming to visual thinking. Language needs change, too. Maybe it's time for some assistive technology using an iPad. Once kids are communicating with regularity, enrich vocabulary and focus on social-emotional language skills such as knowing when it is your turn to talk, making conversation, asking for what you need, and knowing how to phrase what you want to say.

In the motor areas, once-clumsy children and teens can become young adults who enjoy simple sports such as soccer, basketball, skating, swimming, and bike riding. Equipment is now available for almost any size and body. Large tricycles, smaller playing courts, easy-to-manipulate balls, and other adaptive physical education equipment make fitness fun and non-competitive.

Martial Arts

Several experts have explored ancient and Eastern movement and mind-body techniques[21] for improving the sensory, balance, and coordination issues, as well as the resultant anxiety and undesirable behaviors for individuals with autism. These interventions focus on posture and breath, and since deep breathing is known to lessen anxiety, their success is not surprising.

While this section could have been included earlier in this book, it is placed here because mind-body techniques help with body control and promote "mindfulness."[22] They can also be a godsend for younger kids who can learn where their bodies are in space by moving through the motions of a martial art.

Sports such as yoga, aikido, karate, tae kwon do, t'ai chi, and judo can all benefit those with autism, young and old. A study by Boston-area doctors combined yoga with music therapy and dance for 24 children with autism ages 3–16. Subjects showed significantly fewer inappropriate behaviors and unusual visual perceptions after eight sessions.[23]

A more recent study by New York occupational therapists utilizing a classroom yoga program called Get Ready to Learn also showed significantly fewer maladaptive behaviors in the treated group.[24] Several OTs and yoga studios are now offering classes with specific poses and moves for students on the spectrum.

Aikido is a Japanese martial art that is both a practical and effective form of non-violent self-defense, and a means of compassionate conflict prevention. It is also a way to relax and get physical exercise. On its deepest level, aikido is a path of mind-body-spirit awareness and integration.

In Columbus, Ohio, Paul Linden, PhD is a somatic educator and martial artist. He developed Being In Movement®, a mind-body training program he is using successfully with individuals on the autism spectrum. His specific body-awareness training methods help with self-monitoring and self-regulation. He sees improvement in managing aversive stimuli, as well as better focus even in over-stimulating, distracting environments. In addition, his students have learned more graceful, effective styles of movement.

Qigong massage for those with and without autism is showing some promise. A randomized trial over four months on 38 children showed improvements in self-regulation and sensory processing.[25] One of the authors in this study, a physician, has published a book with an accompanying DVD that provide comprehensive instructions for parents on "how to implement a program in their home."[26]

The core part of the program is a 15-minute massage that parents give their child once a day for at least five months. The program has been shown to help children sleep better, have less aggression, transition more easily, decrease self-injurious behaviors, and improve eye contact, language, and social skills. This massage can be given to typically developing children as well as children on the autism spectrum.

Look for local resources that have experience with individuals with special needs and martial arts. These wholesome activities may help your child learn control over multiple facets of his or her body and become a source of ongoing healing from the inside out.

Annual Evaluations

After a student has left the school system, the need for periodic review of physical, emotional, and mental status are still necessary. Reviews can take place quarterly, semi-annually, or annually at the least. Team members can meet in person or using technology. Each should be very familiar with the latest services offered, status of the adult with special needs, and reports of progress.

Take-Home Points

The time to start planning for the future is now! Any educational, vocational, and financial decisions should look beyond the day after tomorrow. Work with experts in transitioning to learn what options are in your geographical area. Get acquainted with key people so that you know whom to go to when the time comes. Make every effort to encourage independence, even when it seems like a real reach for your family member with ASD to accomplish a goal without support. Living in the world of autism can be full of surprises, and some of them are good ones!

The Future of Center 21

The plan for Kuwait is that Center 21 will expand to 100 young adults with special needs by 2015, and relocate to a renovated school building. Eventually it will become a lively mall-like campus that includes villas, shops, cafes, a medical center, therapy rooms, art studios, a sports complex, and more, serving over 1,000 individuals and their families. A huge undertaking? You bet! And if anyone can accomplish this enormous feat it is these dedicated, determined parents.

I have now been to Kuwait four times and hope to return soon, "In sha Allah" (*God willing*), as the Kuwaitis often say. Center 21 parents and their extended families have been such generous hosts. We part in tears with promises to stay in touch. My team's mission is to help the Kuwaitis understand the relationships between health, sensory processing, and behavior. I think if we can accomplish that, our work will be rewarded by seeing these beautiful young adults become more functional.

Additional Resources

Books, websites, organization's materials, webinars, conferences, and other sources abound for those working with teens transitioning to adulthood. In addition to those mentioned in this chapter, here are some others that are excellent.

• *Preparing for Life: The Complete Guide for Transitioning to Adulthood for Those with Autism and Asperger's Syndrome,* by Jed Baker, 2005.

• *A Full Life with Autism: From Learning to Forming Relationships to Achieving Independence,* by Chantal and Jeremy Sicle-Kira, 2012.

• **Autistic Self-Advocacy Network (ASAN):** a 501(c)(3) nonprofit organization run by and for people with autism. Provides support and services to individuals on the autism spectrum while working to educate communities and improve public perceptions of autism. See www.autisticadvocacy.org.

• **"Autism Transition Handbook":** an online support resource sponsored by Devereaux. See www.autismhandbook. org.

[1] Ocean Heaven. Edko Films Limited, 2010.

[2] www.pbs.org. Accessed Oct 14, 2013.

[3] www.brainyquote.com. Accessed Oct 23, 2013.

[4] Individuals with Disabilities Education Improvement Act (IDEIA). 20 U.S.C. § 1401 (3) (26) §300, 2004.

[5] Halpern AS. The transition of youth with disabilities to adult life: A position statement of the division on career development and transition. The Council of Exceptional Children, Fall 1994, 17:2, 117.

[6] Robison JE. Look me in the eye. New York: Random House, 2007.

[7] Grandin T, Dufy K. Developing Talents: Career Planning, Including Higher Education, for Students with Autism and Asperger Syndrome. Shawnee Mission, KS: AAPC Publishing, 2004.

[8] Endow J, Mayfield M. The Hidden Curriculum of Getting and Keeping a Job: Navigating the Social Landscape of Employment: A Guide for Individuals With Autism Spectrum and Other Social-Cognitive Challenges. Shawnee Mission, KS: AAPC Publishing, 2012.

[9] The Center for Special Needs Trust Administration, Inc. http://centersweb.com/ SNT. Accessed Oct 16, 2013.

[10] Gilmour L, Schalomon PM, Smith V. Sexuality in a community based sample of adults with autism spectrum disorder. Research in Autism Spectrum Disorders, Jan–Mar 2012, 6:1, 313–18.

[11] Edmonds G, Worton D. The Asperger Love Guide: A Practical Guide for Adults with Asperger's Syndrome to Seeking, Establishing and Maintaining Successful Relationships. UK: Sage Publications, 2005.

[12] Kerr K. Romantic Relationships and Autism Spectrum Disorder. http://www. amaze.org.au/uploads/2011/08/Fact-Sheet-Romantic-Relationships-ASD-Aug-11. Accessed Oct 23, 2013.

[13] Bererot S, Humble MB, Gardner A. Endocrine Disruptors, the increase of autism spectrum disorder and its cormorbidity with gender identity disorder—a hypothetical association. Int Jrl of Andrology, 2011, 34, e350.

[14] Swan SH, Liu F, Hines M, Kruse RI, et al. Prenatal phthalate exposure and reduced masculine play in boys. Int J of Andrology, 2010, 33, 259–269.

[15] Hellemans H, Colson K, Verbracken C, Verbracken R, et al. Sexual behavior in high-functioning male adolescents and young adults with autism spectrum disorder. J Autism Dev Disord, 37, 260–269.

[16] Geier DA, Geier MR. A prospective assessment of androgen levels in patients with autistic spectrum disorders: Biochemical under-pinnings and suggested therapies. Neuro Endrocrinal Lett, 28, 565–573.

[17] Lemaire M, Thomazeau B, Bonnet-Brilhault F. Gender Identity Disorder and Autism Spectrum Disorder in a 23-Year-Old Female. Archives of sexual behavior, Jul 9, 2013, 1573–2800.

[18] deVries ALC, Noens ILJ, Noens J, Cohen-Kettenis PT, et al. Autism Spectrum Disorders in Gender Dysphoric Children and Adolescents. Jrl Autism and Dev Disorders, Aug 2010, 40:8, 930–36.

[19] Tateno M, Ikeda H, Saito T. Gender dysphoria in pervasive developmental disorders. Psychiatr Neurol Jpn, 2011, 113:12, 1173–83.

[20] Gilmour L, Schalomon PM, Smith V. Sexuality in a community based sample of adults with autism spectrum disorder. Research in Autism Spectrum Disorders, Jan–Mar 2012, 6:1, 313–18.

[21] Rubio R. Mind/Body techniques for Asperger's syndrome. Philadelphia: Jessica Kingsley Publishers, 2008.

[22] Mitchell C. Asperger's syndrome and mindfulness. Philadelphia: Jessica Kingsley Publishers, 2009.

[23] Rosenblatt LE, Goranthla S, Torres JA, Yarmush, RS, et al. Relaxation Response-Based Yoga Improves Functioning in Young Children with Autism: A Pilot Study. J Altern Complement Med, Nov 2011, 17:11, 1029–1035.

[24] Koenig KP, Buckley-Reen A, Garg S. Efficacy of the Get Ready to Learn Yoga Program among Children With Autism Spectrum Disorders: A Pretest–Posttest Control Group Design. American Journal of Occupational Therapy, Sep/Oct 2012, 66:5, 538–546.

[25] Silva L, Schalock M, Gabrielsen K. Early Intervention for Autism with a Parent-delivered Qigong Massage Program: A Randomized Controlled Trial. American Journal of Occupational Therapy, 2011, 65:5, 550 –559.

[26] Silva L. Helping Your Child with Autism: A Home Program from Chinese Medicine. Guan Yin Press: 2010.

CHAPTER 16

Preventing Autism

If autism is treatable . . . if we can actually recover kids from autism . . . if we know the risk factors for autism, then the obvious question is this: Is autism preventable? According to Maureen McDonnell, RN, who for over 10 years planned programs for parents of children diagnosed with autism and their providers, it is! "We now know enough to encourage couples who are contemplating pregnancy, have conceived or who have an infant, to implement certain precautionary principles to minimize the risk of having their child develop autism."[1] Many physicians, researchers, and parents agree. McDonnell states that "we now have a pool of wisdom, good science and common sense from which to draw safe, effective and practical recommendations for preventing autism.

Why, despite our state-of-the-art medical technology, does the United States have one of the highest maternal and infant mortality rates among developed countries?[2] Why, despite billions of dollars spent on research, is autism still a "mystery"?[3]

Because getting pregnant, staying pregnant, giving birth, and raising babies is big business! Jennifer Margulis, PhD, tells it all in *The Business of Baby: What Doctors Don't Tell You, What Corporations Try to Sell You, and How to Put Your Pregnancy, Childbirth, and Baby BEFORE Their Bottom Line.*[4]

"Life can only be understood backwards; but it must be lived forwards."[5] This profound statement most assuredly describes what many parents of children with autism must feel. "If only . . ." are two words they repeat over and over. So many have confided, "If only I knew then what I know now. I would have made very different choices."

Cam Baker Pearson, a.k.a. "Mountain Mama," is one of the founders of the Thinking Moms Revolution (TMR). In February 2013 she bared her heart and soul to the world by bravely posting "How I Gave My Son Autism" on the TMR site.[6] She takes full responsibility for her son's autism.

I don't know if she has read my first book,[7] but clearly Mountain Mama subscribes to Total Load Theory. She believes that her son's autism resulted from the accumulation of assaults on his nervous, sensory, and other systems, not from a single trigger. Some of the culprits she blames—ultrasounds, acetaminophen, and vaccines—are included in this chapter. The actions she took were mostly recommended by well-meaning health care professionals. She, and probably the rest of the "thinking moms," strongly believes that autism is preventable. That is why this book ends with this chapter.

It's too late to cancel the exterminator who sprayed the house with pesticides, retract the needle from the third MMR booster, and eat only organic food during pregnancy for those already diagnosed. But it's not too late to educate the next generation of parents so they can learn from our mistakes, and we have the responsibility to do so! Hopefully this chapter can help fulfill Mama's hope of saving other children by educating prospective parents.

Education is the goal of parent Beth Lambert, author of *A Compromised Generation,*[8] and cofounder of the nonprofit Epidemic Answers. Education is the goal of environmental advocate Justin Valley, author of *Healthy from Day 1*, a tiny e-book written for expectant parents.[9] Education is the goal of Sarah Lane, OD, RYT, HBCE, founder of Natural Beginnings NJ, who offers autism prevention workshops in New Jersey. Eventually these should be available nationwide.

Ideally, young women would become aware of the significance of physical and mental health in high school and college. I would love to see a mandatory course in personal health in every school in America!

A year pre-conception, couples should start thinking about cleaning up their environments, changing their lifestyles, and getting rid of their body burdens. Limiting their exposure to toxins while maximizing nutrition and health prior to conceiving, during pregnancy, and while breastfeeding, as well as learning when to trust the body's healing wisdom, recognizing when a medical professional is imperative, and understanding how lifestyle choices can support rather than undermine health are all vital to having a healthy baby! Why? Because they improve fertility and discourage miscarriage, pregnancy complications, and problems during delivery.

A full year out? Yes, because that's how long it takes to replace the bad stuff, to learn about the good stuff, and for the body to detoxify safely. If you are that prospective parent and are reading this, congratulations! Keep track of your family load factors, and think about how you might reduce them. Now, let's get started!

Pre-Conception

Run Laboratory Tests

I love tests. For over 30 years I administered diagnostic tests to help parents understand and make informed decisions about their children's education, health, and functioning. Tests only give you information; what makes information powerful is your decision to educate yourself about what to do with that information.

Here are some tests to consider *before* becoming pregnant. None are routine; in most cases, you must discuss them with your doctor.

Toxic elements. The earlier in gestation toxic exposures occur, the more detrimental they can be to development. Every woman should know what toxins her body is holding before she gets pregnant, and detox appropriately to ensure that her baby isn't exposed in those early weeks before a positive pregnancy test. Doctor's Data Lab (www.doctorsdata.com) offers a hair analysis of over 30 potentially toxic elements to which we are all exposed, including lead, mercury, arsenic, aluminum, copper, antimony, and cadmium. This inexpensive test is very predictive of the toxic load a pregnant woman dumps into her unborn baby, according to Phillipe Grandjean, MD, an internationally recognized environmental health expert and author of the extraordinary book *Only One Chance: How Environmental Pollution Impairs Brain Development — and How to Protect the Brains of the Next Generation.*[10] *Every* woman should have this test!

Thyroid function. Refer back to chapter 6 to learn about the vital importance of the thyroid gland and the hormones it secretes. A low-functioning thyroid in the mother is a known cause of endocrine disruption in her offspring. Low levels of T4 or marginally elevated levels of thyroid-stimulating hormone (TSH) can affect the unborn baby.[11]

Environmental toxins are endocrine disrupters that affect thyroid function. If a woman is toxic, her thyroid probably is not working properly. In the very early weeks of pregnancy, often before she is even aware she is pregnant, a couple of hours of insufficient thyroid can do subtle damage.[12] Damage may also occur to the hypothalamus, impeding its ability to produce oxytocin and vasopressin, the bonding hormones.

Jared Skowron, ND, describes the cascade of endocrine responses in autism, which can start prenatally with endocrine disruption in the egg or sperm.[13] A sluggish thyroid gland can result in insufficient thyroid hormone during the second and third trimesters of gestation.[14] Low levels or even a mild drop of thyroid hormone in the mother at critical stages of brain development can affect cognitive function in her baby.[15]

Testing for and treatment of thyroid dysfunction is complicated and controversial. All tests and supplements are not created equal. Blood tests for thyroid function, which measure TSH, T4, and T3, frequently fail to detect a problem. New York thyroid specialist

Raphael Kellman, MD, believes that the TSH reference range is too wide, with the upper boundary of "normal" being too high; it thus fails to detect marginally low thyroid in many patients.

Kellman recommends an alternative: the TRH stimulation test, which he has used in over 15,000 patients. This test employs a hormone called TRH to stimulate the pituitary gland, which, in turn, produces TSH to stimulate the thyroid and produce thyroid hormones. When the thyroid is sluggish, the pituitary must produce more TSH. However, frequently, in those with hypothyroidism, high levels of TSH do not show up in the blood, rendering the routine thyroid blood test inadequate in a significant percentage of patients. However, even when the blood levels of TSH are normal in hypothyroidism, unequivocally TSH is high in the pituitary gland. Upon stimulation with TRH, TSH is released on the spot, causing levels to rise and allowing physicians to make a proper diagnosis and treat the patient accordingly. Learn more at www.raphaelkellmanmd. com.

Israeli researchers have shown that many women with fertility issues have hypothyroidism, even though routine blood testing shows they have normal TSH levels. When evaluated using the TRH stimulation test, a significant percentage showed abnormal results.[16]

Vitamin D levels. Every day we are learning about the importance of vitamin D in health. Vitamin D regulates thousands of genes in the human genome. The importance of prenatal, neonatal, and postnatal vitamin D supplementation cannot be underestimated. Vitamin D during gestation and early infancy is essential for normal brain functioning. In 2009 researchers concluded that vitamin D deficiencies in pregnant women should be considered a risk factor for neuro-developmental disorders such as autism.[17]

Insufficient vitamin D is a universal problem.[18] You want your number to be over 30, even though 25 is considered "normal." 40 is even better! If your level is low, start taking supplements at 2000–5000 units of D_3 per day. Recheck in 3 months. High doses are sometimes necessary for a short time to elevate levels.

To learn more about vitamin D, go to www.vitaminDCouncil.org.

An ELISA test for food sensitivities. Look for gluten, casein, soy, egg, garlic, and other intolerances. Discomfort after eating, such as gas or bloating, minor skin irritations, or more serious issues such as constipation or asthma could be a result of food sensitivities. Once you know the problematic foods, you can rotate and eliminate those with moderate to severe reactions.

Genetic profile. Go to www.23andme.com and do a quick gene screening to pinpoint possible difficulties with detoxification. Work with a health care professional to identify supplements that can remediate glitches called single-nucleotide polymorphisms, or SNPs.

Antibody titers. Ask your doctor to run blood titers to find out which diseases you are immune to. Make sure that you are not a hepatitis carrier. Put that in writing to prevent your baby from getting the Hep B shot at birth.

Remove Mercury-Containing Amalgams

The severe toxicity of mercury is explained in depth in earlier chapters. If you have any mercury-containing amalgams in your mouth, strongly consider having them removed safely by a biological dentist at least six months before getting pregnant, and follow up with a mercury detoxification program for at least a couple of months. Even one or two "silver" fillings off-gas into the mouth with brushing, chewing, and drinking hot or cold liquids.[19]

A mother's mercury load off-gases and crosses the placenta, landing in the liver and kidneys of the fetus. It also shows up in her breast milk.[20] Infants' mercury levels correlate with the number of amalgams in the mother.[21]

Heal the Gut

Health begins in the gut. Read chapter 4 to understand the importance of our microbiome, the variety of organisms that live inside us. Caring for the gut is a lifelong priority. Becoming aware of how your gut works and noticing triggers for improper function are keys to establishing a healthy gut. Normalize digestion by eliminating problematic foods identified by the ELISA test. Take digestive enzymes and probiotics. Test for candida, parasites, and other gut bugs. Use natural products to kill them, if present. Make sure that you poop daily. Consider colon hydrotherapy.

Detoxify the Body

Once tests have identified what toxins make up a potential mother's body burden, mercury amalgams are removed, and the gut is working well, it is time to detoxify. **Detoxification with mercury amalgams and abnormal digestion is dangerous!**

No baby is born today without toxic exposure in the womb. Mothers dump a good part of their body burden into their unborn babies through the umbilical cord and into the placenta. The lower a mother's toxic load, the lower the baby's.

The Environmental Working Group (EWG) and Commonweal performed a joint study of 10 children born in August and September of 2004 in US hospitals. Researchers found an average of 200 industrial chemicals and pollutants in umbilical cord blood. Tests revealed a total of 287 pesticides, consumer product ingredients, and wastes from burning coal, gasoline, and garbage, 180 of which are carcinogenic, 217 of which are toxic to the brain and nervous system, and 208 of which can cause birth defects or abnormal development.[22]

Fathers' toxicity can also affect fertility and conception. Toxins in the sperm can lower testosterone levels, which can damage the quality of the sperm and cause birth defects. Poor sperm motility is often related to toxicity.[23]

Detoxification can remove heavy metals and chemicals, normalize digestion, reduce inflammation, heighten energy, and increase circulation to the reproductive system, thus supporting the production of healthy sperm and eggs, and increasing fertility. Many detoxification protocols are available. Work with a health care professional to find one that you like. One easy way to detox is by using a sauna and sweating out the toxins. This was the method of choice for first responders from 9/11 to help them rid their bodies of asbestos and other poisons.[24] Another is a homeopathic detox program that clears out chemicals, metals, parasites, bacteria, viruses, and radiation. Refer back to chapter 7 for more information on detoxification.

Detoxify the Mind and Spirit

Pre-conception is a good opportunity to repair broken relationships and clean the skeletons out of your relationship closet. Pregnancy is a time to focus on only positive, supportive interactions and relationships. If you have a history of family problems, consider a family constellation, also described in chapter 7.

Improve Your Diet

Eat organic, gluten-free, in-season, vegetables galore, with no white foods, colors, flavors, or preservatives. Eliminate or greatly reduce alcohol and caffeine; eliminate tobacco. Minimize consumption of large fish (for mercury levels of fish check www.gotmercury.org). Buy a Vitamix or other juicer and juice organic vegetables. Consume fermented foods like sauerkraut and kimchi daily. Follow Donna Gates's guidelines for the Body Ecology Diet (BED).

Decrease Exposure to Electromagnetic Fields (EMFs)

Get all electronics, including computers, TVs, wireless phones, iPads, Blueray devices, and cell phones out of the bedroom. Use cell phones only with headsets; keep the cell in a purse, never in the bra or pocket. Turn off Wi-Fi at night.

Exercise and Breathe Good Air

Up your exercise program to strengthen muscles and increase stamina. Attend a class two or three times a week. Stretch to increase flexibility. Walk—outside whenever possible. Open the windows; outdoor air is cleaner than indoor air. Use air filters at home and in the office.

Green Your Environment

Gradually switch to nontoxic cleaners (no dry cleaning!), laundry soaps, detergents, pest removal, gardening, and personal care products. If you are doing any renovations, be mindful of which products you are choosing for paint (no VOCs), flooring (consider cork or bamboo), insulation, and other building materials. Cabinetry often contains toxins such as formaldehyde. The extra money you spend on being "green" is worth it long term for your family's health. Go to www.GreenBuildingSupply.com for ideas.

Take Quality Prenatal Supplements

Be sure your supplements include omega-6 fats and a multiple vitamin complex.

Stay Hydrated

Carry water wherever you go in a glass, stainless steel, or safe plastic water bottle. Drink only filtered water.

Say "No Thank You" to Vaccines

Avoid the flu or any other shots at least a year prior to conception.

Pregnancy

Decisions a mother-to-be makes during pregnancy and about her baby's birth are crucial to the baby's healthy future. Consider how much time and energy people spend on planning a wedding or deciding what house, car, or computer to purchase. Your unborn child deserves at least as much consideration.

Diet

The old saying, "Eat for two," is correct. Make nutrient-rich, not high-caloric choices. Say "yes" to 75–100 grams of protein, organic fruits, vegetables, beans, lentils, asparagus, spinach, nuts, and free-range, antibiotic-free animals. Say "no" to sugar and its substitutes, wheat, dairy, and hydrogenated fats. Say "once-in-a-while" to small cold-water fish and soy products. Take the time to sit down and eat slowly, chewing well. The more times you chew your food, the less work the rest of your digestive system has to do, and the more access your body has to the nutrients. Consider five or six smaller meals instead of three large ones. Snack on protein, including smoothies made with protein powder, lean grass-fed meats such as turkey, organic chicken, or fresh nuts.

Drink at least eight cups of good-quality water a day. No alcohol, sodas (especially diet sodas), or caffeinated beverages. Consider consulting with a herbologist and trying some herbal teas and infusions. Many have medicinal qualities and nutrients that can strengthen you.

Supplements

While the right, good-quality foods can provide much-needed nutrition, eating adequate amounts of some nutrients is simply impossible. Contraceptives and other medications can deplete minerals. Continue to take a good comprehensive, natural, and easily absorbed multivitamin. Take ample vitamin D_3, mercury-free omega-3 fish oil, and probiotics. Work with a health care professional to determine the right products, ingredients, and dosages.

Exercise

Doctors sometimes recommend avoiding too much exercise during pregnancy to avoid injury. However, movement is beneficial to both the mother her unborn baby. Finding a good fit between the exercise you like and movement that you can do may take time. Prenatal yoga is a good choice because most instructors are familiar with modifying poses during pregnancy. See more about yoga below under "Relaxation and Sleep."

Dental Care

Avoid all dental work while pregnant. This includes cleaning, root canals and the removal or insertion of fillings.

Chiropractic Care

Find a chiropractor who works with pregnant women and make periodic visits. A chiropractic adjustment during pregnancy is different that an adjustment when you are not with baby. Carrying around a baby the size of a bowling ball is hard on the spine, hips, and structure of the body. Keeping the spine aligned during pregnancy is essential to an easy pregnancy, birth, and quick postpartum recovery. Receive weekly chiropractic care throughout pregnancy to keep your structure balanced in preparation for birth.

Chiropractors trained with the Webster® technique have advanced training in techniques of gentle body and muscle manipulation to properly position a baby for birth. The birth process is intense, and working with a chiropractor can help eliminate any structural stress created by the birthing process. The earlier these adjustments take place, the more likely they can prevent concerns from arising later.

Ultrasounds

Ultrasound is energy in the form of sound waves vibrating at approximately a hundred times the frequency of normal sound. When amplified through the amniotic fluid, this is akin to the assault of a jet engine to the baby's ears. In addition to emitting vibrations of up to 100 decibels, ultrasounds emit heat. Both sound and heat can stress the fetus.

Routine ultrasounds are in vogue, even though a research study of over 15,000 pregnant women published in the *New England Journal of Medicine* showed that they do not improve fetal outcome.[25] Some doctors prescribe them monthly, and even more often if a pregnancy is "high risk" because of the mother's age or multiples. Some pregnant women have as many as a dozen! Just because we know how to look into the womb doesn't necessarily mean we should! British consumer activist Beverly Beech called repeated ultrasounds in pregnancy "the biggest uncontrolled experiment in history."[26]

Prenatal ultrasound may have a negative effect on brain development. Recent research shows a potential relationship between ultrasounds and autism. Manuel Casanova, MD, a neurologist who teaches at the University of Louisville, contends that ultrasound exposure is the main environmental factor contributing to the exponential rise in autism.[27]

Reflexes

Read Chapter 9 on the importance of reflexes, the foundation for our movement patterns. Overactive or underactive reflex patterns can contribute to dysfunction in the body and mind. A birthing mother must have well-integrated reflexes. The Spinal Gallant and Asymmetric Tonic Neck Reflex (ATNR) assist the baby in maneuvering through the birth canal. Mothers who retain either of both of these reflexes may have difficulty giving birth naturally. The baby may not "drop," may be breech, or require a Cesarean section. Simple reflex integration activities prior to birth can help the birth go more smoothly.

Medications

The safety of all prescription *and* nonprescription drugs during pregnancy has not been fully tested. This warning includes antidepressants.[28] If you get sick, drink more water, rest, and take vitamin C up to bowel tolerance; try to avoid antibiotics and other over-the-counter and prescription medications. Look for natural approaches such as herbs, acupuncture, or homeopathy.

Relaxation and Sleep

Learn to meditate. Practice yoga to improve digestion and circulation, and to keep the bowels moving. During pregnancy, yoga can be supremely supportive emotionally; it prepares body, mind, and spirit for the big event. Find a yoga instructor and class for pregnant women. Avoid hot yoga and vigorous vinyasa yoga due to the excess heat.

Prenatal yoga is unique and can be challenging physically. Some poses are energetic, some restorative. Others focus on stretching and strengthening muscles used for birthing, as well as the upper back, shoulders, and arms to prepare the body for holding a growing infant. All focus on breathing, a fundamental skill for birthing.

Prenatal yoga classes include a "check-in" to share experiences, as well as activities focused on centering, breathing, visualization, and relaxation. Most importantly they provide a community of like-minded women who can be supportive throughout pregnancy. This group can evolve into a postpartum "mommies" group. If you cannot find a class, buy a DVD for doing yoga at home during pregnancy.

Practice deep breathing daily. Oxygenation of cells enhances their function. Releasing stress allows the body to put its energy into growing a healthy baby.

Sleep is restorative. Turn in before 10:00 p.m. and sleep at least nine hours every night during pregnancy. Get your zzzs while you can!

Vaccines

Despite your doctor's suggestions, try to avoid any vaccinations, including the flu shot, while pregnant. Even if the vaccines are mercury-free, they contain other toxins. Avoid getting the flu by using immune-boosting foods, vitamins, and herbs instead.

Prepare Your Nipples for Nursing

Two to four weeks before you are to give birth, begin conditioning your nipples with oil or an over-the-counter ointment, such as Lansinoh. You will be happy you did!

Surround Yourself with Supportive People

Spend time with those who are encouraging of your choices. Minimize contacts with those who are negative.

Put Together Your Birthing Team

Speak with friends who have children to learn what practitioners in your area have philosophies consistent with yours. Interview doulas, midwives, and obstetricians. Ask a gazillion questions until you find people you like. If midstream you feel that you made the wrong choice, switch—it's not too late! Surrounding yourself with calm, educated professionals is key to a positive birth experience.

A doula can be a valuable birth support for the birthing mother while the OB or midwife attends to the well-being of the baby. An experienced doula who has seen hundreds of births can help interpret your sensations, evaluate how labor is progressing and determine when it is time to go to the hospital. Doulas cannot make medical decisions; they are your advocate.

Shop Around for a Childbirth Education Class

Many of the classes associated with hospitals focus on preparation for a medicalized birth, not for one that emphasizes the involvement of birthing parents. Consider options such as Hypno-birthing® and the Bradley Method®, both of which focus on cultivating trust in a woman's body to birth normally. Another possibility is home birth, which has been proven safe and has a lower rate of medical interventions for mother and child than hospital birth, as long as it occurs with a certified practitioner.[29]

Make a Birth Plan

A birth plan anticipates and addresses recommendations for intrusive procedures such as induction, an epidural, use of forceps or vacuum extraction, C-section, and clamping the cord prematurely, so that you do not have to make decisions about them in a crisis mode.

These and other medical interventions could torque a baby's spine and affect future function. Labor induction and C-sections are load factors for autism. In one study, Cesarean delivery was associated with a 26% increased risk for autism.[30]

Talk to your team about positioning. Being on your back may not be the best choice. Sitting upright or crouching on all fours for pushing and delivery could enhance your ability to birth with greater ease.

Interview Pediatricians

Shop around for a pediatrician with whom you are philosophically compatible. Maybe a family doctor is a better choice. Sometimes Doctors of Osteopathy (DOs) are more flexible, especially about vaccination schedules. Choose someone who supports health instead of treats illness.

Stock Your Library

Invest in books such as the classic *How to Raise a Healthy Child in Spite of Your Doctor*,[31] *Smart Medicine for a Healthier Child*,[32] *Holistic Baby Guide: Alternative Care for Common Health Problems*,[33] and *Naturally Healthy Babies and Children: A Commonsense Guide to Herbal Remedies, Nutrition, and Health*.[34] These great references advise parents on home treatments for routine childhood illnesses, allergies, and fevers, with clear-cut instructions for determining when a child needs medical intervention. *Most* importantly, recognize when you need expert medical help. Then you could always go to the nearest urgent care center, a brilliant modern convenience. Consider if *you* really need a pediatrician to tell you that your baby is thriving!

Prepare the Baby's Room

Spend more money on an organic mattress than on a fancy crib. If you can find a used crib in good shape, that's even better because it has already off-gassed. Use nontoxic products, such as no-VOC paints and natural flooring. Consider alternative sleeping options for the newborn, such as a safe co-sleeper. Watch those baby monitors; some emit EMFs, which are not good for baby.[35]

Labor and Delivery

Labor is an intense process—nothing like you have ever experienced. No two women, no two pregnancies are the same.

Fear is a terrible motivator! Fear of pain, labor, and problems are ingrained in today's health care model. Even though it may be tempting to think of avoiding labor, moving through the stages of labor and delivery are important learning experiences for both mother and baby. Without fear, birthing can be joyful and even orgasmic.

For the baby, passing through the birth canal exercises reflex patterns that function automatically, without consciousness. A baby who has not used reflexes to get through the birth canal may need help later in development to organize the reflex system. A natural vaginal birth also enhances neurological function and exposes a newborn to bacteria from the mother's vagina.

Antidote fear with knowledge! Knowledge is power! Immerse yourself in learning about natural alternatives to use during labor and delivery. Approach birthing as you would studying for the most important final exam you have ever taken, times ten! Know your options. A stressless, fearless, and trauma-free birth is a wonderful gift you can give your child.

Newborn and First Months of Life

Take Care of Yourself First!

Sleep when the baby sleeps. When awake, touch, move, talk, laugh, emote, and exaggerate interactions. Maintain good dietary habits including ample fruit, vegetables, high-quality protein, and fiber to keep your bowels moving. Make bone broth to replenish minerals, and soups and stews with root vegetables. Use warming spices like cinnamon, cloves, turmeric, and curry. Get a massage once a month or more often if finances permit.

If you are feeling depressed, work with a nutritionist or health care practitioner familiar with postpartum issues to adjust diet and supplements. An interesting method of preventing postpartum depression is placental encapsulation, which involves saving and preparing tissue from the placenta as a supplement. For more information on this fascinating option, go to www.placentalbenefits. info.

Chiropractic Care

Both mother and baby should be evaluated by a qualified chiropractor shortly after birth. Spinal alignment is essential for mom's healthy recovery and continued stamina. The baby's cranial and spinal development affects nervous system function forever. This step is imperative! Some chiropractors want to be in the delivery room to mold a newborn's head within hours of delivery to ensure proper blood flow to the brain.

Consider chiropractic care for your newborn baby, too! A baby with acid reflux, colic, torticollis, or ear infections should be seen by a chiropractor regularly. Many of these common problems can be healed with routine chiropractic care and other lifestyle adjustments. To learn more, read *Kids First: Health With No Interference*.[36]

Feeding

Bottle or breast? Research is overwhelmingly supportive of mother's milk! Nursing is one of the best ways to provide optimal nutrition and to ensure quality bonding time between mother and child. Babies who are breast-fed have lower incidence of sudden infant death syndrome (SIDS), fewer illnesses, and healthier gastrointestinal systems.[37]

Milk takes up to four days to come in. Immediately following birth, nursing babies get colostrum, a clear substance that is very beneficial for their immune systems. If you decide not to nurse, purchase colostrum as transfer factor and give it to your baby. Read about this remarkable product in chapter 5.

While breastfeeding, keep lubricating your breasts. Remember to stay well hydrated. Keep water with you at all times! Nurse often, as a baby's stomach is small and can hold only a few tablespoons of fluid at a time.

Having trouble nursing? Support is key to success! Hire a lactation consultant, join groups, or call La Leche League. Get a breast pump, especially if your baby is sick or hospitalized; breast milk is good medicine! Use a nipple shield to help baby latch on. Read books. Go online. Lactation consultant Nancy Mohrbacher, the "Breastfeeding Reporter," offers a website, books, and interactive app for smart phones. Go to www.nancymohrbacher.com.

How long should a mother nurse? It depends on so many factors! The longer the better, up to a point. For a good year seems to be what most doctors recommend to support a baby's developing brain, immune, and digestive systems.

When is the right time to introduce solid food, and what foods are best? Only you and your health care provider can determine that. Most doctors are now recommending postponing solid food until three to six months. Feeding your baby solid food too early can compromise gut health, the immune system, and trigger food allergies. Some professionals use the emergence of teeth as an indicator that the baby's gut is ready to digest foods.

Avocado is a popular "first food" because it is already mushy and contains excellent nutrition. Steam organic vegetables and puree them, or buy an organic brand of prepared vegetables without sugar or other additives. Introduce one food at a time to minimize allergic reactions. Red cheeks, dark circles under the eyes, tummy problems, a cough, or runny nose can all indicate food reactions. No early cow's milk, soy, or grains. If you insist on rice cereal, make sure it is organic, but even organic rice could contain arsenic!

Diapers, Bottles, and Other Baby Products

Oh dear, another area that requires research! Cloth or disposable? With chemicals or without? Glass or plastic? All diapers, powders, lotions, creams, and bottles are not created equal.

Did you know that what makes disposable diapers so absorbent, lotions so smooth, and bottles so colorful is toxic chemicals and plastics? Choosing to diaper with organic diapers, smother your baby with organic oils, and buy glass instead of plastic is similar to choosing to eat, clean, and decorate with nontoxic products.

Sarah Lane, OD, of Natural Beginnings NJ has developed a checklist to help you decide:

Is this product free of volatile organic compounds (VOCs), Bisphenol-A (BPA), and other chemicals?

Do I feel 100% comfortable with all the ingredients in this product? Am I choosing this product because it's cute or because it's safe? Is this product going to off-gas?

Do your homework and make decisions that are consistent with your values, philosophy, and finances.

Bonding with Baby

You cannot spoil a newborn! Hold, talk to, and wear your baby. Even though a baby does not yet understand words, tone and facial expressions speak volumes! Keep baby close by utilizing an on-the-body baby carrier. Wearing baby while you cook, vacuum, and move around the house offers the vestibular system much-needed stimulation. As you and the baby move in space, neurons myelinate and grow. Babies *must* move for their brains to develop.

So many different types of baby carriers exist! Make sure that newborn legs are not dangling; baby's hips should be in a supported sitting position. Try on many carriers, and find one that is comfortable for both you and baby. If money allows, purchase a different one for each parent, allowing baby to be held in different positions.

Movement is food for a baby's nervous system. Limit time in popular seats, walkers, carriers, jumpers, and buckets that keep a baby on its back at a 45-degree angle, inhibit movements, and put their reflexes in "jail." Lifting the head from this position is extremely difficult. One very popular seat that has recently gotten bad press from physical therapists for its inhibition of an infant's movement is the Bumbo Baby Seat.[38]

Avoid electronic devices of all kinds! Babies do not benefit from videos, television, phones, iPads, or other electronic games. Their eyes and ears are not ready for that type of stimulation, and using these technological marvels could interfere with development.

Sleeping Position

In the past 20 years, doctors have recommended back-sleeping to lower the risk of SIDS. Before SIDS most babies slept on their tummies. Barry Richardson, a British expert in materials degradation, and T. James Sprott, a New Zealand chemist and forensic scientist, believe that SIDS is the result of accidental poisoning due to toxic gases released from baby mattresses. These gases are produced by the interaction of common household fungi with phosphorus, arsenic, and antimony, chemicals which are either present naturally in the mattresses or which have been added as flame-retardant chemicals.[39] If this is true, many cases of SIDS could be preventable also!

Babies on their backs are neurologically upside-down. From that position they can barely raise their heads, much less put weight on their arms and hands or begin to crawl and creep. Many of them have flattened heads with bald spots. Although back-sleeping babies usually appear to developing normally, lack of early lower-brain development from spending too much time on their backs may translate into later learning and behavior challenges. Clearly the advantages of tummy sleeping outweigh the risks.

Tummy Time

Antidote back-sleeping with tummy time! Tummy time promotes the development of strong head and neck muscles by allowing the baby to hold up the head against gravity. During tummy time, babies bear weight on their arms and hands, learn to reach with the eyes and the hands together, strengthen their cores, and eventually move through space to explore.

Place newborn babies on their tummies on the floor or on a blanket several times a day after naps, eating, and diaper changes, when they are awake and content. Once a baby has head control, all waking hours should be spent prone. This position is so important for hand development, the emergence and integration of primitive reflexes, and bilateral and binocular integration.

As babies gain strength in the third month, tummy time becomes more fun. Their first random movements enhance posture and coordination, eye tracking, arm rotation, and hand strength. The result is a firm foundation for crawling, creeping, manipulating toys, and later drawing with a pencil.

Four- and five-month-old babies are more purposeful, scooting and pivoting to reach toys. If you place a rolled up towel under a baby's chest and armpits, allowing him to be slightly inclined, he will smile and then reach out for stimulating objects.

Crawling and creeping organize important parts of the central nervous system that provide the foundation for all future growth and learning. When the lower brain develops appropriately, higher-level cognitive skills emerge naturally and easily. Disorders involving self-regulation, sensory integration, and learning could signal a lack of appropriate development in these key areas.

Babies who do not experience adequate tummy time sometimes show a propensity to turn or hold their heads predominately to one side. If neck muscles contract too much, medical help may be necessary to restore the full motion needed for normal development. Untreated, this condition, called "torticollis," can require extensive therapy or even surgery. To avoid torticollis,

- switch arms frequently when feeding;
- frequently reverse the baby's position on the diaper table;
- carry the baby in a variety of ways, allowing him to experience different head positions;
- in a baby carrier or car seat, keep the neck straight with head supports;
- avoid equipment that holds the baby in a semi-reclining position;
- provide baby with adequate vestibular stimulation through swaying, dancing, and dipping upside-down to encourage eye movement development (all of these movements should be slow and controlled).

Vaccinations

Of all the subjects to research, this one is the *most important!* Read *everything* you can to educate yourself on the pros and cons. Learn about vaccine ingredients, called adjuvants, which potentiate the pathogen. Adjuvants include aluminum, formaldehyde, and MSG. Even though the media shouts that no cause-and-effect relationship exists between vaccines and autism,[40] many believe that vaccination can be a load factor in genetically vulnerable children. Learn the laws of your state; the 50 states differ markedly in requirements. Go to the extremely informative website of the National Vaccine Information Center (NVIC) to find out how your state interprets vaccine law.

In a majority of states parents are required to make their first vaccination decision within 24 hours of a baby's birth. The hepatitis B shot is often given at birth. Unless a mother is positive for hepatitis B, a newborn need not receive this vaccine because the disease is transmitted primarily through sexual activity.

Your choice of pediatrician will determine how much flexibility you have in vaccine decision-making. The law states that infants with immune defects should not be vaccinated; however, few pediatricians test for immune deficiency before giving shots. One pediatrician I know says she does not vaccinate until "I know who is in there!" The American Academy of Pediatrics has a one-size-fits-all vaccination schedule. A 26-week preemie struggling for life could get the same shots as a robust, full-term baby. That doesn't make sense to me.

The NVIC has established guidelines to help parents make informed vaccine decisions. A "yes" to questions one through three is reason to reconsider vaccination carefully. Everyone should be able to answer "yes" to questions four through eight before vaccinating.

1. Is my child sick right now?
2. Has my child had a bad reaction to a vaccination before?
3. Does my child have a personal or family history of:
   • previous vaccine reactions
   • convulsions or neurological disorders
   • severe allergies
   • immune system disorders
4. Do I know if my child is at high risk of reacting?
5. Do I know how to identify a vaccine reaction?
6. Do I know how to report a vaccine reaction?
7. Do I know the vaccine manufacturer's name and lot number?
8. Do I know I have a choice?

In order to make an informed decision about vaccination, parents must consider a child's birth history and genetic background. How many load factors does a child already have? Could a vaccination today be "the straw that breaks the camel's back"?

If you have *any* reservations about vaccinating a child, postpone, spread out, or avoid vaccines based on a family history or current illness. *No* long-term studies show that giving multiple vaccines at once is safe. *Never* allow a doctor to administer more than one shot on a given day. Some, like the MMR or DPT, already contain three pathogens. Three is two too many for some kids.

Never vaccinate a sick child or one who is on or just coming off of an antibiotic. The child's immune system may not be able to handle the insult of the vaccination while trying to fight off the infection. Did you know that many doctors and health departments us multi-dose vials? Ask for single-dose vials. Protocol requires that the health care provider shake the vial vigorously to ensure even distribution of pathogens and adjuvants. Is it even possible that each and every one of the ten doses is identical? Unlikely.

Never give acetaminophen (Tylenol®) before or after a vaccine. William Shaw, PhD, at Great Plains Lab has shown a relationship between acetaminophen use and autism.[41] Instead, use vitamin C or echinacea drops and cod liver oil to boost a baby's immune system for a few days prior to and after vaccinating. Also consider using homeopathic vaccination before and after the first shot of any pathogen. This lessens the likelihood of shocking the immune system.

Vaccine waivers are available in every state if you decide not to vaccinate:

- *Medical Exemption:* All 50 states allow a medical exemption to vaccination. Proof of medical exemption from an MD or DO is a signed document stating that administering one or more vaccines would be detrimental to the health of an individual. Some states accept a private physician's written exemption without question. Others ask the state health department to review the doctor's statement; accepting or revoking it are options.

- *Religious Exemption:* All states allow a religious exemption to vaccination except Mississippi and West Virginia. The religious exemption is intended for people who hold a sincere religious belief opposing vaccination to the extent that if the state forced vaccination, it would be an infringement on their right to exercise their religious beliefs. Some state laws define religious exemptions broadly to include personal religious beliefs, similar to personal philosophical beliefs. Other states require an individual who claims a religious exemption to be a member of a state-recognized religion with official tenets that prohibit invasive medical procedures such as vaccination. Some laws require a signed affidavit from the pastor or spiritual advisor of the parent exercising religious exemption that affirms the parent's sincere religious belief about vaccination, while others allow the parent to sign a notarized waiver.

• *Philosophical, Personal, and Conscientious Belief Exemption:* The following 18 states allow exemption to vaccination based on philosophical, personal, or conscientiously held beliefs: Arizona, Arkansas, California, Colorado, Idaho, Louisiana, Maine, Michigan, Minnesota, New Mexico, North Dakota, Ohio, Oklahoma, Texas, Utah, Vermont, Washington, and Wisconsin. In some of these states, individuals must object to all vaccines, not just a particular vaccine in order to use the philosophical or personal belief exemption.

If parents believe a child is at high risk for suffering vaccine-induced injury or death, they have the moral right to protect their child from harm. If they choose to selectively vaccinate a child or use no vaccines at all, they should be prepared to hire a lawyer if charged with child medical neglect for failing to vaccinate a child with all state required vaccines.

All vaccines offer only temporary immunity, which is why more than one dose and boosters are recommended. A blood test from a private laboratory, costing about $55, can determine whether a child has sufficiently high antibody titers to prove existing immunity to a specific disease. Some children have proof of immunity after a single shot, which lasts for many years, and others cannot show proof of immunity even after many boosters.[42]

Duration of vaccine-induced immunity varies from person to person, just as the risk for vaccine reactions varies from person to person. Consider asking your doctor to draw a titer before administering a booster. He or she probably won't like this and will tell you that your insurance probably won't cover the cost. Do it anyway! Inoculating your child with a dose of a pathogen to which his or her body already has immunity unnecessarily exposes him to other toxins also included in the vaccine.

Vision Development

Neuroscientist Karen Pierce, PhD, at UC San Diego Autism Center of Excellence has been interested in gaze patterns in infants as predictive of later autism. In late 2010 she discovered that babies at-risk for autism as young as 12-months spend greater time visually examining geometric patterns than they do social patterns. This newly described attribute of babies at-risk for autism received worldwide press.[43]

Babies have predictable visual milestones, just as they do in the areas of movement and language. By six weeks, a baby should look at you and smile. Eyes should work together, as if a string is attached to them: if one eye looks left, the other eye should look left. Any variation of this is of concern and requires an immediate evaluation by an eye care professional.

Even if no eye or vision problems are apparent, the American Optometric Association (AOA) recommends scheduling your baby's first eye assessment between six and twelve months. InfantSEE®, a public health program managed by Optometry Cares®—The AOA Foundation, is designed to ensure that eye and vision care becomes an essential part of infant wellness care to improve a child's quality of life. Under this program, participating optometrists provide a comprehensive infant eye assessment as a no-cost public service. The doctor looks for excessive or unequal amounts of nearsightedness, farsightedness, or astigmatism, as well as eye movement ability and eye health problems. To find a doctor near you, go to www.infantsee. org.

Take-Home Points

Autism is preventable! Can we guarantee that by following the guidelines in this chapter we will wipe out autism? No! However, we know the risk factors, and by being mindful of decisions we make along the way, we can ensure healthier babies by reducing the load factors that accumulate. For more information, several excellent books cover the topics in this chapter in greater depth:

- *Brighton Baby: The Complete Guide to Preconception and Conception* by Roy Dittmann, OMD, MH
- *Healthy from Day 1*, an e-book by Justin Valley
- *Preventing Autism & ADHD: Controlling Risk Factors Before, During and After Pregnancy* by Debby Hamilton, MD
- *Preventing Autism: What You Can Do to Protect Your Children Before and After Birth* by Jay Gordon, MD

Now is the time to continue to advocate for the next generation of children, our grandchildren. Join organizations such as Epidemic Answers and Saving Our Kids, Healing Our Planet (SOKHOP), and fund education and research on the importance of a toxin-free, stress-free world for conception and birth. Support the Prevent Autism Now campaign to improve education and awareness of the lifestyle choices we can make to minimize toxicity and therefore reduce the risk of developing autism and other developmental delays. Future generations of kids cannot wait for tomorrow's research! We must act *now*! It is possible and we can do it!

---

[1] McDonnell M. Getting Healthy Before Getting Pregnant. www.sokhop.com. Accessed Nov 12, 2013.

[2] http://en.wikipedia.org/wiki/List_of_countries_by_infant_mortality_rate. Accessed Dec 9, 2013.

[3] Murray P. Autism Rate Rises To 1 In 50 Children — Cause Still A Mystery. www.singularityhub.com. Apr 8, 2013. Accessed Dec 9, 2013.

[4] Margulis J. The Business of Baby: What Doctors Don't Tell You, What Corporations Try to Sell You, and How to Put Your Pregnancy, Childbirth, and Baby BEFORE Their Bottom Line. New York: Scribner, 2013.

[5] Kierkegaard S. www.BrainyQuote.com. Accessed Nov 12, 2013.

[6] Pearson CB. How I gave my son autism. Feb 2013. http://thinkingmomsrevolution.com. Accessed Dec 6, 2013.

[7] Lemer P. Envisioning a Bright Future: Interventions that work for children and adults with autism spectrum disorders. Santa Ana, CA: OEPF, 2008.

[8] Lambert B. A Compromised Generation. Boulder, CO: Sentient Publications, 2010.

[9] Valley J. Healthy from day 1. Amazon, 2011.

[10] Grandjean P. Only One Chance: How Environmental Pollution Impairs Brain Development—and How to Protect the Brains of the Next Generation. New York: Oxford University Press, 2013.

[11] Román G, Ghassabian A, Bongers-Schokking JJ, Jaddoe VW, et al. Association of gestational maternal hypothyroxinemia and increased autism risk. Annals of Neurology, Aug 13, 2013.

[12] Molloy CA, Morrow AL, Meinzen-Derr J, Dawson G, Bernier R, Dunn M. Familial autoimmune thyroid disease as a risk factor for regression in children with Autism Spectrum Disorder: A CPEA Study. J Autism Dev Disord, Apr 2006, 36:3, 317–24.

[13] Skowron JM. Autism and the Endocrine Response. http://www.naturopathydigest.com/archives/2006/oct/skowron.php. Accessed Dec 24, 2013.

[14] Nagayama, et al. Concentrations of organochlorine pollutants in mothers who gave birth to neonates with congenital hypothyroidism. Chemosphere, Jun 2007, 68:5, 972–76.

[15] Zoeller R, et al. Thyroid disruption and brain development: What is it that we don't know? Neurotoxicology and Teratology, 2008, 30:3, 248.

[16] Eldar-Geva T, Shoham M, Rosler A, Margalioth E, et al. Subclinical hypothyroidism in infertile women: The importance of continuous moniotorin and the role of the thyrotropin-releasing hormone stimulation test. Gynecological Endcrinology, 2007, 23:6, 332–37.

[17] Grant WB, Soles CM. Epidemiologic evidence supporting the role of maternal vitamin D deficiency as a risk factor for the development of infantile autism. Dermatoendocrinol, Jul–Aug 2009, 1:4, 223–28.

[18] deBorst MH, de Boer RA, Stolk RP, Slaets JP, et al. Vitamin D deficiency: Universal risk factor for multifactorial diseases. Curr Drug Targets, Jan 2001, , 97–106.

[19] Mercola J. Still Carrying around this potent neurotoxin next to your brain? http://articles.mercola.com/sites/articles/archive/2011/09/04/mercury-poisoning-from-silver- fillings.aspx. Accessed Apr 8, 2014.

[20] Williams F. Toxic breast milk. New York Times Magazine, Jan 9, 2005.

[21] Mercola J. Still Carrying around this potent neurotoxin next to your brain?

[22] Environmental Working Group. The Pollution of Newborns: A benchmark investigation of industrial chemicals, pollutants and pesticides in umbilical cord blood. Jul 14, 2005. www.ewg.org. Accessed Dec 9, 2013.

[23] Hauser R. The environment and male fertility: Recent research on emerging chemicals and semen quality. Semin Reprod Med, Jul 2006, 24:3, 156–67.

[24] Boyers B. New York Rescue Workers Detoxification Project. www.OrganicConnecting.com. Accessed Apr 8, 2014.

[25] Ewigman BG, Crane JP, Frigoletto FD, Lefevre ML, et al. Effect of Prenatal Ultrasound Screening on Perinatal outcome. NEJM, Sep 1993, 12, 329.

[26] Buckley S. Ultrasound Scans: Cause for Concern. Nexus, Oct–Nov 2002, 9:6.

[27] Williams EL, Casanova MF. Ultrasound and autism: How disrupted redox homeostasis and transient membrane porosity confer risk. In Dietrich-Muszalska, Gagnon, Chauhan, ed. Studies on psychiatric disorders. New York: Humana Press, 2013.

[28] Lund N, Pedersen LH, Henriksen TB. Selective serotonin reuptake inhibitor exposure in utero and pregnancy outcomes. Archives of Pediatrics & Adolescent Medicine, 2009, 163, 949–54.

[29] Johnson K, et al. Outcomes of planned home births with certified professional midwives: Large prospective study in North America, BMJ, Jun 2005, 330, 1416.

30 Gardener H, Spiegelman D, Burka SL. Prenatal Risk Factors for Autism: A Comprehensive Meta-analysis. Br J Psychiatry, Jul 2009, 195:1, 7–14.

[31] Mendelsohn R. How to Raise a Healthy Child in Spite of Your Doctor. New York: Ballantine Books, 1987.

[32] Zand J, Rountree R, Walton RM. Smart Medicine for a Healthier Child. Garden City Park, NY: Avery, 2003.

[33] Neustaedter R. The Holistic Baby Guide: Alternative Care for Common Health Problems. Oakland, CA: New Harbinger Publications, 2010.

[34] Romm AJ. Naturally Healthy Babies and Children: A Commonsense Guide to Herbal Remedies, Nutrition and Health. New York: Celestial Arts, 2003.

[35] http://www.magdahavas.com/dect-baby-monitors-dangerous/. Accessed Jan 13, 2014

[36] Ressel O. Kids First: Health With No Interference. Garden City Park, NY: Square One Publishers, 2013.

[37] Schanler RJ. Infant benefits of breastfeeding. www.uptodate.com. Accessed Dec 8, 2013.

[38] Deardorff J. Therapists see no developmental benefits from seats. Chicago Tribune, Mar 15, 2012.

[39] Franklin H. Could chemicals in mattresses combined with fungus cause crib death? www.johnleemd.com. Accessed Dec 9, 2013.

[40] Krans B. CDC: Still No Evidence to Support Autism-Vaccination Link. Mar 29, 2013. www.healthline.com. Accessed Dec 9, 2013.

[41] Shaw W. Evidence that Increased Acetaminophen use in Genetically Vulnerable Children Appears to be a Major Cause of the Epidemics of Autism, Attention Deficit with Hyperactivity, and Asthma. Journal of Restorative Medicine, 2013, 2, 9–16.

[42] http://www.historyofvaccines.org/content/articles/top-20-questions-about-vaccination#5. Accessed Apr 8, 2014.

[43] http://neurosciences.ucsd.edu/faculty/Pages/karen-pierce.aspx. Accessed Dec 8, 2013.

INDEX

Page numbers followed by f indicate figures; t, tables.

casein
  in camel milk, 140
  in edible reinforcers, 398
  eliminating foods containing, 86, 87, 96
  intolerance to, 93
  problems digesting, 92–94
case managers, role of, 24, 25
Cassily, James, 299
Cat and Cow pose, 254
Catching Fire (Wrangham), 67
"cat's whiskers" test, 345
CEASE therapy, 195–196
celiac, 130
cellular immunity
  humoral immunity dominance over, 131, 136–137
  overview of, 124
  vaccination bypassing, 126
  vaccination weakening of, 130
Center 21 (Kuwait), 459, 486
Center for Autism and Related Disorders, Inc. (CARD), 398–399
Center for Discovery, 471–472
centering dimension, 230
central vision, 324, 325, 328–329
cerebellum, 41–42
cerebral cortex, 242
cerebral palsy, 241
cerebrospinal fluid flow, 219
cervical vertebra, first, 217–218
chaining, 395
Chapel Haven, 470–471
Cheatum, Billye Ann, 268–269
checkbook, balancing, 466
chelation, 199–202, 206
chemical and environmental stressors, 12f, 55–62, 79–80, 132
Chemical Safety Improvement Act (CSIA), 38
chemokines, 131
Chessen, Eric, 304–305
chewing, 256
chicken pox, 147
childbirth education classes, 501
Childhood Disintegrative Disorder (CDD), 8, 9
children with autism
  capabilities, optimism about, 377
  differences in, xvii–xviii, 42, 48

feeling comfortable with, 377
  future, hope for, 377
  observing, 386–387
  potential of, 378
Children with Starving Brains (McCandless), 87
child's lead, following, 360, 364
Child with Special Needs, The (Greenspan and Wieder), 361
Chinese parsley. See cilantro
Chinitz, Judy, 108
chiropractic care, 214–217, 233, 498, 504
chiropractic neurology, 214
chlorella
  detoxification role of, 182, 189, 190–191, 193
  laser energetic detoxification combined with, 198
chlorella growth factor (CGF), 190, 191
Chlorine Dioxide (CD), 144–145
Chretien, Kristina, 382
chronic cerebro-spinal venous insufficiency (CCSVI), 201–202
chronic health problems, 92
cilantro, 182, 189–190
circadian rhythms, 164, 167
classical homeopathy, 194–195
classroom performance, 465
Classroom Visual Activities, 347
class size, increase in, 73
cleaning products, 56, 60
cleansing, principle of, 112
clostridia, 89
clostridum dificile (C. diff), 106
clothing, 61, 79, 280t
Coalition of Safe Minds, The, 36
coconut kefir, 112
coconut pudding, 112
cod liver oil, 186, 327
cognition, 368
Cognitive Affective Training, 390, 402–403
cognitive-behavioral therapies, 390, 402–404
cognitive enhancement programs, 435–437
cognitive function, 307
cognitive perceptions, 361

electro-smog, 57, 66
Eli Lilly, 128
elimination diets
  in absence of known allergy, 97
  allergy elimination diet, 103
  gluten and casein, 93
  leaky gut and, 91–92
  medications compared to, 96
  overview of, 87
  studies of, 96
  supplements combined with, 144
  week-long, 86
ELISA test (Enzyme-Linked
  Immunosorbent Assay), 97, 494
Elmiger, Jean, 196–197
EMFs. *See* Electro-magnetic fields
emotional attunement, 371
emotional bonding, 277
emotional competence, 383
emotional development, 368, 372
emotional ideas, 363, 369
Emotional Intelligence (Goleman), 387
emotional interactions, 362
emotional issues, unresolved, 206
emotional reactions versus cognitive
  perceptions, 361
emotional stressors, 12f, 76–77, 78–80
emotional thinking, 363, 369
emotional well-being, 410
emotions
  as cognition component, 368
  managing, 463
  neurophysiological basis for, 384
  understanding, importance of,
    361–362
  empathy
  oxytocin link to, 167, 168
  play role in, 357
  understanding, 358
employers, identifying potential, 467
employment, 464-472
  deficits impeding, remediating, 371,
    387
Enayati, Albert, 35–36
encephalopathy (term defined), 139
*Encyclopedia of Dietary Interventions for
  Autism* (Seroussi and Lewis), 94
Endangered Minds (Healy), 70–71
endocrine disruption
  in autism, 164–165

cerebrospinal fluid flow blockage,
  219
  dealing with, 159, 171
  toxin role in, 36, 37
Endocrine Disruption Exchange Inc.,
  The (TEDX), 37
endocrine system, 48, 160–163, 171
endotoxins, 38
energy blockages, releasing, 213
engagement, 363, 369
Engaging Autism (Greenspan and
  Wieder), 361
environment
  adapting to, 422
  autism role of, 14–15, 16, 30
  greening, 496
  healthy practices, 79–80
  pests in, 356
  progress in right, 377
  sensory needs, meeting, 464, 468
  situations as teaching moment, 396
  stimuli, modifying, 397
  toxic, 30, 491–492, 495
  vision-enhancing changes in,
    345–346
environmental and chemical stressors
  assaults, 132
  categories, 55–59
  eliminating and reducing, 59–62,
    79–80
  overview of, 12f
environmental toxins, 36–38
enzymes, 87
epidemic (defined), 2
epigenetics, 16
epinephrine, 162
episodic memory, 374
epsom salt baths, 198
Epstein-Barr, 147
equal employment opportunity, 6,
  467
ergonomics and lighting, 451
Erwin, Brian, 279
essential fatty acids (EFAs), 118,
  186–187, 288
Essential Glutathione™, 189
essential oils, 312–313
estrogen, 160, 163, 169
ethylmercury, 45
evidence-based literature, 402